MANAGEMENT GUIDELINES FOR PEDIATRIC NURSE PRACTITIONERS

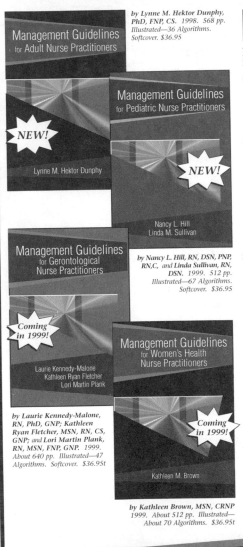
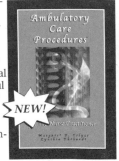

MANAGEMENT GUIDELINES FOR PEDIATRIC NURSE PRACTITIONERS

Nancy Herban Hill, RN, PNPC, APN
Formerly Professor and Director
Graduate Program in Nursing
Mississippi University for Women
Columbus, Mississippi
Consultant
Delta State University
Cleveland, Mississippi
Consultant
Arkansas State University
Jonesboro, Arkansas
Pediatric Nurse Practitioner
Mountain View, Arkansas

Linda Sullivan, RN, CS, DSN, FNP
Nurse Practitioner
Children's Health Center, Inc.
Columbus, Mississippi
Professor
Mississippi University for Women
Columbus, Mississippi

 F. A. DAVIS COMPANY • Philadelphia

F. A. Davis Company
1915 Arch Street
Philadelphia, PA 19103

Printed in the United States of America

Last digit indicates print number: 10 9 8 7 6 5 4 3 2 1

Acquisitions Editor: Joanne P. DaCunha, RN, MSN
Production Editor: Michael Schnee
Cover Designer: Louis J. Forgione

As new scientific information becomes available through basic and clinical research, recommended treatments and drug therapies undergo changes. The authors and publisher have done everything possible to make this book accurate, up to date, and in accord with accepted standards at the time of publication. The authors, editors, and publisher are not responsible for errors or omissions or for consequences from application of the book, and make no warranty, expressed or implied, with regard to the contents of the book. Any practice described in this book should be applied by the reader in accordance with professional standards of care used with regard to the unique circumstances that may apply in each situation. The reader is advised always to check product information (package inserts) for changes and new information regarding dose and contraindications before administering any drug. Caution is especially urged when using new or infrequently ordered drugs.

Library of Congress Cataloging-in-Publication Data

Hill, Nancy L., 1934-
    Management guidelines for pediatric nurse practitioners/Nancy L. Hill, Linda M. Sullivan.
        p. cm.
    Includes bibliographic references and index.
    ISBN 0-8036-0230-8 (alk. paper)
    1. Pediatric nursing. 2. Nurse practitioners. I. Sullivan,
Linda, 1947– . II. Title
    [DNLM: 1. Pediatric Nursing—methods. WY 159 H6475m 1998]
    RJ245.H55 1998
    610.73'62—dc21
    DNLM/DLC
    for Library of Congress   98-5907
                                                                CIP

DEDICATION

To pathfinders and visionaries who "saw the Vision of the world, and all the wonder that would be."

Alfred, Lord Tennyson
Locksley Hall

PREFACE

Pediatric clients are not small adults, but persons with unique needs—developmentally, physically, and emotionally. The practice of the nurse practitioner deals not only with the identified client but also with the parent or guardian to elicit a history of the illness as well as the meaning of the illness for that client and family. The degree of difficulty, because of the lack of verbal ability in the majority of pediatric clients, presents nurse practitioners with a unique opportunity as they listen to presenting complaints, elicit signs and symptoms, evaluate information in light of current knowledge, and arrive at diagnoses and treatment plans. The process is often much like swimming in deep, murky water, with only glimpses of daylight.

Therefore, pediatric nurse practitioners and students have a need for a concise manual to assist in their assessment, evaluation of signs and symptoms, and initiation of treatment. The purpose of this book is to meet that need. The material presented has been drawn from a variety of sources—both medical and nursing—which is appropriate, because the nurse practitioner is both a nurse and a primary provider of health care.

ACKNOWLEDGMENTS

Our heartfelt gratitude goes to those who "aided and abetted" this endeavor: with special regard to our editor, Joanne DaCunha, who has patiently seen us through all the "misadventure" of the past 4 years; to our husbands and families, who have waited, watched, wondered, and encouraged; to Drs. Jacob Skiwski, James Zini, and David Burnette, who welcomed us to their practices and have encouraged us in our professional endeavors; to other mentors, students and colleagues, including Dr. Barry McCraw, who have added comments and given support.

A special thank-you to Drs. Beverly Bowns and Shirley Burd, who introduced me to teaching 25 years ago. To Linda Sullivan, who believed in me when I decided to replace the theoretical with the practical as I entered retirement: a special thanks from Nancy.

N. H.
L. S.

BIOGRAPHICAL

SKETCHES

Nancy H. Hill, RN, DSN, APN, is a retired professor from Mississippi University for Women in Columbus, Mississippi, where she initiated the family nurse practitioner program in 1975. She is a graduate of Missouri Valley College in Marshall, Missouri, with a joint BSN (1956) and a diploma in nursing from St. Luke's Hospital School of Nursing (1955), St. Luke's Hospital, Kansas City, Missouri. She holds graduate degrees from Tulane University in New Orleans, Louisiana (1967), and the University of Alabama at Birmingham (1982, 1986), as well as a postmaster's certificate as a pediatric nurse practitioner from M.U.W. (1994). She has been a consultant in nursing education, and, since her retirement in 1994, has taught part time at Delta State University and been in practice as a pediatric nurse practitioner in Mountain View, Arkansas. She holds national certification as a pediatric nurse practitioner and a license in Arkansas as an advanced nurse practitioner. Among her publications is *Community Health: A Systems Approach* (1976, with Carrie Braden). She is married, has one son, and since retirement occupies her time with writing and painting.

Linda Sullivan, RN, CS, DSN, is a professor at Mississippi University for Women in Columbus, Mississippi, where she teaches part time in the family and pediatric nurse practitioner program. She also maintains a full-time collaborative pediatric practice in Columbus with Dr. Jacob Skiwski. Dr. Sullivan graduated from Hunter College in New York City in 1969, where she received her Bachelor of Science in Nursing. In 1986, she received her master's degree from M.U.W. She holds national certification as a family nurse practitioner, along with certification from the state of Mississippi. She received her Doctorate in Nursing from the University of Alabama at Birmingham in 1993. Among her publications is her latest book, titled *The Impact of Homelessness on Children*. She serves on multiple statewide and community committees and is an advisor and primary caregiver for several shelters in the area. She also works closely with local law-enforcement agencies on the care of abused and neglected children. Dr. Sullivan is married and has three children and one granddaughter.

CONSULTANTS

Terry A. Hall Buford, RN, MN
Clinical Instructor
University of Missouri
Kansas City, Missouri

Gail M. Kiechhefer, RN, PhD
Assistant Professor and Coordinator,
   FNP Program
University of Washington
Seattle, Washington

Mary Ann Krammin, RN, PhD, PNP
Professor of Nursing
Oakland Community College
Waterford, Michigan

Mary Ann Ludwig, RN, PhD, PNP
Clinical Associate Professor
University of Buffalo School
   of Nursing
Buffalo, New York

CONTENTS

UNIT III
TREATING ILLNESS

HOW TO USE

THIS BOOK

This book focuses on ambulatory care pediatrics and the conditions most often encountered in such a pediatric practice. The format assists the nurse practitioner in the diagnosis and treatment of such conditions.

The book is organized by systems. The inclusion of the flow charts and diagrams will assist the nurse practitioner in the diagnostic and treatment process. The resource section in Appendix 1 is an aid to locating resources for the nurse as well as the family.

UNIT I

THE
HEALTHY
CHILD

CHAPTER **1**

GROWTH AND

DEVELOPMENT

Health-care providers must be aware of normal parameters of growth and development of a child from the fetal through the young adult stages. These norms are representative of the majority of cases seen in clinics; they can help the pediatric nurse practitioner when assessing, caring for, and developing a plan of care for the child and family. This chapter presents the physical, neurological, and psychological growth parameters for each age group. Nutrition requirements are addressed in Chapter 3.

Fetal Growth

PHYSICAL DEVELOPMENT

Cell division occurs as the primary activity during the first week of intrauterine life. During the next few weeks, the ectoderm, entoderm, and mesoderm are formed as the embryo continues to grow, reaching an essentially human form between the fourth and eighth week of intrauterine life. By the eighth week, the fetus weighs only about 1 g; at 16 weeks, it weighs about 100 g and is about 17 cm long. During the second trimester, the fetus undergoes more rapid growth: It weighs about 1000 g and is about 35 cm long. During the third and last trimester the fetus continues to grow, primarily increasing its subcutaneous tissue layer until it is mature and ready for delivery. Although respiratory development can begin as early as the 18th week, survival outside the uterus is not possible until about the 24th to 26th week. Although as medicine continues to improve in its ability to care for the premature infant, 500 g is considered the lowest weight at which viability is possible. Survival of these infants is often tempered by the presence of multiple long-term problems that will affect both the infant and the family for a lifetime to come.

When the child is born, fetal circulation gradually changes to normal circulation; the infant's blood type is predominantly hemoglobin F. Congenital problems, such as sickle cell disease or trait, can be detected at the time of newborn screening. If problems are indicated by the results of the initial test, the results should be validated by hemoglobin electrophoresis after 3 months of age.

NEURODEVELOPMENT

By the eighth week of intrauterine life, neurological development can be seen in muscle contractions of the fetus, which can be elicited by a local stimulus. By the ninth week of gestation, all areas of the body, with the exception of the spine, the back of the head, and the vertex, can be measured in terms of neurological response. These movements, which can also be felt by the mother, are often the first evidence of "another life within" for the mother.

The fetus is capable of habituation by late pregnancy. For example, the fetus increases its activity in response to loud noises or other sensory stimulus. Although little is truly known about the effects of maternal stimulation on the fetus, some newborns respond to the same types of music, singing, or other soothing measures that their mothers used during pregnancy.

In general, one factor that needs to be stressed to the mother during the prenatal period is the importance of regular check-ups by the health caregiver, who can be a general practitioner, nurse midwife, or obstetrician. These check-ups are essential to both the mother and unborn child's life. Regular activity, adequate rest, and good nutrition on the part of the mother all have profoundly positive effects on the fetus; deficits in these areas may lead to extremely detrimental outcomes for both mother and fetus. Although there are other congenital or acquired problems that can affect the infant and mother, the importance of good health care can often help either to remediate these problems or identify them early enough so that adequate preparations can be made to allow for the optimal condition of both the infant and mother at delivery.

The Newborn

PHYSICAL GROWTH

Currently, the average weight of the newborn infant is about 7.5 lb (range, 5.5–10 lb); male infants are slightly heavier than their female counterparts. The average length of an infant is approximately 20 inches; most infants (95%) are 18–22 inches long at birth. The average head circumference is about 14 inches. The body shape of the newborn is different from that of the child:

The head is disproportionately larger than the body.
The face is more rounded and the jaw smaller.
The extremities are shorter.
The abdomen is protuberant.
The chest is round or barrel-shaped.

Birth traumas or other abnormalities may be noted at birth. The most common include:

- Conjunctival hemorrhages from the effort of a vaginal delivery.
- Molding of the head, the degree of which is proportionate to the time the head spends in the birth canal.
- Occasionally, for a very large baby, a fractured clavicle from a vaginal birth.
- Minor bruises and abrasions due to a difficult or traumatic delivery or the use of forceps.

Parents should be reassured that these minor problems will resolve rapidly.

The primary need of the newborn is to establish efficient, effective respiratory effort and gas exchange. Respirations range from 35 to 50 breaths/min on average for the newborn. Occasionally, a newborn will exhibit periodic breathing—periods of rapid respirations followed by sharp declines in the respiratory rates. As long as these periods are relatively infrequent and not prolonged, they are considered normal.

Cardiac changes from fetal to newborn circulation are necessary to avoid persistent fetal circulation, which can prove deadly for the newborn. Should persistent fetal circulation be suspected, the nurse practitioner (NP) needs to refer the newborn quickly to a pediatric cardiologist. A relatively new protocol of treatment with nitrous oxide is the most likely treatment for this condition. Cardiac rates for the normal newborn range from 120 to 160 beats/min.

One can meet the nutritional needs of the infant, who expresses hunger by crying at regular intervals, by feeding the child at 2- to 3-hour intervals or on demand (if not greater than 5 hours between feedings). Rooting, a response elicited when the cheek is stroked or when the child turns its head toward the nipple, is present at birth. The swallow and gag reflex, which are also present, make meeting nutritional needs possible. Establishing a pattern of feeding often takes several weeks, because sleep patterns often go hand in hand with feeding.

The newborn should pass a meconium stool within the first 24 hours. If no stool is passed, two problems should come to mind: (1) imperforate anus and (2) cystic fibrosis. Other problems may also be associated with the lack of a stool, but these two are the most common and should be given immediate attention.

Because body temperature falls rapidly following delivery, the infant should be kept on a warmer until the temperature stabilizes. This process usually takes 4–8 hours. If the body temperature is unstable, infection is the most likely cause, provided the infant was not premature.

Because extracellular fluids constitute about 35% of the newborn's body weight, the normal loss of these fluids causes a 6–10% loss of body weight during the first 2 weeks of life. If the loss exceeds 10%, dehydration should be suspected; measures to correct this should be quickly instituted.

The hemoglobin for a newborn is 17–19 g/dL; the number of leukocytes will be 10,000/mm^3, increasing over the next 24 hours to as high as 20,000/mm^3. Although this is still considered normal, one should still continue to observe for other signs of a potential infection.

The newborn's digestive system is best suited for the digestion of carbohydrates and proteins; fats are generally poorly handled. When the liver is incapable of conjugating bilirubin, a condition called hyperbilirubinemia ensues, manifested by increasing jaundice of the skin and sclera. Phototherapy may be instituted either in the hospital or at home, depending on the reason and levels of the elevated bilirubin.

Physical development is rapid as the newborn progresses into the infancy period. At this point, the need for sleep and adequate nutrition is of vital importance to the infant (Fig. 1–1). Nutritional needs now average 110 kcal/kg per day, and sleep requirements average 16–18 hours/day.

NEURODEVELOPMENT

The newborn can fix its gaze on objects from the moment of birth. It is capable of following objects, lights, or movements, and it also reacts to certain environmental stimuli, such as noxious odors, and a resultant accelerated heart rate may be noted when the newborn is exposed to such stimuli. The Neonatal Behavioral Assessment Scale, composed of four parts, is a very efficient tool currently used to assess the newborn's neurodevelopmental level. Interactive and motor processes, control of the physiological state, and reaction to stress are evaluated.

PSYCHOSOCIAL DEVELOPMENT

Bonding, attachment, and imprinting are all theories on how the relationship between the parent(s) and the infant can best be established. If these are accomplished early on, generally the baby feels safer and more stable in its new environment. The mother's attitude and actions should be assessed both right at birth and shortly afterward to determine whether the family is achieving the goals of bonding and attachment. When bonding and attachment are not achieved, the NP needs to observe for emotional and resultant physical problems for both the infant and mother. Maternal depression, and neglect and/or abuse of the infant, are often results of poor bonding.

Many changes have taken place in the latter half of this century, including the belief that childbirth is more than a medical activity. Childbirth is also a social event that involves the family and child along with the medical team. The family and infant benefit most when the process allows for meeting family-centered needs to ensure good psychosocial development of both the infant and family.

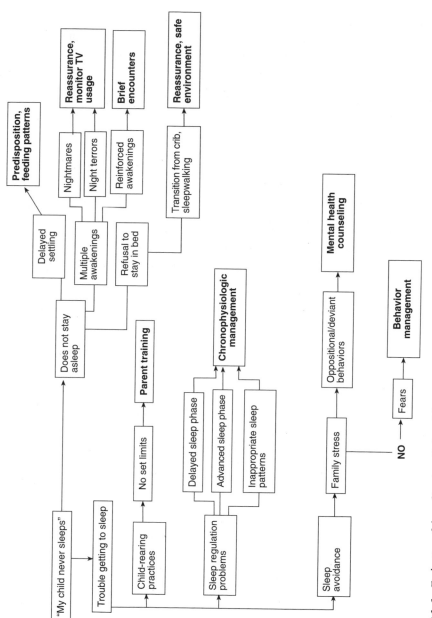

FIGURE 1–1 Evaluation of sleep disorders. (Adapted from Berman, S: Pediatric Decision Making, ed 2. BC Decker, Philadelphia, 1991, with permission.)

Infancy

GROWTH

By 10 days of age, most full-term infants return to their birth weight. Generally, between 5 and 6 months, the infant should double its birth weight. By 1 year, the birth weight triples. On average, length increases by about 1 inch/month, with an average yearly increase in height between 10 and 12 inches.

At birth, the head circumference is greater than the chest circumference, but by the end of the first year, these two measurements should be about the same. The head increases from the newborn average of 34–35 cm to about 44 cm at 6 months and 47 cm by age 1.

The anterior fontanel increases in size up to age 6 months, when a gradual decrease in size is noted. The anterior fontanel closes between the ages of 9 and 18 months, whereas the posterior fontanel closes by age 4 months.

In infants, the eruption of teeth occurs during the first year. Eruption can start by 5 months up to 9 months on average for first teeth, but parents should be reassured if teeth do not appear by 9 months. See Table 1–1 for the schedule of eruption of teeth. Most infants have six to eight teeth by the end of the first year.

The development of fine and gross motor skills (Table 1–2) progresses from simple head lifting and palmer grasp at 1 month to standing alone and stroking with a crayon at 12 months of age. A complete list of developmental milestones can be found in Table 1–3. Neurological development is summarized in Table 1–4.

TABLE 1–1   ERUPTION OF TEETH

Primary Teeth	Age of Eruption in Months
Central incisor	6–7.5
Lateral incisor	7–9
Cuspid	16–18
First molar	12–14
Second molar	20–24

Permanent Teeth	Age of Eruption in Years
Central incisor	6–8
Lateral incisor	7–9
Cuspid	9–12
First bicuspid	10–12
Second bicuspid	10–12
First molar	6–7
Second molar	11–13

TABLE 1–2 NORMAL PATTERN OF DEVELOPMENT

Gross Motor Skills

Birth	Reflex head turn; moves head side to side
1 mo	Lifts head when prone
3 mo	Lifts shoulders up when prone
4 mo	Lifts up on elbows; head steady when upright
5 mo	Lifts up on hands; rolls from front to back; no head lag when pulled to sitting from supine position
6 mo	Rolls back to front
7 mo	Sits alone 30 seconds or more
8 mo	Crawls/sits well
9 mo	Pulls to stand
10 mo	Cruises
13 mo	Walks
30 mo	Walks backwards
2 yr	Runs; kicks a ball
2.5 yr	Walks up and down stairs (taking one step at a time and holding on; stands on one foot [2.5 yr])
3 yr	Walks up stairs alternating steps; rides a tricycle
4 yr	Walks down stairs alternating steps/hops on one foot
3 yr	Skips

Fine Motor/Adaptive Skills

1 mo	Tracks horizontally to midline
2 mo	Tracks past midline/tracks vertically
3 mo	Unfisted for >50% of the time; tracks 180 degrees; visual threat; discovers midline
3 mo	Reaches for bright object; brings object to mouth
4 mo	"Rakes" at bright object
5 mo	Transfers object from one hand to the other
8 mo	Three-finger pincer grasp
9 mo	Neat pincer grasp; bangs cubes in midline
15 mo	Tower of two cubes; scribbles spontaneously
18 mo	Tower of four cubes
2 yr	Copies vertical and horizontal line; tower of six cubes
3 yr	Copies circle
4 yr	Copies "+" (3.5 yr)
4.5 yr	Copies square; draws person with three parts (4.5 yr)
5 yr	Copies triangle; draws person with six parts

Personal/Social Skills

Newborn	Regards face
6 wk	Spontaneous social smile
6 mo	Discriminates social smile
7 mo	Displays stranger anxiety; plays peek-a-boo (7–9 mo)
12 mo	Drinks from a cup
15–18 mo	Uses a spoon, spilling a little
2 yr	Washes and dries hands
3 yr	Uses a spoon well; uses buttons
4 yr	Washes and dries face; engages in cooperative play
5 yr	Dresses without assistance

Language Skills

Newborn	Alerts to bell
2 mo	Cooing; searches with eyes for sound
4 mo	Turns head to sound of voice or bell; laughs (3 mo)
6 mo	Babbles
8 mo	Mama/dada nonspecific
9 mo	Understands the word "no"
12 mo	Mama/dada specific; follows one-step command with gesture/3–5 word vocabulary
14 mo	Follows one-step command without gesture
16 mo	Can point to several body parts
2 yr	50-word vocabulary; two-word sentences; uses pronouns indiscriminately
2.5 yr	Gives first and last names; uses plurals
3 yr	250-word vocabulary; three-word sentences; speech intelligible to strangers 75% of time; uses pronouns discriminately

Cognitive Skills

Newborn–2 yr	Sensorimotor
2–6 yr	Preoperational
6–11 yr	Concrete operational
>11 yr	Formal operations

Miscellaneous Cognitive Milestones

24 mo	Concept of today
30 mo	Concept of tomorrow
36 mo	Concept of yesterday
7 yr	Concept of right and left

Source: Berkowitz, C: Pediatrics: A Primary Care Approach. WB Saunders, Philadelphia, 1996, with permission.

TABLE 1–3   MILESTONES OF DEVELOPMENT—A SUMMARY*

Newborn	When prone, pelvis is high, knees are under abdomen
2–4 wk	Watches mother intently as she speaks to him
1 mo	Ventral suspension (held prone, hand under abdomen)—head up momentarily, elbows flexed, hips partly extended, knees flexed
4–6 wk	*Smiles at mother in response to overtures*
6 wk	*Ventral suspension—head held up momentarily in same plane as rest of body; some extension of hips and flexion of knees and elbows*
	When prone, pelvis is largely flat, hips mostly extended (but when sleeping, the baby lies with pelvis high, and knees are under abdomen, like a newborn)
	Pulls to sit from supine position—much head lag, but not complete; hands often open
	When supine, follows object 90 cm away over angle of 90°
2 mo	Ventral suspension—maintains head in same plane as rest of body
	Hands are largely open
	When prone, chin is off couch; plane of face is 45° to flat surface (e.g., bed or floor)
	Smiles and vocalizes when talked to
	Eyes follow a moving person
3 mo	Ventral suspension—holds head up long time beyond plane of rest of body
	When prone, plane of face is 45–90° from flat surface
	When pulled to sit, there is only a slight head lag
	Hands loosely open
	Holds rattle placed in hand
	Vocalizes a great deal when talked to
	Follows object for 180° (lying supine)
	Turns head to sound (3–4 months) on a level with the ear
4 mo	When prone, plane of face is 90° to flat surface
	Hands come together
	Pulls dress or shirt over face
	Laughs aloud
5 mo	When prone, weight is on forearms
	When pulled to sit, there is no head lag
	When supine, feet come to mouth; plays with toes
	Able to go for object and get it
6 mo	When prone, weight is on hands; extended arms
	When pulled to sit, there is no head lag
	When supine, lifts head spontaneously
	Sits on floor, hand forward for support
	When held in standing position, full weight is on legs
	Rolls, prone to supine
	Begins to imitate (e.g., a cough)
	Chews
	Transfers cube from one hand to another
7 mo	*Sits on floor seconds, no support*
	Roll, supine to prone
	When held standing, bounces
	Feeds self with biscuit
	Attracts attention by cough or other methods
	Turns head to sound below level of ear
8 mo	Sits unsupported; leans forward to reach objects
	Turns head to sound above level of ear

Continued

9 mo	Stands, holding on; pulls to stand or sitting position
	Crawls on abdomen
9–10 mo	*Uses index finger approach*
	Uses finger-thumb apposition—picks up pellet between tip of thumb and tip of forefinger
10 mo	Creeps on hands and knees; abdomen off flat surface
	Can change from sitting to prone and back
	Pulls self to sitting position
	Waves goodbye
	Plays pat-a-cake
	Helps to dress—holding arms out for coat, foot for shoe, or transferring object from one hand to another for sleeve
11 mo	Offers object to mother, but will not release it
	Utters one word with meaning
	When sitting, pivots around without overbalancing
	Walks, holding on to furniture; walks with two hands held
12 mo	Utters two to three words with meaning
	When prone, walks on hands and feet like a bear
	Walks, one hand held
	Casting objects, one after another, begins
	Gives object to mother
13 mo	*Walks, no support*
	Mouthing of objects stopped
	Slobbering largely stopped
15 mo	Creep up stairs; kneels
	Makes tower of two cubes
	Takes off shoes
	Feeds self, picking up an ordinary cup, drinking, putting it down
	Imitates parent in domestic work ("domestic mimicry")
	Jargon
18 mo	*No more casting*
	Gets up and down stairs, holding rail
	Jumps, both feet
	Seats self in chair
	Makes tower of three to four cubes
	Throws ball without falling
	Takes off gloves and socks; unzips
	Manages spoon well
	Points to three parts of body on request
	Turns pages of books, two or three at a time
	Points to some objects on request
	Toilet control—tells parent that he wants to go potty; largely dry by day
21–24 mo	*Spontaneously joins two or three words together to make sentence*
24 mo	Picks up object from floor without falling
	Runs
	Kicks ball
	Turns doorknob
	Makes tower of six or seven cubes
	Puts on shoes, socks, pants; takes off shoes and socks

Continued on following page

TABLE 1–3 *Continued*

Points to four parts of body on request
Imitates vertical and circular strokes with a pencil
Turns pages of a book singly
Is mainly dry at night
Climbs stairs, two feet per step

Motor
   Gross: Runs well, no falling
   Walks up and down stairs alone
   Kicks large ball on request
   Fine: Turns pages of book singly

Adaptive
Builds tower of six to seven cubes
Aligns cubes for train
Imitates vertical and circular strokes with pencil

Language
Uses pronouns
Uses three-word sentences; jargon discarded
Carries out four directions with ball ("on the table," "to mother," "to me," "on the chair")

Personal-social
Verbalizes toilet needs consistently
Pulls on simple garments
Inhibits turning of spoon in feeding
Exhibits domestic mimicry

30 mo   *Motor*
   Gross: Jumps up and down
   Walks backward
   Fine: Holds crayons in fist

Adaptive
Copies crude circle, closed figure
Names some drawings: house, shoe, ball, dog

Language
Refers to self as "I"
Knows full name

Personal-social
Helps put things away
Unbuttons large buttons

3 yr   *Motor*
   Gross: Alternates feet going upstairs
   Jumps from bottom step
   Rides tricycle, using pedals

Continued

Fine: Holds crayon with fingers
Pincer grasp

Adaptive
Builds tower of 9–10 cubes
Imitates three-cube building
Names own drawing
Copies circle and imitates cross

Language
Uses plurals
Names action in picture book
Gives sex and full name
Obeys two prepositional commands (e.g., "on" and "under")

Personal-social
Feeds self well
Puts on shoes

4 yr   *Motor*
Walks downstairs alternating feet
Does broad jump
Throws ball overhand
Hops on one foot

Adaptive
Draws person with two parts
Copies cross
Counts three objects with correct pointing
Imitates five-cube gate
Pick longer of two lines

Language
Names one or more colors correctly
Obeys five prepositional commands (e.g., "on," "under," "in back," "in front," "beside")

Personal-social
Washes and dries face and hands; brushes teeth
Distinguishes front from back of clothes
Laces shoes
Goes on errands outside of home

5 yr   *Motor*
Skips, alternating feet
Stands on one foot more than 8 sec
Catches, bounces ball

Adaptive
Builds two steps with cubes

Continued on following page

TABLE 1–3 *Continued*

Draws unmistakable person with body, head, etc
Copies triangle
Counts 10 objects correctly

Language
Knows four colors
Names penny, nickel, dime
Gives descriptive comment on pictures
Carries out three commands (e.g., "go under the table, get the penny, and give it to me.")

Personal-social
Dresses and undresses without assistance
Asks meaning of words
Prints a few letters

6 yr   *Motor*
Has advanced throwing
Stands on each foot alternately, eyes closed
Walks line backward, heel-toe

Adaptive
Builds three steps with blocks
Draws person with neck, hands, and clothes
Adds and subtracts within 5
Copies drawing of diamond

Language
Uses Stanford-Binet items (vocabulary)
Defines words by function or composition (e.g., "house is to live in")

Personal-social
Tie shoelaces
Differentiates AM from PM
Knows right from left
Counts to 30

*Most important milestones in italics.
Source: Adapted from Palmer, FB: Streams of development. In Oski, FA, et al (eds): Principles and Practice of Pediatrics. JB Lippincott, Philadelphia, 1990, pp. 606–615,

Between the ages of 6 and 8 months, the child can repeat sounds such as ma-ma and da-da. By age 1, a child can demonstrate some familiarity with the meaning of a word.

By age 6 months, the infant shows a preference for the mother; at age 6–8 months, the infant develops separation anxiety when away from the mother. By 9 months, this dependence decreases.

TABLE 1-4 NORMAL REFLEXES IN INFANTS AND CHILDREN

Response	Age at Time of Appearance	Age at Time of Disappearance
Reflexes of Position and Movement		
Moro reflex	Birth	1–3 mo
Tonic neck reflex (unsustained)	Birth	5–6 mo (partial up to 2–4 yr)
Neck righting reflex	4–6 mo	1–2 yr
Landau response	3 mo	1–2 yr
Palmar grasp reflex	Birth	4 mo
Adductor spread of knee jerk	Birth	7 mo
Plantar grasp reflex	Birth	8–15 mo
Babinski response	Birth	Variable
Parachute reaction	8–9 mo	Variable
Reflexes to Sound		
Blinking response	Birth	
Turning response	Birth	
Reflexes to Vision		
Blinking to threat	6–7 mo	
Horizontal following	4–6 wk	
Vertical following	2–3 mo	
Optokinetic nystagmus	Birth	
Postrotational nystagmus	Birth	
Lid closure to light	Birth	
Macular light reflex	4–8 mo	
Food Reflexes		
Rooting response—awake	Birth	3–4 mo
Rooting response—asleep	Birth	7–8 mo
Sucking response	Birth	12 mo
Handedness	2–3 yr	
Spontaneous Stepping	Birth	
Straight Line Walking	5–6 yr	

Toddler Years

PHYSICAL GROWTH

During the second and third year of life, the toddler period, there continues to be an accelerated growth rate, the average toddler gaining between 5 and 6 lb and about 5 inches. Although there is a somewhat decreased appetite, the loss is apparent in decreased subcutaneous tissue as the child begins to become more lean and muscular. Between the second and third year, the abdomen remains protuberant, while a mild lordosis is noted in the stance of the toddler. The head circumference increases only about 2 cm during the second year, and the brain reaches about 80% of the size of the adult brain. The teeth continue to erupt, with an average total of 14–16 teeth at the end of the second year.

NEURODEVELOPMENT

Table 1–2 lists fine and gross motor skills and Table 1–3 presents appropriate developmental milestones during this period. The major accomplishment is walking and increased fine motor control. The child becomes very capable of exploring the environment at this age, so care must be taken to ensure safety. Cognitively, toddlers begin to recognize themselves as separate from others. They begin to make choices independent of their adult caregivers. Their language skills continue to increase, and by 18 months they have a vocabulary of 10–12 words. Play is generally solitary, and there is no significant interaction with other children. Toilet needs can now be verbalized. The earliest age at which toilet training should be initiated is 18–24 months. Parents need to understand that the child must be able to verbalize needs, walk, and manipulate clothing before starting toilet training. During this period, the child can exhibit temper tantrums, frustration, and anger. Parents should manage these behaviors in a firm but loving way, as this approach is the most effective.

The phenomenon of magical thinking is first seen during this period. Toddlers tend to believe that if they think something will happen, it *will* happen, and if it does happen, then they *caused* it to happen.

By age 2–3, toddlers have a 300-word vocabulary, which increases by the end of the third year to approximately 900 words. Speaking often occurs concurrently with walking. This progressive understanding of speech includes recognition and repetition of both their first and last names, the identification of colors, and recognition of size differences.

By age 18 months, they can recognize pictures in books; by age 2, their vision is normally 20/40. Between the ages of 2 and 3, they can jump, hop on one foot, pedal a bicycle, and stop a ball successfully. They can also now climb stairs one at a time. Their drawing skills continue to improve, and they can draw stick figures representing people, make pictures more proportionate to real life, and by the age of 4, can copy figures. Other fine and gross motor skills and developmental milestones can be seen in Tables 1–2 and 1–3.

Preschoolers

PHYSICAL GROWTH

During the preschool years, ages 3–5, both height and weight gains are predictable at about 4–5 lb and 2.5–3.5 inches/year. The body mass becomes leaner, and the lordosis in the stance becomes less pronounced. The protuberant abdomen disappears by age 4, and normal arches now appear on the feet, as the fat pads that once hid them are now gone. The face and jaw grow proportionately, and approximately 20 teeth are now visible. Sleep requirement is generally 12 hours at night, with at least one nap per day.

School-Age Children

PHYSICAL GROWTH

Height generally increases during the school-age years at a rate of about 2.5 inches/year. Weight increases by approximately 5 to 7 lb/year. The head circumference increases in size very slowly at this point, with the brain achieving adult size by age 12.

There is less body fat, and organ development is complete. The facial bones continue to develop rapidly. During this period, the nasal accessory sinuses develop (by 7 years of age).

The spine becomes straighter, and if there have been any noticeable leg abnormalities (e.g., knock-knee, or bowleg), these usually are improved because the legs are now straighter. During this period in life, the lymphatic system is most active and the tonsils are the largest.

The heart rate ranges from 60–100 beats/min, respirations from 18–30 breaths/min, and the blood pressure from 90/60 to 108/60 mmHg. Activities requiring specific motoric and muscular skills are now being mastered, as the child can now direct his or her actions with improved accuracy.

The first permanent teeth, molars, are seen after age 6; as these arrive, the primary teeth usually begin to shed in the same order in which they arrived. About four teeth per year are shed and subsequently replaced.

Puberty begins at ages 10–13 in girls and 11–14 in boys. Both delayed and precocious puberty require special attention from the NP. Gender identity undergoes refinement at this time. Sexually oriented play is common, and masturbation or self-exploration is normal for this age group. As the child matures, he or she will have an increasing sense of modesty.

Nutritional needs can be met in accordance with the food pyramid (see Chapter 3, Fig. 3–1), and the approximate number of calories required of a child is calculated by adding 1000 plus 100 × the child's age. See Chapter 3 for further information about nutritional requirements.

School-age children should get about 10 hours sleep per night.

NEURODEVELOPMENT

Refinement of language and motor skills continues during this period. Gross motor and fine motor skills become increasingly refined. Cognitively, the child is in a concrete operational stage and can now differentiate right from left. Handedness is developed by age 6.

Between ages 6 and 7, eye-hand coordination improves, and the ability to dress oneself develops. The child can hop, skip, jump, run, climb, wrestle, and ride a bicycle. Between ages 7 and 8, the child has improved conscious and cognitive skills, a longer attention span, and improved physical coordination. Between ages 8 and 10, strength, endurance, and increased precision with hand movements all increase.

Adolescence

PHYSICAL GROWTH

The physical, psychological, and social states of well-being are intimately linked during adolescence. Physical, psychological, and social developmental changes can make this a tumultuous time for the adolescent and a difficult time for parents and health-care providers who wish to provide support and guidance. Biological changes that occur during this period are referred to as puberty. Girls experience a growth spurt at about age 12 and boys at age 14.

Weight generally increases by about 5 lb/year, and a 2.5- to 3.0-inch increase in height per year is normal. During early adolescence, girls increase their body-fat content, whereas boys become more muscular. In middle adolescence, girls grow 3 inches taller and boys 4 inches taller per year. There is a distal-to-proximal progression of skeletal growth, with an increase in foot size noted. By late adolescence, growth slows and the femur, humerus, and sternoclavicular epiphysis fuse.

Heavier girls generally begin menarche earlier than thinner girls. Other factors that influence the onset of menarche are eating disorders, chronic illness, and the mother's age at the time of onset of menarche.

In males, facial hair begins to grow at the corners of the upper lip and spreads. As axillary hair appears, so does body odor; thus, special attention should be given to teaching proper hygiene.

Sexual maturity of both males and females can be evaluated by Tanner staging (see Chapter 11, Table 11–1). Physical sexual maturity is completed during this period. The males voice deepens.

Dentition continues as primary teeth erupt up through ages 18–22 (third molars).

NEURODEVELOPMENT

In general, no gross changes occur in the brain or neurological system during this period. There is, however, a period during middle adolescence in which an increase in daytime sleepiness is noted.

Cognitively, concrete, formal operations can be achieved. Abstract thinking is accomplished. Adolescents should also be able to perceive the consequences of their behaviors. In early adolescence there is an increase in risk-taking behaviors, but by late adolescence there is more conformity to societal and family norms. Psychosocial development for boys is dominated by the need for achievement and independence, whereas girls seek to improve interpersonal skills and love relationships. By late adolescence, career choices are made and family cohesiveness returns.

General Information

Growth and development should be assessed at each visit. To assess important growth parameters accurately, height, weight, and head circumference should be plotted on growth charts. Serial measurements are required for accurate evaluation, especially when a problem exists. (Growth charts for boys and girls.)

Dentition follows a relatively predicable pattern, as noted in the previous section (see Table 1–1). When fluoride is not available in water, it should be supplemented in the following manner:

- Birth to 6 months: No additional supplement is necessary.
- 6 months to 3 years: Give only if the water concentration is less than 0.3 ppm (0.25 mg/day).
- 3–6 years:
  - If the concentration is less than 0.3 ppm, give 0.5 mg/day.
    If the concentration is greater than 0.3 ppm, give 0.5 mg/day.
    If the concentration is 0.3–0.6 ppm, give 0.25 mg/day.
- 6–16 years:
  - If the concentration is less than 0.3 ppm, give 1 mg/day.
    If the concentration is 0.3–0.6 ppm, give 0.5 mg/day.

Brushing with a soft-bristle toothbrush should begin when the first tooth erupts; the child should be brought to the dentist by age 2.

Diet is intimately linked to growth and development, so close attention should be paid to eating patterns from the time of birth. The food pyramid provides guidance for health-care providers and parents, but flexibility and special considerations for the vegetarian should be made.

Sexual maturity occurs during adolescence and Tanner staging allows the health-care provider to evaluate appropriate anticipatory guidance during each stage. The NP should, however, be alert to any sexually transmitted diseases occurring at *any* period of time and should consider sexual abuse as an etiology in children who have not achieved sexual maturation.

Immunizations are essential to an adequate health-care program. These begin at birth and continue through adulthood. Tables 1–5 and 1–6 provide guidelines for immunizations.

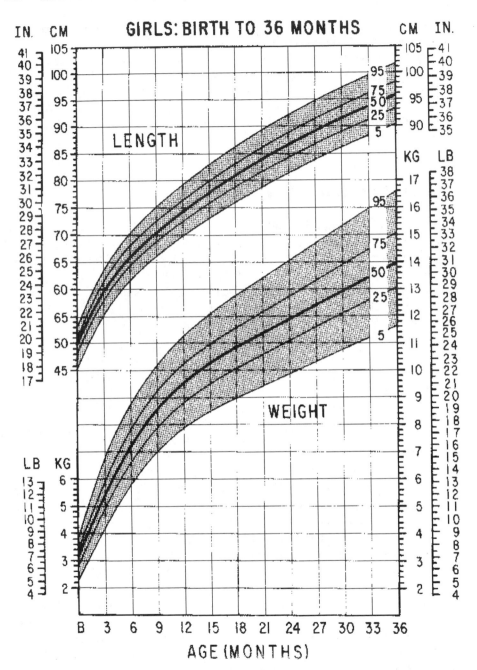

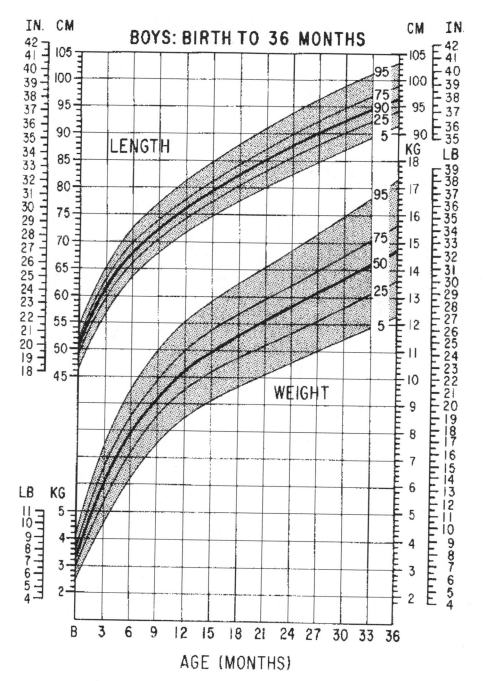

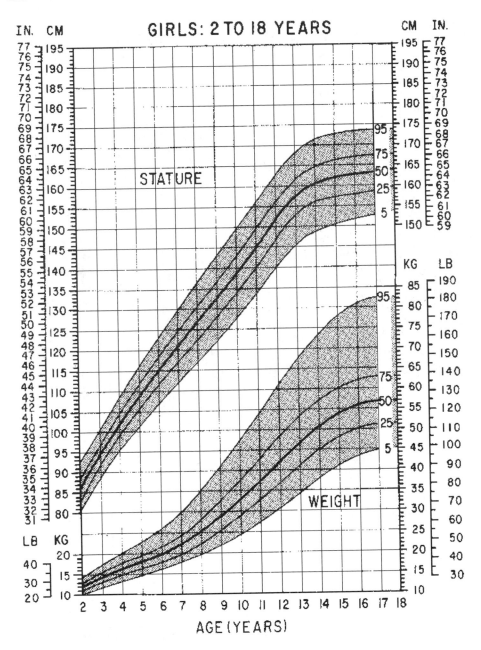

GIRLS: 2 TO 18 YEARS

STATURE

WEIGHT

AGE (YEARS)

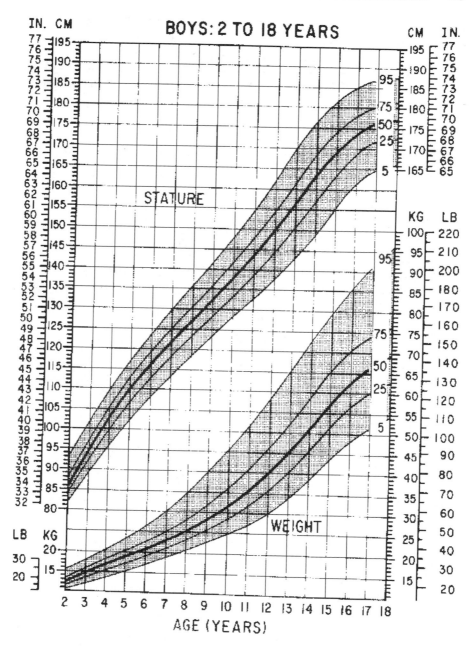

TABLE 1-5   RECOMMENDED CHILDHOOD IMMUNIZATION SCHEDULE

Vaccine	Recommended Age	Comments
Hepatitis B.		Given at 11–12 yr visit if child has not previously had all three doses.
Dose 1.	Birth to 2 months.	
Dose 2.	1–4 mo.	
Dose 3.	6–18 mo.	
Booster.	11–12 yr.	
Diphtheria, tetanus, and pertussis (DPT).	2, 4, and 6 mo. Dose 4 may be administered at 12 months if at least 6 mo have elapsed since last DPT dose.	Tetanus and diphtheria toxoids, adsorbed (Td) is recommended at ages 11–12 if at least 5 years have elapsed since the last dose of DPT, DTaP, or DT.
DPT or diphtheria and tetanus toxoids and acellular pertussis (DTaP).	4–6 yr.	
Haemophilus influenzae type B (HIB).	2, 4, and 6 mo.	If PRP-OMP (Pedavax-HIB) is administered at 2 and 4 mo, no dose is required at 6 mo.
Booster.	May be administered at 12–15 mo.	
Polio.	2, 4, and 6 mo after dose 2.	Inactivated poliovirus vaccine is recommended for persons with a congenital or acquired immune deficiency disease or altered immune state.
Measles, mumps, and rubella.	12–15 mo. Dose 2 is recommended at age 4–6 yr or 11–12 yr.	
Varicella zoster virus.	After 12 mo.	Should be administered to unvaccinated children at 11–12 yr.

An important consideration for any good growth and developmental assessment is the ability of the health-care provider to be open to a discussion of a variety of lifestyle choices and to be knowledgeable about these choices. Each child should be included in the process of health care and, by adolescence, should begin to assume some responsibility for his or her own care. The issue of privacy during exams and discussions should be considered. It is important to allow the adolescent time alone with the health-care provider; physical exams should be conducted without the parent present.

Counseling regarding all aspects of care should be provided at each visit. When abnormalities are noted, referrals should be made to the appropriate expert. Hearing, vision, and speech should be evaluated at appropriate intervals,

TABLE 1–6 SCHEDULE OF IMMUNIZATIONS FOR CHILDREN
NOT IMMUNIZED WITHIN THE FIRST YEAR OF LIFE

Children Under 7	Immunization
First visit to provider	HB, DPT, OPV, MMR, Hib (if child is 15 mo or <6 yr)
1 mo after first visit	HB, DPT
2 mo after first visit	DTP, OPV, Hib
>8 mo after first visit	DTP, or DTaP, HB, OPV
4–6 yr	DTP or DTaP, OPV, MMR
11–12 yr	MMR (if not received at 4–6 yr)
14–16 yr	Td (repeat every 10 yr)

Children Over 7	Immunization
First visit	HB, Td, OPV, MMR
2 mo after first visit	HB, Td, OPV
8–14 mo after first visit	HB, Td, OPV
10 yr	Td (repeat every 10 yr)
11–12 yr	MMR

and when deficiencies are noted, the patient should be referred and treated promptly.

Certain factors have an impact on growth and development (Fig. 1–2). Genetics, cultural influences, physical and emotional health and well-being, negative environmental influences (e.g., poverty), learning disorders, and chronic illnesses are among the many problems that affect growth and development. These factors can either foster or detract from the normal patterns of growth expected within a certain age group. When evaluating the growth and development of a child, the NP should weigh all these factors while appreciating his or her uniqueness.

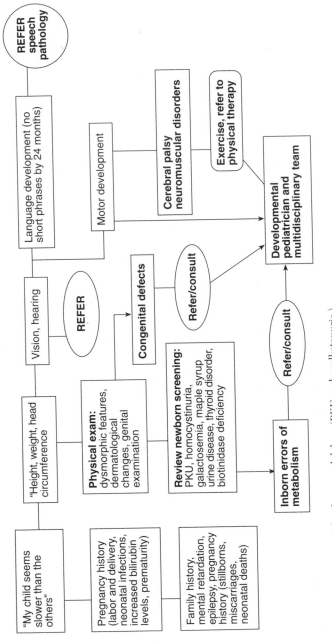

FIGURE 1–2 Evaluation of developmental delays. (PKU = phenylketonuria.)

CHAPTER **2**

PROMOTING HEALTH

Health-care activities comprise the triad of illness care, illness prevention, and health promotion. Health promotion entails facilitating each child to achieve maximum health potential by way of age-appropriate health-education activities that also include anticipatory guidance.

Several conceptual frameworks have been developed and have evolved to assist the nurse practitioner (NP) in understanding the behavior of parents and patients. These frameworks can assist the NP in planning appropriate individual activities. The models considered most useful in assisting the NP in encouraging patients to engage in positive health activities are the Health Belief Model (HBM), the Self Efficacy Model (SEM), and the Health Promotion Model (HPM).

The HBM is designed to explain why a person does not engage in positive health activities. This model provides the background for understanding what might motivate a child, adolescent, or parent to engage in, or begin to practice, healthier lifestyle activities.

The SEM empowers patients by allowing them to act effectively and independently toward achieving the goal of a healthy lifestyle.

The HPM can assist in assessing a person's beliefs regarding health promotion, rather than disease prevention, by identifying the cognitive, perceptual, and modifying factors operational in a patient's life. When collaboratively designing a health-promotion plan, the NP should discuss the family's understanding and beliefs regarding health. Furthermore, the community's beliefs and resources must be understood. Multiple factors influence behaviors and personal beliefs. Community resources and beliefs, cultural influences, developmental stage, and knowledge level of the patient and family must all be assessed when discussing health promotion within the context of family and community.

An important factor crucial to the promotion of health is the family's relationship with a regular primary care giver. The development of this relationship is important when establishing a plan for long-term health maintenance. This relationship can provide stable contact with a person who is familiar with the child and the family and thus may facilitate quicker access to the health-care network in cases where the child requires special, acute, or long-term care.

Activity/Rest

With regard to physical activity, the NP should remain cognizant of developmental skills and levels of the child. It is important to encourage parents to set limits, provide safe daily activities, and encourage participation in a variety of activities including aerobic physical exercises. Passive activities such as watching television should have reasonable, allowable limits, but excessive participation in these activities should be discouraged.

Patterns of sleep and rest should be discussed. Regular sleep patterns are essential for the growing child. A variety of sleep rituals become important to the child; these should be monitored and respected by the parent. New parents should be advised that the average neonate sleeps an average of 16 hours/day. By age 3 months, the child still sleeps approximately 15 hours/day, but in a slightly more organized pattern, with more consistent nighttime sleep being had by all members of the family. By age 6 months, most infants sleep through the night and continue to have two naps per day. Between ages 12 and 24 months, the morning nap is no longer a part of the infant's regular pattern, although the afternoon nap generally continues until age 4 or 5 years. By age 2 years, the child sleeps approximately 11 hours per night, which gradually decreases until, at age 18, the adolescent needs about 8 hours of sleep per night.

Sleep position for the newborn should be supine or on the side on a firm mattress with no pillows in the crib. This newer practice has significantly reduced the incidence of sudden infant death syndrome (SIDS).

Ego Integrity

Understanding the self-concept of the child is critical to developing positive health-promotion strategies. Even parents whose child is in the infancy stage need to be encouraged to view the child as a separate entity, whose personality develops from the moment of birth.

There is a need to encourage all parents to provide positive feedback to children on their achievements and to relate to them in an accepting, nonpunitive manner. As children mature, the parents need to allow them to begin to make choices and express themselves while at the same time setting safe and acceptable limits. Positive reinforcement is the best tool toward developing a child with a healthy self-esteem. Children at all ages should be allowed a degree of privacy, but should be encouraged to maintain an active role in family activities.

Elimination

Activities of elimination should be discussed, and the parents of the newborn should be made aware of the wide range of normal elimination patterns for stool and urine in infants. Although elimination patterns vary from one child to the next, regular bowel patterns established without the use of enemas, medications, and suppositories should be encouraged.

As the child matures, toilet training is the next major challenge facing the child and parent. The NP should encourage the parent to wait until the child is physically, developmentally, and emotionally ready to be trained before attempting this significant developmental task. Often the child who has a traumatic experience while being toilet trained develops problems related to encoporesis (psychogenic megacolon) and can have difficulty establishing normal elimination patterns.

For the adolescent, a concern of caregivers is that the preoccupation with body image may lead to overuse of laxatives in an effort to lose weight.

At all ages, the child should be taught the importance of good hygiene and handwashing.

Food/Fluid

During the prenatal period, concerns regarding breastfeeding versus bottle feeding need to be discussed with the mother. Feeding techniques, whether via bottle or breast, need to be demonstrated to the mother so that she develops at least a modicum of comfort at feeding time. Generally, the NP should stress to parents that they are responsible for providing adequate amounts of nutritious foods to the child in a pleasant atmosphere. Parents need to realize that they serve as role models for the child. The family's eating habits are usually mimicked by the child. Specifics regarding which foods to provide the developing child, caloric needs, the proper time to introduce certain foods, and providing lifelong guidelines for proper nutrition are discussed in Chapter 3.

Hygiene

Hygiene and infection control should be addressed at each visit. Infants should be bathed no more than once per day. For the neonate, umbilical cord care should be explained to the parents. Cord care consists of the application of alcohol to the stump with each diaper change. The parents should take care to prevent contamination of the healing cord with either feces or urine.

As children enter the toddler and preschool stage, they should be encouraged to bathe regularly and change their clothes as needed. One of the concerns of older children, especially adolescents, is acne, which can be controlled to some extent by stressing proper hygiene.

Safety

Safe practices at all ages should be encouraged. Issues of safety are related to issues of transport, environment, and recreational activities:

Transport: Car seats graduating to seat belts are essential for providing safe transportation. The newest standards indicate that a young child should ride only in the rear seats of automobiles. Air bags have been known to cause injury and death to young passengers placed in the front seat.

Environment: School nurses have the opportunity to assess and assist school programs in playground safety, including equipment, and observing for the use of appropriate gear for sporting events.

Recreational activities: Safe practices regarding bicycles (helmets), roller blades, and roller skates (helmets and padding) pertain to older age groups. Water-safety instruction should be a part of the parents' responsibility for safeguarding the child.

The home environment should be child-proofed depending on the age of the child. Parents need to be aware of hazards such as electrical outlets and safe storage of toxic substances, including medicines. The presence of lead in older homes is a particularly important issue in older inner-city neighborhoods and rural areas.

Fire safety should be taught, and every home should have an escape plan. Children, because of their natural curiosity, are fascinated by fire, but they should be taught not to play with cigarette lighters or matches.

Safe practices regarding the use of guns, both personal and hunting, need to be taught. The proper storage of guns in the home should be discussed.

Sexuality

Sexuality is often a sensitive issue for parents to discuss, but the NP who seeks to help the family develop a healthy lifestyle needs to begin to discuss and be open to questions related to the sexual development of the child. Discussing the natural sense of physical comfort and pleasure that even young children derive from genital stimulation and the family's own beliefs about sexuality are important.

During the preschool years, parents should understand the natural curiosity children have about sexuality, and how it will be important to provide appropriate information as their child matures. Adolescents need to be encouraged to keep the lines of communication open with their parents regarding their development of an individual sexual identity. Counseling, which should be available for this age group, should be centered around responsibility toward self and others, how to say "no," prevention of sexually transmitted diseases, and the way to deal with sexual abuse.

Social Interaction

Providing the family with information by which they gain insight into the family's role relationships is important. For self-esteem to be nurtured, each child must feel that he or she belongs in a family and should be allowed to assume a certain place or role within that family unit. Understanding how siblings feel regarding the newest member of the family is also important.

Discussing discipline strategies, participation in family activities, responsibility of each family member, and the ways in which the child interacts with friends when outside the home may often reveal an emerging problem that needs to be addressed. As the child enters adolescence, the parents need to understand that his or her dependence on the family decreases while positive peer relationships become critical to the child's well-being. At this time, the lines of communication need to be kept open between adolescents and their peers, parents, and other family members.

Summary

Health-promotion activities and responsibilities lie within the boundaries of the family, the patient, and the community. Health-care providers can best serve their patients when they operate under the belief that they can help patients maximize their health potential by serving as a guide and facilitator who designs and oversees ways to achieve that goal.

The American Academy of Pediatrics provides recommendations for preventive pediatric practices that should be incorporated into the NP's plan of care for each child. See Tables 1–5 and 1–6 for a list of recommendations for immunizations for children from birth and for children not immunized within the first year of life.

CHAPTER 3

NUTRITION

Normal growth and development depend on good nutrition. Health-care providers need to be knowlegeable in all areas of nutrition when assessing their clients. The nurse practitioner (NP) should ask about the nutritional habits of the child or infant, feeding preferences, and feeding problems, and they should be able to evaluate their patients within expected parameters of growth.

The principal food source for all infants during the first year of life is either formula or breast milk. Although many parents question the wisdom of delaying solid foods, they are unnecessary before the age of 4 to 6 months; in fact, early introduction of solid foods may increase the frequency and severity of food allergies. During the first 1–2 months infants should consume 2–3 ounces of milk every 2–3 hours for a total of 16–24 ounces of milk per day. For those infants who breastfeed, a good guide to follow is 10 minutes on each breast every 2–3 hours per day. Breastfed infants need to be fed more frequently because breast milk is digested in about 1½ hours, whereas formula takes about 4 hours to digest. When the infant is about 6 months old, 22–26 ounces of formula (or breast milk equivalent) per day is sufficient for adequate growth. Breastfeeding is preferred for infants up to age 6 months; maternal HIV infection is the only contraindication for this method of feeding. Although there are subtle differences among formulas, all sufficiently meet the growth needs of infants. For a comparison of these differences, see Table 3–1. Although the iron content of formula is higher than that of breast milk, a sufficient amount of iron exists in breast milk to make supplements unnecessary. Fluoride (0.25 mg/day) should be given to all breastfed infants.

Solid foods are generally introduced at age 4–6 months. Some signs that the child is ready for solid food include:

- More than 32 ounces of formula is required per day.
- Current weight has already doubled the birth weight.
- There is an increased demand for feedings (8–10 per day).

Persistent hunger indicates that the infant is not being satisfied by formula or breast milk alone. Generally, the first solid food introduced is rice cereal, followed by single-grain cereals. Fruits and vegetables should be introduced one at a time; no more than two new foods per week should be introduced. Meats are generally not given before age 6 months.

Juices, starting with apple juice, are given at age 4–6 months. Initially, no more than 2 ounces of juice per day should be given. The child can gradually increase consumption to 4–6 ounces of juice per day. The NP should encourage parents to give water from birth on because water can sometimes regulate the infant's bowel patterns, particularly if the infant has been constipated. Care should be taken, however, not to give more than 4 ounces per day until after age 2 months, due to the danger of increasing sodium levels in infants.

The parent should be encouraged to use a spoon to feed the child, *not* to put solid foods in a bottle or feeder. Therefore solid foods should not be given before the child is capable of eating from a spoon. Initially, 1 tbsp cereal is mixed with 2–3 ounces of liquid. Gradually, this mixture is thickened so that by age 7 months, the child is eating up to 6 tbsp cereal mixed with the same amount of liquid.

Weaning the child from breast milk or formula can be done by age 1 year, at which time homogenized Vitamin D–enriched milk can be given. By age 2 years, skim or 2% milk can be introduced. Table 3–2 lists the suggested caloric intake for children.

As children grow, table foods appropriate for their age should be introduced. Finger foods, low-fat snacks, and easily digestible foods should be included in the toddler's diet. For school-age and adolescent children, simple guidelines can be followed that can help ensure a healthy diet. First, children's eating habits are set early in life. Second, the family's patterns of nutrition will be the model for the child's pattern. The American Health Association has made the following recommendations for a healthy diet for the child and adolescent:

- Each meal should consist of one high-quality protein.
- Milk and other low-fat dairy products should be a part of each meal.
- Vegetables and fruits high in vitamins A and C should also be included in at least two meals per day.
- Whole grain, enriched breads, or cereals should be consumed daily.
- Meat should be included in four servings per week (4 ounces per serving).
- Fish and poultry should be consumed one to two times per week.
- Dark green, leafy, or deep yellow vegetables should be consumed each day, but at a minimum of four times per week.
- A maximum of four eggs per week should be consumed.

Ideally, the Daily Food Guide Pyramid can help parents plan their children's meals each day (Fig. 3–1).

The formula-fed infant does not need vitamin supplement unless the water used to mix the formula does not contain fluoride. A fluoride dose of 0.25–0.50 mg/day is needed. Because the breastfed infant does not receive all the neces-

TABLE 3–1 APPROXIMATE COMPOSITION OF INFANT FORMULAS*

	Kilocalories/ Ounce	Protein		Fat	
		Source	g/dL	Source	g/dL
Human Milk					
Mature human milk	20	Human milk	1.0	Human milk	4.4
Premature Formulas (Hospital and Transitional)					
Enfamil Human Milk Fortifier (3.8 g) added to 100 mL preterm milk (Mead Johnson)	24	Preterm human milk plus fortifier, whey and caseinate	2.3	Preterm human milk fat	3.5
Enfamil Premature (Mead Johnson)	24	Nonfat milk, whey	2.4	Soy, MCT (40%), coconut oils	4.1
Similac NeoCare (Ross)	22	Nonfat milk, whey	1.9	Soy, coconut, MCT (25%) oils	4.1
Similac Natural Care Human Milk Fortifier (Ross)	24	Nonfat milk, whey	2.2	MCT (50%), soy, coconut oils	4.4
Similac Special Care (Ross)	24	Nonfat milk, whey	2.2	MCT (50%), soy, coconut oils	4.4
SMA-Preemie (Wyeth Ayerst)	24	Whey, nonfat milk	2.0	Coconut, oleic, oleo, soy, MCT (10%) oils	4.4
Cow's Milk–based Formulas					
Bonamil (Wyeth Ayerst)	20	Nonfat milk	1.5	Soy, coconut, soy lecithin oils	3.6
Enfamil (Mead Johnson)	20	Whey, nonfat milk	1.4	Palm olein, soy, coconut, high-oleic sunflower oils	3.8
Gerber (Gerber)	20	Nonfat milk	1.5	Palm olein, soy, coconut, high-oleic sunflower oils	3.7

Carbohydrate Source	g/dL	Sodium (mEq/dL)	Potassium (mEq/dL)	Phosphorus (mg/dL)	Calcium (mg/dL)	Osmolality (mOsm/kg water)
Lactose	6.9	0.7	1.3	14	32	300
Preterm human milk, lactose, fortifier, corn syrup solids	10.1	1.5	1.7	60	117	410–440
Corn syrup solids, lactose	9.0	1.4	2.1	67	134	310
Corn syrup solids, lactose	7.7	1.0	2.7	46	78	290
Lactose, polycose	8.6	1.5	2.7	85	171	280
Lactose, polycose	8.6	1.5	2.7	73	146	280
Lactose, glucose polymers	8.6	1.4	1.9	40	75	280
Lactose	7.1	0.8	1.6	36	46	290
Lactose	7.0	0.8	1.9	36	53	300
Lactose	7.2	0.9	1.9	39	51	320

Continued on following page

TABLE 3–1 *Continued*

	Kilocalories/ Ounce	Protein		Fat	
		Source	g/dL	Source	g/dL
For Special Feeding Problems					
Portagen (Mead Johnson)	(Ross) 20	Sodium caseinate	2.4	MCT (86%), corn oil	3.3
Monodisaccharide-free diet powder Product 3232A (Mead Johnson)	13 Using 81.0 g powder and water to make 1 quart	Casein hydrolysate with added amino acids	1.9	MCT (85%), corn oil	2.9
Protein Vitamin Mineral Formula Component (Ross)	Add 30 g powder, CHO, and fat to 900 mL water	Casein	2.2	Coconut oils: may add corn, soy, safflower, MCT oils	Tr
RCF CHO-Free Formula Base	12 Dilute 1 : 1 without added CHO	Soy protein isolate with L-methionine	2.0	Soy, coconut oils	3.6
For Feeding Beyond 4 to 6 Months of Age with Solids Added to Diet					
Follow-Up (Carnation)	20	Nonfat milk	1.8	Palm olein, soy, coconut, high-oleic safflower oils	2.8
Follow-Up Soy (Carnation)	20	Soy protein isolate with L-methionine	2.1	Soy oil	3.7
For Feeding Beyond 1 Year of Age					
Whole cow's milk	20	Cow's milk	3.3	Cow's milk	3.7
Next Step (Mead Johnson)	20	Nonfat milk	1.8	Palm olein, soy, coconut, sunflower oils	3.4
Next Step Soy (Mead Johnson)	20	Soy protein isolate with L-methionine	2.2	Palm olein, soy, coconut, high-oleic sunflower oils	3.0
Similac Toddler's Best (Ross)	20	Nonfat milk	2.4	High-oleic safflower, coconut, soy coils	3.2

Carbohydrate Source	g/dL	Sodium (mEq/dL)	Potassium (mEq/dL)	Phosphorus (mg/dL)	Calcium (mg/dL)	Osmolality (mOsm/kg water)
Corn syrup solids, sucrose	7.8	1.6	2.2	48	64	230
Modified tapioca starch, may add 59 g CHO/ quart, corn syrup solids, sucrose, glucose, fructose	2.8 6.3	1.2	1.9	43	64	Dependent on additional CHO source: 250 without CHO source
May add sucrose, polycose, dextrose, fructose	Tr	1.6	2.5	51	72	Dependent on source and amount of CHO
May add sucrose polycose, dextrose, fructose	—	1.3	1.9	50	70	Dependent on source and amount of CHO
Corn syrup, lactose	8.9	1.2	2.3	61	91	326
Sucrose, tapioca dextrin	6.8	1.2	2.0	61	91	270
Lactose	4.7	2.1	3.9	93	119	288
Corn syrup solids, lactose	7.5	1.2	2.2	57	81	270
Corn syrup solids, sucrose	8.0	1.3	2.6	61	78	260
Sucrose, lactose	7.4	1.2	2.6	64	105	360

Continued on following page

TABLE 3–1 *Continued*

	Kilocalories/ Ounce	Protein		Fat	
		Source	g/dL	Source	g/dL
Nutrient Dense					
Kindercal (Mead Johnson)	30	Calcium caseinate, sodium caseinate, milk protein concentrate	3.4	Canola, high-oleic sunflower, corn, MCT (20%) oils	4.4
PediaSure (Ross)	30	Caseinate, whey proteins	3.0	High-oleic safflower, soy, MCT (20%) oils	5.0
PediaSure with Fiber (Ross)	30	Caseinate, whey proteins	3.0	High-oleic safflower, soy, MCT (20%) oils	5.0

*This dietitians' guide provides pertinent information to dietitians, physicians, and other members of the health-care team who care for infants and children. Specifically, it outlines the type and variety of formulas available for feeding infants and young children. Nutritional composition is provided for comparison because of the many products available commercially. Each product includes brand name; caloric content; source and amount of protein, fat, carbohydrate, amount of sodium, potassium, phosphorus, calcium; and osmolality. Product information is subject to change. The most current information regarding formula ingredients, label claims for nutrient amounts, and directions for preparation and use can be obtained by referring to product labeling. CHO = carbohydrates; MCT = medium-chain triglyceride; RCF = Ross carbohydrate free.
From Hattner, J., & Kerner, J. (1995). *Infant formula composition.* Stanford, CA: Department of Nutrition and Food Services. Stanford University Medical Center.
Source: USDA Handbook No. 8-1. Values are based on liquid formula unless otherwise indicated.

sary vitamins present in formula, a vitamin supplement is usually recommended. If iron supplements are prescribed for the breastfed infant, a dose of 1–15 mg/kg per day, in two to three divided doses, is advised. Because of the variability of children's eating patterns and unmet nutritional requirements, a chewable daily vitamin supplement may be needed once children reach school age. Girls who have begun menses should be given a vitamin with iron.

Because nutrition is so vital to good health, the NP should assess the child's growth at each visit and discuss with the parent and child, when appropriate, how the child's dietary needs are being met. Great care should be taken to detect eating abnormalities; the NP should begin by identifying the problems and working with the families to correct them. Although it is important to attempt to meet all required guidelines, the NP should be flexible and creative when helping families establish good eating habits.

Carbohydrate Source	g/dL	Sodium (mEq/ dL)	Potassium (mEq/dL)	Phosphorus (mg/dL)	Calcium (mg/dL)	Osmolality (mOsm/kg water)
Maltodextrin, sucrose, soy fiber	13.5	1.6	3.4	85	85	310
Corn syrup solids, sucrose	11.0	1.7	3.4	80	97	310
Corn syrup solids, sucrose, soy fiber	11.0	1.7	3.4	80	97	345

TABLE 3–2 SUGGESTED CALORIC INTAKE FOR CHILDREN

Age	cal/day
Newborn	300
1 year	600
2 years	875–900
3–4 years	1000–1100
5–7 years	1140–1240
Actual caloric needs of children are as follows:	
6–7 years	90 cal/kg per day
7–10 years	70 cal/kg per day
Boys over 10	2500–3000 cal/day
Girls over 10	2200 cal/day

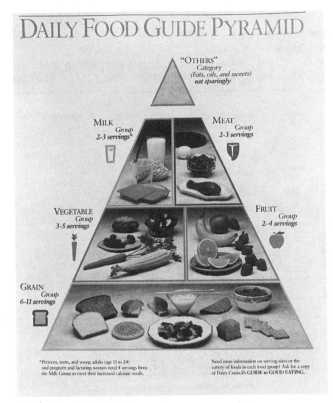

FIGURE 3–1   Daily Food Guide Pyramid.

UNIT II

ASSESSMENT

CHAPTER **4**

HISTORY TAKING

While taking the patient's history, the astute nurse practitioner (NP) can often obtain the most important clues toward making an accurate diagnosis. The components of a complete health history should include:

- Chief complaint or reason for the present visit.
- History of the present illness.
- Past medical history.
- Review of systems.
- Family history.
- Socioeconomic history.

The interview is a time for building rapport with the child and the caregiver, as well as for the collection of pertinent data leading to a diagnosis. Other clues that assist the NP can also be observed. The interaction between parent and child, the tone of voice used, and the posture of both child and parent during the interview, as well as the effect of giving information on either the child or parent should be noted. The NP should note his or her overall impression of the parent and child, including their general appearance, cleanliness, and status of clothing and grooming. The credibility of the informant should be gauged. (For example: Is this person knowledgable about the child, interested in the child and the illness, and able to communicate effectively?)

Client Information

Initially, the patient's and guardian's name, as well as the patient's birth date, address, insurance, and any other identifying information, should be obtained.

Chief Complaint

The chief complaint, including what the problem is, when it started, what may have precipitated the problem, and the signs and symptoms related to the problem should all be ascertained from either the child or the child's caregiver. The following is a list of other information needed: exposure to an illness either in the home or community, previous similar episodes, attempted remedies and their degree of success, and whether any other family members are also ill with the same or similar symptoms.

Past History

When obtaining information related to past medical history, both prenatal and perinatal information should be gathered. Prenatal history should include whether the pregnancy was planned, whether prenatal care was obtained, and the month in which the care began. The NP should also seek to obtain information related to the course of the pregnancy—that is, whether there were any problems during the pregnancy, including a history of any illnesses or accidents. Another important question to ask is whether any drugs (including prescription medications), alcohol, or tobacco were used during the pregnancy. An overall impression of the pregnancy should also be obtained from both the mother and father when possible. It is important to ascertain how the parents perceived the pregnancy when evaluating their reaction to the child and his or her illness.

Next, a perinatal history should be obtained, including where the child was born, who delivered the baby, and the type of delivery (vaginal versus cesarean section). Information related to the length of labor, type of anesthesia, and problems with either the mother or neonate at birth should also be explored. If possible, the Apgar score should be obtained. The birth weight and the height, and chest, and head circumferences should also be noted. The gestational age of the infant should be obtained. Finally, any neonatal complications and follow-up should be discussed.

Developmental Information

Developmental information should be collected. The NP needs to identify when developmental milestones were met. Any specific problems related to the emotional well-being of the child, parent, or family unit should be explored. The family history of health and disease should be evaluated. The age of the parents and the presence of siblings and others in the home should be explored. Familial diseases need to be identified and, when possible, a genogram constructed. The rank order of the children should be noted.

Past Health Problems

When investigating past health problems, the NP should explore the types of problems the child has had, the treatments given, and the outcomes. Any previous hospitalizations should be discussed; when possible, those records should be obtained.

Other health problems should be disclosed. Asthma, sickle cell disease, diabetes, cancer, chronic otitis, and pharyngitis are a few of the chronic illnesses that may have an impact on the present problem or treatment regimens. Previous hospitalizations and surgeries should be recorded along with any past injuries and accidents. Allergies to food, environmental factors, and current medications should be identified. Growth patterns, including careful plotting of height, weight, and head circumferences, should be recorded at each visit. Growth and developmental concerns, along with problems in these areas, should also be discussed.

Current Medications

Current medications and the reason prescribed should also be charted. Dosage, length of time on the medication, and the response to each medication should also be identified. Finally, an immunization history should be obtained, including any problems ever encountered following an immunization. Laboratory data should be recorded and discussed with the child and his or her guardian.

Additional Information

As part of the history, the NP should ask some form of the following open-ended question: "Is there anything else you would like to share or ask regarding your child at this time?" This type of question gives the child or parent an opportunity to offer information, ask questions, or voice concerns, often providing vital information to the NP.

In the next phase of taking the child's history, a review of systems (ROS) should be done (see Chapter 5).

Following the ROS, the following can be identified: the child's health-maintenance patterns, nutritional history, activities, sleep patterns, elimination patterns, temperament, cognitive or perceptual problems, self-perceptions, and sexual development; and the parents' discipline philosophy, perceptions, spirituality, or beliefs.

Health maintenance patterns should be discussed, and the NP should ask the parent and child (if appropriate) what, if any, usual primary care have they received. Other areas to explore are: whether dental care has been obtained regularly; whether there have been regular visits to primary-care facilities, eye doctors, and dentists; and whether any recommended safety measures are used, such as car seats, seat belts, smoke alarms, and other home safety measures.

Nutrition

Nutritional patterns should be explored, and the NP should inquire about the types of foods eaten and preferred, any problems with tolerating certain foods, or any problems with swallowing. Concerns about being too heavy or too thin should also be discussed. Whether an infant is breastfed or bottle fed and what type of formula has been tolerated best should also be noted in the history. Finally, the NP should question the child and/or parent about the need for any special nutritional foods or supplements, or whether any other unique nutritional needs or problems exist.

Physical Activity

Physical activities including the amount, type, and duration of exercise, either aerobic or anaerobic, should be noted. The amount of time a child watches television per day should be ascertained. The NP should ask whether any activities are limited because of health problems. Types of activities, including sports, exercise classes, and organized play should also be identified.

Sleep

Sleep patterns and problems should be identified.

Cognitive/Perceptual

The NP should identify any hearing, vision, learning, attention, or sensory problems.

Sexual Development

Sexual development and concerns should be discussed with both parents and children. When providing care to the adolescent, the NP should be sure to allow time for the adolescent to address concerns and give information in private, without the parent present. This privacy allows the adolescent an opportunity to share information or ask questions that he or she might be hesitant to ask otherwise.

Other Problems

Problems with elimination, including daily toileting habits, toilet training history, bed wetting (nocturnal or diurnal), or bowel problems (constipation or diarrhea), should be discussed. The NP should inquire about the child's temperament, reaction to stressful events, anxiety, and response to environmental changes.

The parents' discipline strategies and philosophy should be discussed. When possible, the NP should evaluate the child's perception of disciplinary measures in the home.

Although spirituality is an individual and personal affair, it is often helpful to identify spiritual beliefs and any effect they may have on health problems. These beliefs often have a great impact on treatment choices and health behaviors.

Summary

The NP needs to be open to allowing the parent or patient the opportunity to discuss freely, in an accepting, nonjudgmental environment, anything he or she has to say. The history taker needs to be empathetic and accepting of all that is revealed during this part of the examination. Some sources state that 80% of all the information one needs to know about a patient and his or her problems is obtained during this part of the examination—the history.

CHAPTER 5

REVIEW OF SYSTEMS

When performed in an organized manner, the review of systems (ROS) ensures that the nurse practitioner (NP) obtains information about the function or dysfunction of each system that may be important in both determining the presence of a problem and developing an overall plan for health promotion.

The most common approach to reviewing system function is to take a head-to-toe approach; however, in children flexibility is the general rule. Areas of distress should always have the first priority.

Routine physical examination includes collection of vital signs and overall health and well-being. It then proceeds to examination of each system in an organized fashion using inspection, palpation, percussion, and auscultation.

Vital Signs

Normal vital signs change as the child ages (Table 5–1). Temperature variations in children may be the result of exercise, fever, stress, and the environment,

TABLE 5–1 VARIATIONS IN VITAL SIGNS BY AGE

Age	Temperature (°F)	Pulse (beats/min)	Respiration (breaths/min)
3 mo	99.4	130	30–80
1 yr	99.7	115	20–40
3 yr	99.0	105	20–30
5 yr	98.6	95	20–25
9 yr	98.1	95	17–22
13 yr	97.8	85	17–22

including wearing too many clothes for the air temperature. Pulse and respiratory variations are an indication of exercise, anxiety, or illness.

General Health

Ask the parent or caregiver about the state of the child's overall health and well-being, including physical, emotional, and developmental status and any congenital anomalies that have been identified previously. Also, note whether the child is frequently fatigued, because this may be an indication of a problem (Fig. 5–1).

Skin

Inspect the skin and determine the color, turgor, and texture, or the presence of rashes, birthmarks, lesions, or tattoos along with other evidence of skin conditions. Inquire about frequent itching of the skin. Note the texture of hair, which could indicate a problem with nutrition or the endocrine system.

Head, Neck, Face

Assess head growth, circumference at birth, and any history of trauma. Note any history of headache. Note vision or hearing problems, difficulty inspiring because of nasal obstruction, or frequent sore throats.

Ask about routine dental care and any dental problems.

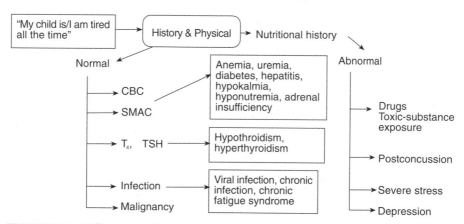

FIGURE 5–1 Differentiating fatigue. (CBC = complete blood count; SMAC = Sequential Multiple Analyzer Computer; T_4 = thyroxine; TSH = thyroid-stimulating hormone.)

Chest

Ask about problems with breathing, frequent infections, and chronic respiratory illness. Note known cardiac problems, including congenital anomalies, murmurs, irregular heart rhythms, or activity intolerance.

Genitourinary

Ask about past urinary tract infections, known structural problems, and if applicable, menstrual history. In particular, note any increased urinary frequency, burning, irregular urinary stream, enuresis, and perineal itching.

Musculoskeletal

Determine the presence of any pain, limitations in movement, gait abnormalities, past fractures, or joint problems.

Neurological

Note the presence or history of any seizures, tremors, tics, or problems with loss of consciousness.

Hematological

Note history of anemia, blood loss, transfusions, or other signs of bleeding disorders.

Summary

The ROS can be a revealing and important part of the examination and should always be thorough. The ROS may provide information not gathered during any other part of the examination and therefore should not be overlooked when obtaining a complete history.

TREATING

ILLNESS

CHAPTER **6**

ASSESSING THE SKIN
AND LYMPHATICS

When assessing the skin and lymphatics, the history is an important tool used to collect diagnostic clues and to help narrow the number of potential causes of presenting signs and symptoms. Certain medications, exposure to chemicals or other environmental substances, and several medical diseases and disorders can cause symptoms evidenced on the skin and in the lymph nodes. In fact, many skin problems are indications of other disease processes within the body (Flowers & Hacker, 1994). When assessing the skin, there are four important questions to address:

1. Is a lesion or rash present?
2. Is there a change in skin color?
3. Is pruritus present?
4. Has there been a change in hair or nails?

The lymphatic system is observed for:

- Palpable nodules.
- The presence of systemic infections.

Assessing the Skin

To assess the skin, the nurse practitioner (NP) needs to look and feel. Therefore, inspection and palpation are the techniques that provide the most useful information.

INSPECTION

Initially, observe the four factors of color, turgor, texture, and the presence and distribution of lesions. Normal skin has large variations in shades of color, depending on the amount of pigmentation. Any deviation from the patient's normal pattern may indicate a problem. Notice whether the pigmentation is consistent. Any areas of hyperpigmentation or hypopigmentation may need further investigation. For example, during pregnancy, it is normal for areas of darker pigmentation to appear on the face or in a medial line on the abdomen. A butterfly distribution on the face is suggestive of systemic lupus erythematosus. Absence of color in localized areas, indicating decreased pigmentation, is referred to as vitiligo. Total absence of pigmentation is termed albinism.

In assessing the skin, the NP should remember that the areas of skin affected by hormones (i.e., genitalia, nipples, areolae) will be darker in dark-skinned persons compared to those of lighter skin. These darker skinned groups include Native Americans, African-Americans, and Asians. Because these people have increased amounts of melanin, which protects the skin against ultraviolet (UV) rays, they have a lower incidence of skin cancer compared to whites. Cultural differences are also apparent in body odor (e.g., Asians and Native Americans have little to none, whereas whites and African-Americans tend to have a stronger body odor) and in the amount of chloride excreted (e.g., African-Americans excrete less in the sweat, as do Ashkenazi and Sephardic Jews).

The NP should note any evidence of cyanosis, jaundice, or pallor. These signs may be observed first in the sclera or nail beds and may be the most useful areas in which to assess dark-skinned patients. The presence of any of these signs warrants further investigation of the cardiopulmonary and hepatic systems.

Localized areas of skin-color variation may be indicative of skin tumors. The size and configuration of such variations are important. Note that any skin tumor larger than 6 mm is indicative of malignant melanoma (Table 6–1).

Skin texture normally has a soft, pliable texture, much like that of a baby's abdomen. The texture of the skin may reveal roughness, perhaps a result of the ambient environment, or the presence of sweating or dryness, which may be normal for the individual but could also indicate systemic diseases, such as fever, neoplasms, nephritis, or myxedema. The presence of excoriations should lead to questions about itching. Systemic disease processes evidenced by changes in skin texture:

"Soft": secondary hypothyroidism, hyperpituitarism, and eunochoid states.
"Hard": scleroderma, myxedema, and amylidosis.
"Velvety": Ehlers-Danlos syndrome.

Skin turgor is one of the best ways to estimate the hydration and nutritional status in the infant and child. When lifting a piece of skin and then releasing it, normal turgor is evident if the skin promptly resumes the normal contour. In cases of dehydration, this response is delayed.

Edema, increased fluid in the tissues, may indicate nephritis. Often the presence of edema is noted first in the eyelids. It may precede the onset of generalized edema, or facial edema may herald rapidly deteriorating problems, such as a severe allergic reaction. Peripheral edema may warrant further investigation of the cardiopulmonary system, whereas abdominal edema may suggest hepatic disease.

TABLE 6-1 SKIN TUMOR COMPARISONS

Color	Texture	Probable Tumor Type
Normal	Corrugated	Warts
	Smooth	Cysts
	Irregular	Keloids
	Varied, flat, verrucoid, smooth	Nevi
Pink or red	Flat, rough, smooth	Hemangiomas
	Varied, flat, verrucoid, smooth	Nevi
Brown	Crumbly, "pasted on"	Seborrheic keratosis
	Varied, flat, verrucoid, smooth	Nevi
	Smooth, sharply marginated	Lentigines
	Indurated	Dermatofibromas
Tannish yellow	Hard	Xanthomas
	Plaques	Xanthelasmas
	Corrugated	Warts
	Irregular	Keloid
Dark blue or black	Crumbly, "pasted on"	Seborrheic keratosis
	Flat, rough, smooth	Hemangiomas
	Flat	Blue nevi
	Indurated	Dermatofibromas

TABLE 6-2 CATEGORIZING SKIN LESIONS

Type	Description
Primary	
Macule	A flat hypopigmented or hyperpigmented lesion up to 1 cm in diameter, such as a freckle
Patch	A macule >1 cm in diameter
Papule	An elevated lesion up to 0.5 cm in diameter, such as an elevated nevus
Nodule	Large, elevated papule approximately 0.05–2 cm in diameter; may be in the epidermis, dermis, or subcutaneous tissue
Plaque	Elevated flat, circular lesions 0.3 cm or larger in diameter; it may have distinct edges or blend with the adjacent skin
Vesicle	Elevated lesion <0.3 cm in diameter, often transparent and filled with fluid
Pustule	A pus-filled vesicle that may indicate the presence of infection
Bulla	Large, translucent >0.3 cm in diameter, filled with fluid
Wheal	Firm, flat-topped, well-circumscribed elevation of skin from edema of the dermis
Secondary	
Scale	Dry, thin plaques of keratinized epidermal cells
Crust	Dried exudates on the surface of the skin
Lichenification	Shiny surface with exaggerated skin lines and induration from chronic rubbing of the skin

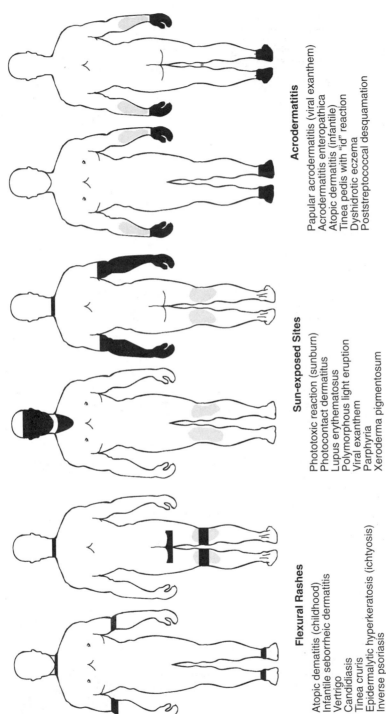

Flexural Rashes

Atopic dermatitis (childhood)
Infantile seborrheic dermatitis
Vertrigo
Candidiasis
Tinea cruris
Epidermalytic hyperkeratosis (ichtyosis)
Inverse psoriasis

A

Sun-exposed Sites

Phototoxic reaction (sunburn)
Photocontact dermatitis
Lupus erythematosus
Polymorphous light eruption
Viral exanthem
Parphyria
Xeroderma pigmentosum

B

Acrodermatitis

Papular acrodermatitis (viral exanthem)
Acrodermatitis enteropathica
Atopic dermatitis (infantile)
Tinea pedis with "id" reaction
Dyshidrotic eczema
Poststreptococcal desquamation

C

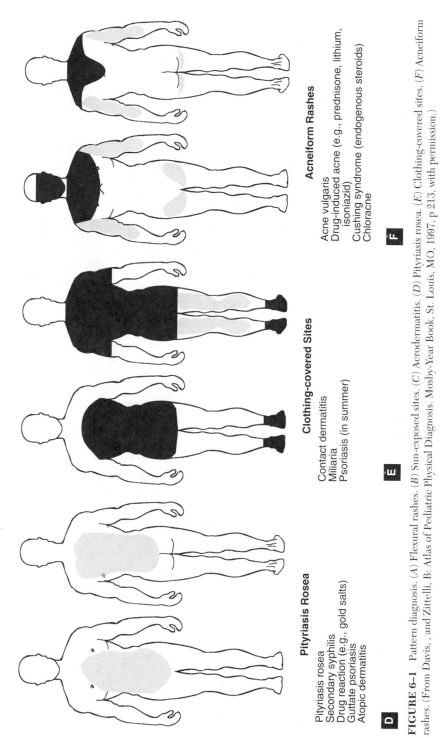

Pityriasis Rosea

Pityriasis rosea
Secondary syphilis
Drug reaction (e.g., gold salts)
Guttate psoriasis
Atopic dermatitis

Clothing-covered Sites

Contact dermatitis
Miliaria
Psoriasis (in summer)

Acneiform Rashes

Acne vulgaris
Drug-induced acne (e.g., prednisone, lithium, isoniazid)
Cushing syndrome (endogenous steroids)
Chloracne

FIGURE 6–1 Pattern diagnosis. (*A*) Flexural rashes. (*B*) Sun-exposed sites. (*C*) Acrodermatitis. (*D*) Pityriasis rosea. (*E*) Clothing-covered sites. (*F*) Acneiform rashes. (From Davis, , and Zittelli, B: Atlas of Pediatric Physical Diagnosis. Mosby–Year Book, St. Louis, MO, 1997, p 213, with permission.)

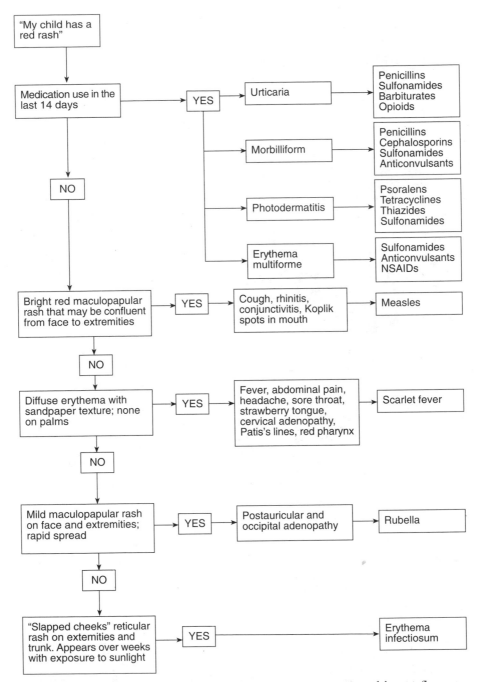

FIGURE 6–2 Determining the cause of a red rash. (NSAIDs = nonsteroidal anti-inflammatory drugs.)

Skin lesions are characterized by distribution, configuration, and color. Note the primary lesion and any secondary changes (Table 6–2; Fig. 6–1). Distribution often provides the first clue in determining the diagnosis of skin lesions. For example, acne vulgaris is commonly seen on the face and shoulders; atopic dermatitis is seen on the neck and the antecubital and popliteal space; pityriasis rosea is noted on the anterior and posterior chest, abdomen, and buttocks, but not on the legs or arms; and psoriasis is noted on the knees, elbows, fingers, scalp, and lower back. Configuration, or the arrangement of the lesions, also provides clues as to specific diagnosis. Serpiginous lesions are seen in parasitic diseases, linear lesions in scabies, and reticulated lesions in fifth disease. Color is another important descriptor. Pinkish yellow lesions are seen in pityriasis rosea and seborrheic dermatitis; dull red, silvery lesions are seen in psoriasis.

Along with the history and presence of other signs or symptoms, skin lesions can suggest an underlying systemic disorder, such as an allergic response or a childhood illness (Figs. 6–2 and 6–3).

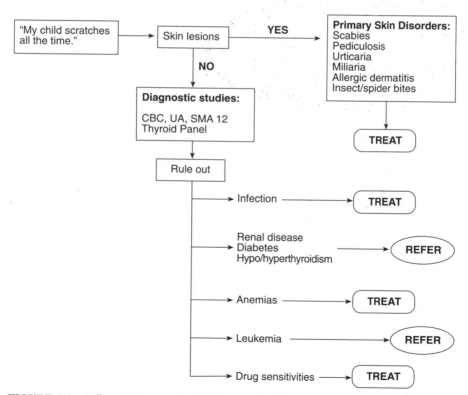

FIGURE 6–3   Differentiating pruritis. (CBC = complete blood count; UA = urinalysis; SMA = Sequential Multiple Analyzer.)

Inspection of the nails can provide clues to an underlying condition. For instance, pallor of the nail beds can indicate anemia, whereas a bluish discoloration (cyanosis) can indicate poor tissue oxygenation, possibly resulting from a cardiovascular or pulmonary disorder. Clubbing is often indicative of cardiovascular problems or cystic fibrosis; pitting may be seen in psoriasis; and lines in the nail beds are often associated with renal or hepatic diseases.

The NP should examine the hair and scalp, particularly the color, texture, and distribution of hair. Racial and cultural differences will be evident. For example, the hair of Asians is fine and straight, whereas the hair of African-Americans is fragile with textures ranging from straight to kinky. African-Americans routinely use oils on their hair and scalp because these tend to be extremely dry. In African-American children, extreme nutritional deficits affect the hair not only in the texture, but also in the color: The hair becomes straighter and turns coppery. Also, inspect the hair for lice or nits, or any abrasions caused by scratching. Areas of hair loss may indicate a fungal infection or trichotillomania—a compulsive twisting or pulling out of the hair, commonly exhibited when the child is stressed.

In summary, skin diseases are common and account for a large number of office visits. In addition, evaluation of the skin can give the first clues to systemic diseases.

Assessing the Lymph Nodes

In children up to the age of 12 years, cervical and inguinal nodes of up to 1 cm in diameter are normal. In all other areas, nodes up to 3 mm are considered normal. The NP should inspect and palpate these lymph nodes to determine their size, mobility, warmth, and tenderness. Acute infections usually result in large, warm, and tender nodes arising either from local infection or from the presence of a generalized disease process. Enlarged, isolated nodes are usually seen with a localized disease process, such as occipital or posterior auricular adenopathy seen in measles, external otitis, and local scalp infections. Enlarged cervical nodes are usually the result of acute infections in the mouth and throat. Enlargement of the left supraclavicular node ("sentinel node") may indicate the presence of Hodgkin's disease in children.

Abscess

An abscess is a pus-filled nodule in the dermis; it is usually self-limiting with effective treatment.

Etiology: The entrance into a superficial skin wound as a result of laceration or puncture wound of a pathogen, usually *Staphylococcus aureus*.

Occurrence: Common.

Age: Occurs at any age.

Ethnicity: Not significant.

Gender: Occurs equally in males and females.

Contributing Factors: Any alteration in the integrity of the skin, such as soft tissue trauma or insect bite.

Signs and Symptoms: Patient may give a history of superficial skin trauma and may have a fever. Examination of the lesion reveals swelling, erythema, and a fluctuant mass with or without drainage.

Diagnostic Tests: Culture of the drainage from the abscess shows offending organism, usually *S. aureus*.

Differential Diagnosis: Abscesses are rarely confused with other entities.

Treatment

Incision and drainage
Antibiotic therapy: Erythromycin or dicloxacillin 250–500 mg tid for 1 week; cefadroxil, 30 mg/kg daily or bid for 7–10 days

Follow-up: Return to clinic for evaluation of treatment efficacy in 7 days.

Sequelae: If not treated promptly and appropriately, bacteremia may occur but osteomyelitis is rare.

Prevention/Prophylaxis: Keep fingernails short and avoid scratching sites of insect bites. Practice good handwashing techniques.

Referral: Refer to consulting physician for cases requiring incision and drainage.

Education: Instruct parents in hygienic measures, such as keeping fingernails short and avoiding scratching lesions, and in the ways of keeping cross-contamination at a minimum.

Acne

Acne is a disorder of the pilosebacious follicles. Lesions present as noninflamed comedones (closed, whiteheads; open, blackheads), inflammatory papules, pustules, nodules, and cysts. Acne is classified as mild, moderate, or severe, depending on the extent of the lesions.

Etiology: Increase in the sebaceous glands due to androgen stimulation, blockage of the follicular canal, and growth of the skin bacterium *Propionibacterium acnes*.

Occurrence: Common.

Age: Neonatal acne, as a response to maternal androgen, appears at ages 2–4 weeks and subsides by ages 4–6 months. Acne vulgaris eruptions begin in preadolescence (50% of boys, ages 9–11); 85% of adolescents will have the lesions. Peak incidence occurs at ages 16–19 for males and 14–17 for females.

Ethnicity: Not significant.

Gender: Occurs in males more frequently, but the lesions are more persistent in females.

Contributing Factors: Increase in sebaceous gland stimulation due to hormonal changes (female exacerbations increase at time of menses). There may be a seasonal variation noted, worse during the winter and better during the summer. Tension, fatigue, and individual foods may trigger an acne flare-up. Washing and drying the skin roughly, as well as squeezing and picking at the lesions, irritate the skin and promote an inflammatory reaction.

Signs and Symptoms: Child presents with a history of skin lesions on the face, neck, chest, upper back, and shoulders, which have been increasing in number. Usually gives a history of trying over-the-counter (OTC) preparations without any benefit.

Inspection reveals mild to severe skin lesions present as noninflamed comedones, inflammatory papules, pustules, nodules, and cysts, which may exist concomitantly.

Diagnostic Tests: None; however, for females with cystic acne who are being considered for treatment with isotretinoin (Accutane), a complete blood count, high- and low-density lipoproteins, liver enzymes, and pregnancy test results should be obtained. If treatment with isotretinoin is initiated, pregnancy test results should be obtained monthly. May culture drainage from lesions if abscess formation occurs.

Differential Diagnosis

Flat warts of the face may be confused with the comedones, but the warts are small, flesh-colored, flat-topped papules with a finely textured surface.

In *bacterial folliculitis*, the presence of visible hairs in the pustules will be noted. If cultured, *S. aureus* will be present.

Treatment

Mild Acne

The patient should use only gentle facial soap, such as Dove or Neutrogena, and pat—not rub—the skin dry. Topical benzoyl peroxide gel (2.5%, 5%, 10%) should be applied to the entire face every morning. Usually treatment is begun with the 5% gel; benzoyl peroxide may cause skin irritation that disappears after the first 2 weeks of use. Topical tretinoin (Retin-A), 0.025% cream or 0.01% gel, is applied nightly 1/2 hour after cleansing skin. Azelaic acid cream (Azelex), applied twice a day, can also be used. Tretinoin may cause skin irritation that will disappear after the first 2 weeks of use. If there is no response after 6 weeks, the concentration should be increased to 0.25% of the gel or 0.05–0.1% of the cream. Improvement should be evident in 5–6 weeks.

Moderate Acne

Treatment is begun in accordance with the regimen outlined above. If there is no response to the benzoyl peroxide and topical tretinoin, or the medication causes significant irritation, a topical antibiotic solution should be substituted for the benzoyl peroxide (e.g., clindamycin, erythromycin, tetracycline, or meclocycline), morning and evening. Oral antibiotics (e.g., tetracycline, 500 mg bid for 1–2 months) can be given. If no response, a trial of erythromycin 250–300 mg bid should be administered.

Severe (Cystic) Acne

Isotretinoin, 1 mg/kg orally for 4 months (initiated by physician only), should be administered.

Follow-up: After initiating therapy, evaluate response at 2 weeks, 1 month, and then every 2 months.

Sequelae: In severe cases, scarring may occur.

Prevention/Prophylaxis: Adolescents should avoid oil-based cosmetics and face creams, oily hair products, and hair spray. In addition, keeping hair off the forehead (i.e., no bangs) and hands off the face should be stressed.

Referral: In cases of severe acne and for recommendation or consideration for the use of isotretinoin (Accutane), refer to a physician.

Education: The adolescent should be instructed to eat a balanced diet; not to restrict diet unless he or she notices that certain foods seem to make the problem worse; to use water-based cosmetics sparingly; not to pick at the lesions; and to have patience, as improvement does not occur overnight. In fact, patients who use tretinoin and isotretinoin may experience redness, peeling, and itching for several weeks as the skin adjusts to the medication. Females taking antibiotics need to be aware of the risk of vaginal candidiasis. In addition, oral antibiotics may interfere with oral contraceptives, thus requiring additional precautions. Patients taking tretinoin or tetracycline should be instructed to avoid excessive skin exposure, particularly during the hours of 10 AM and 2 PM.

Alopecia

Alopecia describes the loss of hair, partial or complete, usually from the scalp, but the condition may affect other areas of the body. The term does not include the loss of hair due to breakage. Normal hair growth progresses in two cycles: the anagen cycle, or growth phase; and the telogen cycle, or resting phase (20% of hair follicles are in this stage). Normal loss of hair during the telogen phase is 50 hairs per day. The several forms of alopecia include:

Androgenetic alopecia (male pattern baldness).
Alopecia areata (noncicatrical alopecia).
Alopecia universalis (loss of all body hair).
Follicular mucinosis or alopecia mucinosa (unknown cause; benign eruptions of lesions on face or scalp).
Telogen effluvium (diffuse hair loss).

Trichotillomania (compulsive, subconscious manipulation of the hair).
Traction alopecia (due to hair style).
Toxic alopecia (a result of ingestion of certain medications).

Alopecia is further classified as scarring or nonscarring. Nonscarring alopecias are reversible, whereas scarring alopecias result in permanent hair loss.

Etiology: The specific mechanism cannot always be determined, but may be a result of intrinsic factors in growth, or an indication of an underlying disorder.

Occurrence: Fairly common.

Age: All age groups.

Ethnicity: Not significant.

Gender: Occurs equally in males and females.

Contributory Factors

Genetic factors, such as progeria.
Metabolic defects, such as homocystinuria, endocrine-related illnesses (e.g., those involving the thyroid, adrenals, pituitary glands), celiac disease.
Infections, tinea, high fevers, seborrheic dermatitis.
Radiation and certain chemotherapeutic agents.
Behavioral patterns.

Signs and Symptoms: The child may present in the clinic with the complaint of hair loss when shampooing or when brushing the hair, or the condition may be discovered during the course of the physical examination. A careful history of drug use, behavior, grooming patterns, and recent illness is helpful.

Inspection reveals a specific pattern of hair loss, the presence of lesions (inflammatory or tumorous), and the presence of scarring.

Diagnostic Tests: Culture and sensitivity studies in cases of suspected infection. Examination under a Woods lamp to identify the presence of fungal infections. Microscopic examination of a hair follicle for the presence of exclamation-point hairs. Biopsy of the site for confirmation of scarring of the follicles.

Differential Diagnosis

Telogen effluvium: Occurs in children ages 2–4 months, children with a history of severe febrile illness, or adolescents in the postpartum period.
Toxic alopecia: History of exposure to radiation or chemotherapeutic agents; also heparin and coumarin may induce shedding of hair.
Trichotillomania: History of habitual twisting or pulling at the hair. Consider alopecia areata and tinea capitis in the differential diagnosis.
Alopecia areata: Round or oval scalp patches and rapid hair loss; usually affects other body sites. Nails should be examined for signs of dystrophy.

Often (20% of cases) there is a family history of the condition. Review history for the presence of stress and systemic diseases such as thyroiditis, anemias, and vitiligo. Assess the child for tinea capitis and seborrheic dermatitis.

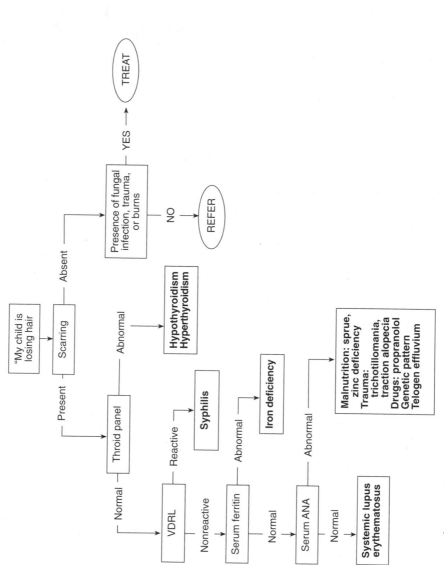

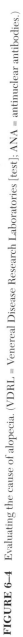

FIGURE 6–4 Evaluating the cause of alopecia. (VDRL = Venereal Disease Research Laboratories [test]; ANA = antinuclear antibodies.)

Treatment: If an underlying illness is found, usually treatment of the illness is sufficient to achieve regrowth. In traction alopecia, an alteration in hair style is sufficient. Satisfactory regrowth depends on the degree to which the hair follicles have been scarred. If extensive scarring has occurred, regrowth of hair does not occur. Behavioral management techniques are useful for adolescents with trichotillomania. Topical steroids may be applied to the scalp in cases of alopecia areata.

Follow-up: Ten days to 2 weeks for evaluation of progress.

Sequelae: Long-term trauma to the follicles results in scarring and permanent loss of hair.

Prevention/Prophylaxis: In cases of traction alopecia, reduction in the severe pulling of the hair resulting in structural damage to the follicles. Observe early the habit pattern of trichotillomania.

Referral: Refer to dermatologist for suspected cases of skin tumors, and to a mental health facility for counseling in cases of severe trichotillomania.

Education: Instruct parents that in most cases the condition is reversible. Instruct parents as to changing their child's hair style in cases of traction alopecia, as well as regarding the importance of treating any underlying inflammatory processes. In severe cases, such as those resulting from radiation or chemotherapeutic agents, the purchase of head coverings such as a wig improves the self-image of the child (most insurance companies cover the cost of the wig if prescribed as a "cranial prosthesis" [Fig. 6–4]).

Atopic Dermatitis

Atopic dermatitis (AD) is characterized as a chronic, relapsing, pruritic, eczematous skin condition. It is part of the "allergic triad" that includes allergic rhinitis and asthma.

Etiology: It is unknown whether there is a genetic predisposition, but it is highly possible: 66% of children have a family history of atopy. An immunologic basis has been proposed because 80% of children with AD have elevated IgE concentrations; therefore, food hypersensitivity needs to be considered as an etiologic factor. Structural differences in the skin have also been proposed (i.e., that the water content of the stratum corneum may have a reduced water-binding capacity as well as reduced water content).

Occurrence: Estimated that 5% of children have AD.

Age: Between 2 months and 5 years.

Ethnicity: Not significant.

Gender: Slightly higher in males (20% in males, 19% in females).

Contributing Factors: Family history of AD, asthma, allergic rhinitis, food allergy, skin infection, irritation from clothing or chemicals, or stress have been considered.

Signs and Symptoms: Parent gives history of lesion distributed in the following manner:

Infants: Head, diaper area, and extensor surfaces of the extremities.
Older children: Neck, face, upper chest, and antecubital and popliteal fossa. The lesions are mildly to severely pruritic. There is often a family history of asthma, allergic rhinitis, or AD.

Physical findings depend on age. Infants present with vesicles and juicy papules, whereas older children present with lichenified plaques on the head, neck, antecubital and popliteal fossa. Depending on the degree of excoriation, secondary infection may be present.

Diagnostic Tests: Elevated IgE concentration have been found in children with AD.

Differential Diagnosis

Rash may appear similar to *scabies*. However, the characteristic distribution on the hands and feet of scabies and the absence of linear burrows facilitate differentiation.

The rash may be confused with *seborrheic dermatitis*. However, the yellow, greasy patches and areas of distribution—the scalp, face, and chest—found in seborrheic dermatitis are exclusionary.

Treatment

Nonpharmacological

Adequate skin hydration should be maintained, including measures such as nightly baths of 15–20 minutes and avoiding the use of abrasive materials. Only gentle soaps (e.g., Dove, Neutrogena) or nonsoap cleaning agents (e.g., Aveeno, liquid cleansers such as Dove, Moisturel, Neutrogena) should be used. A wet dressing may be applied (e.g., tube socks or pajamas applied to body part, using another pair to cover the wet dressing). Do not allow child to become chilled. To prevent loss of moisture, moisturizers such as Vaseline, Crisco, Eucerin cream, or Aquaphor should be used during the day, as needed, for itching or dryness. In cases where moisturizers do not help, the patient should be instructed to use special preparations such as Lac Hydrin or Lacticare, which contain lactic acid, or urea creams such as Carmol or Aquacare Cream. The patient should avoid using perfumed products and bath oils and should keep fingernails short.

Pharmacological

Topical steroids are often used in acute situations. As a general guideline, prescribe the right vehicle and the right potency. Ointments are considered best for use on lichenified or thickened skin, but unacceptable for hairy or moist areas. For moist areas, prescribe creams; for the scalp, prescribe lotion or gels. For lichenified or thickened skin, a moderate-potency steroid ointment should be applied twice daily for 2 weeks. The following areas should be given special attention:

- *Scalp*: Moderate-potency steroid gel or solution applied daily for 2 weeks. Examples of moderate potency steroid ointments are mometasone furoate 0.1% cream or ointment (Elocon), hydrocortisone valerate 0.2% cream or ointment (Westcort), triamcinolone acetonide 0.01% cream or 0.1% ointment (Kenalog, Aristocort).
- *Moist dermatoses:* Low-potency cream applied twice daily for 7–10 days.
- *Face, groin, axillae, scrotum, or eyelids:* Low-potency cream applied three times daily for 7–10 days. Examples of low-potency steroid ointments are hydrocortisone 0.25%, 0.50%, 1%, 2.5% (Hytone, Nutracort, and OTC preparations); fluoromethalone 0.02% cream (Oxylone); and methylprednisolone 1% (Medrol). Tar products such as Estar Gel and T-Gel may be used for minor symptoms. These products may cause burning or skin irritation. Antihistamines may be used at nighttime for their sedative and antipruritic effect. Oral antibiotics should be prescribed if there is further skin breakdown with impetiginization.

Follow-up: The patient should return to the clinic in 1–2 weeks for evaluation of healing process.

Sequelae: In cases of widespread skin breakdown, a secondary infection may develop with vesicles, honey-colored drainage, pain, and increased oozing. Asthma may develop in 50% of the children.

Prevention/Prophylaxis: Modification of the diet has been suggested as a preventive measure in infants; this entails avoiding milk, eggs, and wheat for first 6 months of life, although this has not been proved effective. Identify and avoid environmental and stress factors that may act as "triggers" to exacerbations. Maintaining increased moisture through the use of creams or ointment and avoidance of harsh soaps, perfumes, or additives may be helpful.

Referral: Refer to allergist for a radioallergosorbent test (RAST) if food allergy is being considered as an underlying cause.

Education: Reassure parents that most children will outgrow AD by adolescence. Teach parents to observe child for identification of trigger factors. Stress to parents the importance of good skin care and not allowing the child to get sunburned. Increased compliance may result if parents and child are provided with written instructions related to the therapeutic regime.

Burns

Burns are thermal injuries to the epidermis and dermis. They are classified as:

Superficial (first-degree), involving the epidermis.

Partial-thickness (second-degree), involving the epidermis and dermis.

Full-thickness (third-degree), all epidermal and dermal levels.

Etiology: The destruction of the skin by excessively hot liquids, chemicals, electricity, or radiation; accidents.

Occurrence: Each year, 1% of the population is burned or scalded; 2.3 in 10,0000 die of burn injuries. The upper extremities are involved in 71% of cases; 52% involve the head and neck.

Age: All age groups.

Ethnicity: Not significant.

Gender: Occurs equally in males and females.

Contributing Factors: Lack of knowledge related to proper safety and storage of hazardous substances, a lack of regard for known dangers, and possibility of child abuse.

Signs and Symptoms: Patient provides history of exposure of the skin to a hazardous substance that resulted in injury to the skin. Need to query as to the causative agent, circumstances related to the injury, time elapsed since injury, and tetanus immunization status. In cases of chemical burn, the NP needs to know the type and concentration of the solution, as well as any other pertinent past history.

An examination of the skin reveals the following (Fig. 6–5):

Superficial: Skin is painful, dry, red, hypersensitive.

Partial-thickness: Skin is red, may blister or turn white, is dry, blanches with pressure, has decreased sensitivity.

Full-thickness: Skin is avascular, dry, depressed, leathery, without sensation.

It is important that the percentage of body surface involved be estimated adequately. The palm of a child's hand is approximately 1% of his or her body surface area. Burns on the face, eyes, ears, hands, feet, and perineum are always considered severe, as are those associated with major trauma, inhalation burns, and electrical burns. Children under age 10 have variations of body surface area on the Lund and Browder modification of the Berkow scale (Table 6–3).

Diagnostic Tests: None.

Differential Diagnosis: None.

Treatment: Outpatient treatment is based on the type and degree of burn, as follows:

Superficial: Application of cool compresses. Analgesia may be given for minor discomfort.

Partial-thickness with blisters: Initially, do a septic debridement with antiseptic cleansing using 1–5% povidone-iodine, and rinse with normal saline. Apply topical antibiotic (silver sulfadiazine) and protect with bulky dressing.
Full-thickness: Refer for hospitalization.

Follow-up: The patient should return in 24 hours for evaluation, change of dressing, and further debridement, as required.

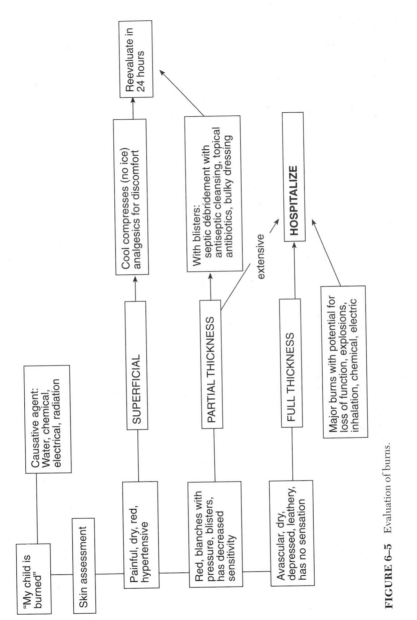

FIGURE 6–5 Evaluation of burns.

Sequelae: Secondary infection is a potential complication of burns. The risk for disability depends on the location of the burn. Burns to the face, eyes, ears, feet, perineum, or hands pose the greatest risk for disability. Superficial and partial-thickness burns do not cause permanent disability; however, full-thickness burns usually leave some impairment. Inhalation injuries can cause permanent respiratory compromise.

TABLE 6–3 VARIATIONS FROM ADULT DISTRIBUTION IN INFANTS AND CHILDREN (IN PERCENT)

	Newborn	1 yr	5 yr	10 yr
Head	19	17	13	11
Both thighs	11	13	16	17
Both lower legs	10	10	11	12
Neck	2			
Anterior trunk	13			
Posterior trunk	13			
Both upper arms	5	These percentages		
Both lower arms	6	remain constant at all ages		
Both hands	5			
Both buttocks	5			
Both feet	5			
Genitalia	1			

Source: After Berkow, as cited in Hay, W, et al: Current Pediatric Diagnosis and Treatment, ed 12. Appleton and Lange, Norwalk, CT, 1995, p 355, with permission.

Prevention/Prophylaxis: Proper use and storage of chemicals, appropriate safety measures for electric current, alertness to the inherent dangers in fire and water, and proper sunbathing methods. Teach safety to the parents of young children.

Referral: Refer for hospitalization in the following cases: full-thickness, inhalation, chemical, and electrical burns, as well as explosions. Report any suspicion of abuse. Refer any patient with a burn that could potentially cause loss of function or scarring (e.g., hands, fingers).

Education: Instruct parents regarding safe practice in the use and storage of chemicals, as well as safety measures for avoiding exposure to electrical current. Instruct parents in ways to monitor substances or elements that are potentially harmful. Instruct parents and children as to the dangers of exposure to the sun, appropriate sunbathing methods, and proper use of sunscreen lotions. Teach young children the dangers of fire.

Candidiasis

Candidiasis is an inflammatory skin reaction resulting from infection with *Candida albicans.*

Etiology: The yeast organism, *C. albicans*, is the offending agent.

Occurrence: Common.

Age: Usually observed in infants; can be seen in other age groups.

Ethnicity: Not significant.

Gender: Occurs equally in males and females.

Contributing Factors: Improper cleansing of the genital area, use of cornstarch as a diaper powder, and occlusion of the genital area by plastic pants or absorbent diapers that are too tight. Patients taking antibiotics or birth control pills, or who have diabetes or HIV, are at higher risk for the development of yeast infections.

Signs and Symptoms: Presenting complaint is the presence of a red rash with accompanying itching and burning of the skin. Inquire as to the area of the body, for although the usual site is the genital area, candidal infections can occur in other moist areas, such as under the breasts, axillae, and in skin folds. Important clinical factors are past medical history, current medical regimen, and in young children, a family history of diabetes. Physical findings reveal a beefy-red, erythematous area with satellite lesions (papules and pustules).

Diagnostic Tests: An examination of the pustules or scales using a potassium hydroxide (KOH) prep that reveals the presence of hyphae is diagnostic. In recalcitrant cases, a blood sugar level should be drawn to identify covert diabetes.

Differential Diagnosis

Contact dermatitis due to chemical irritants is a possibility, but it does not produce the characteristic satellite lesions of candidal infection.

Tinea cruris may be considered, but the lesions in tinea are much better demarcated.

Treatment

Nonpharmacological

General instructions for infants include encouraging frequent diaper changes, allowing the infant's bottom to air-dry during the day, and eliminating plastic pants.

Pharmacological

Topical applications, such as nystatin (Mycostatin) applied every 3–4 hours. Alternatives are clotrimazole (Lotrisone) or miconazole (Micatin), or ketoconazole (Nizoral) applied twice daily.

Follow-up: The patient should return in 1–2 weeks for evaluation of healing process. In recalcitrant cases, order tests to check for diabetes.

Sequelae: Systemic infection may occur in persons who are immunosuppressed. There may be renal, hepatic, pulmonary, or cerebral abscesses, or "cotton wool" retinal lesions.

Prevention/Prophylaxis: Adjusting the factors that keep the person at risk, such as keeping the diaper area dry, or treating concomitant medical problems such as diabetes.

Referral: Refer if systemic infection or diabetes mellitus is suspected.

Education: Instruct parent regarding proper application of topical cream and general hygienic measures.

Cellulitis

Cellulitis is a deep infection of the skin resulting in a localized area of erythema.

Etiology: Entrance into a superficial skin wound as a result of laceration or puncture wound of a pathogen, usually Group A streptococci. In children under age 3 with facial cellulitis, the causative organism is usually *Haemophilus influenzae,* and the infection is associated with otitis media.

Occurrence: Common.

Age: Occurs at any age.

Ethnicity: Not significant.

Gender: Occurs in males and females.

Contributing Factors: Any past alteration in the integrity of the skin, such as soft tissue trauma or insect bite.

Signs and Symptoms: Client may give a history of superficial skin trauma and will usually have a fever. In cases of buccal cellulitis, a history of otitis media or complaints of ear pain may be elicited.

Physical: Examination of the lesion reveals swelling, erythema, local induration and discoloration, tenderness and pain, and minimal drainage and involvement of local lymph nodes.

Diagnostic Tests: Obtaining a culture of the affected area in cellulitis is not usually possible, but a blood culture or culture of skin aspirate may show Group A streptococci.

Differential Diagnosis: Cellulitis may be confused with *contact dermatitis;* however, contact dermatitis is pruritic and there is absence of fever.

Treatment: Application of warm, wet compresses and antibiotic therapy (erythromycin or dicloxacillin, 500 mg qid for 10 days). In cases of facial involvement, prescribe parenteral coverage for *H. influenzae*: ampicillin with chloramphenicol or third-generation cephalosporin, such as cefadroxil (Duricef), (30 mg/kg daily or bid for 7–10 days).

Follow-up: The patient should return to the clinic in 24–48 hours, and again in 10 days, for evaluation of therapeutic response. The fever should respond in 24–48 hours, but the tissue swelling will not resolve for 1–2 weeks.

Sequelae: If the infection is treated promptly and appropriately, the patient will be unlikely to have bacteremia, local abscesses, and osteomyelitis (these are currently rare complications).

Prevention/Prophylaxis: Appropriate cleansing of superficial skin lacerations.

Referral: Refer to consulting physician for cases of facial cellulitis and those requiring incision and drainage.

Education: Instruct parents in practicing proper hygiene, keeping fingernails short, and avoiding scratching lesions.

Contact Dermatitis

Contact dermatitis is the inflammatory, pruritic reaction of the skin to an exogenous chemical. There are two types:

Irritant: The result of a substance that has a directly toxic effect on the skin.
Allergic: The immunologic reaction that causes tissue inflammation.

Etiology: Examples of some of the agents:

Irritant: Acids, alkalis, solvents, and detergents.
Allergic: Metals, plants (e.g., poison ivy and poison oak), medicines, and rubber compounds (Table 6–4).

Occurrence: Common.

Age: All age groups.

Ethnicity: Not significant.

Gender: Occurs equally in males and females.

Contributing Factors: Exposure to offending substances.

Signs and Symptoms: Patient usually presents with an itchy rash. Allergic reactions usually take 24–48 hours, occasionally 8–12 hours, or as long as 7 days to manifest after exposure. Elicit history of exposures, hobbies, and changes in hygienic agents (e.g., soaps, detergents, laundry softeners), makeup, or perfumes. Query as to exposure to plants, animals, and metals.

Clinical presentation varies from acute vesicles to chronic, lichenified, eczematous reactions. For example:

Poison ivy, poison oak, or poison sumac: Linear streaks of papules and vesicles.
Rubber compounds: Eczematous reaction limited to hands, feet, and diaper area.
Chemical irritation (e.g., feces, urine): Extreme redness.

Diagnostic Tests: None.

Differential Diagnosis

In *cellulitis*, the skin is painful rather than pruritic.
In *eczema* and *fungal infections*, the distribution and history helps in the differential diagnosis.

TABLE 6–4 ALLERGENS ASSOCIATED WITH CONTACT DERMATITIS

Location	Possible Allergen
Scalp	Hair dyes
	Shampoos
	Tonics
Eyelids	Eye makeup
	Hair sprays
Neck	Aftershave lotions
	Perfumes
	Soaps
	Washing agents
	Nickel jewelry
Trunk	Clothing
	Washing agents
Axillae	Deodorants
	Soaps
Genitalia	Soaps
	Contraceptives
	Deodorants
	Washing agents
Feet	Shoes
	Sneakers
	Deodorants
	Socks
	Washing agents
Hands	Nickel jewelry
	Soaps
	Dyes
	Plants

Source: Swartz M: Textbook of Physical Diagnosis: History and Examination, ed 2. WB Saunders, Philadelphia, 1994, p 95, with permission.

Treatment

Generalized Contact Dermatitis (Poison Ivy, Poison Oak, Poison Sumac)

For an acute, severe response, give a short course of steroids for a minimum of 5 days, and then taper for a total of 10 days. Astringent dressings (Domboro) and soothing oatmeal baths (Aveeno) may relieve itching. In cases of a milder response, topical steroids may be applied to lesions. Antihistamines may be given to relieve itching; hydroxyzine (Atarax) 10–25 mg or diphenhydramine (Benadryl), 25–50 mg qid. (*Note*: Do not apply diphenhydramine lotion: The lotion is absorbed systemically, and an overdose of medicine can occur.)

Diaper Dermatitis

For mild diaper dermatitis, encourage the mother to make frequent diaper changes, not to use plastic pants, and to clean the diaper area thoroughly after each diaper change. Some time during the day, allow the infant's bottom to air-dry. Trying a different type of diaper might assist in healing. Use powder sparingly, and do not use cornstarch. For more severe cases, try a barrier by applying zinc oxide to the area.

Follow-up: The patient should return in 1–2 weeks for evaluation of the healing process.

Sequelae: Excoriations as a result of the intense pruritus can result in impetiginization. Autosensitization is a generalized subacute dermatitis following a localized dermatitis. It is considered a hypersensitivity reaction to the substance produced by the acute dermatitis.

Prevention/Prophylaxis: Avoidance of the offending substances, shown in Fig. 6–6.

Generalized Contact Dermatitis

Poison ivy (*Rhus radicans*) is a perennial woody climbing vine. There are three leaves that are ovate, thin, bright green, and shiny. Poison oak (*Rhus toxicodendron*) is a low shrub similar to Poison ivy; lobate leaves are thicker, dull green, and hairy on both sides. Poison sumac (*Rhus vernix*) is a deciduous shrub with 7–13 leaves that are elliptical to oblong.

Diaper Dermatitis

Change diapers frequently. Avoid rubber or plastic pants.

Referral: None.

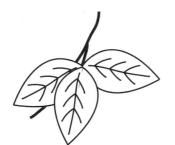

Rhus radicans
Rhus toxicodendron

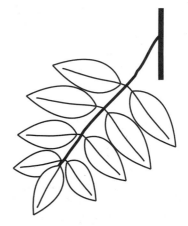

Rhus vernix

FIGURE 6–6   Leaves of Poison Ivy, Poison Oak, and Poison Sumac.

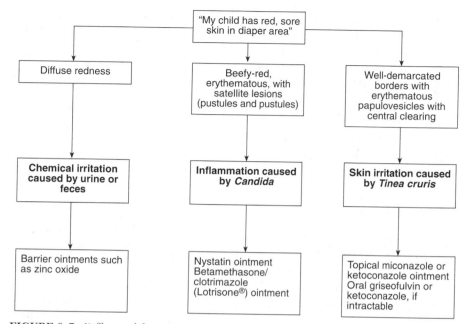

FIGURE 6–7 Differential diagnosis and treatment of diaper rash.

Education: Teach parents and children to recognize poison ivy and poison oak. Poison ivy leaves, stems, and roots are still toxic in the wintertime. In fact, the reaction may be worse: Because the plant is dehydrated, the toxic substance is enhanced. Therefore instruct parents and children to wear protective clothing, gloves, and long sleeves, even in the winter time, when handling the plant.

Teach parents that they need to keep the child's genital area as dry as possible. Teach parents and children to recognize substances that irritate (Fig. 6–7).

Drug Eruptions

There are varied skin eruptions due to administration of a drug. Some eruptions occur immediately, whereas others occur in 7–14 days after administration of the drug; the reaction may even be as long as 2 weeks after the drug is administered. The reaction arises from immunologic or nonimmunologic mechanisms.

Etiology: Immune reactions are of four major types:

Type I (IgE-dependent) reactions, which produce histamine and other vasoactive amines, occur within minutes of administration.

Type II (cytotoxic) reactions are tissue-reactant. Haptenic groups are introduced onto a cell surface, making the tissue susceptible to antibody- or lymphocyte-mediated cytotoxicity. These groups bind to cell surfaces, damaging the cells and thus inducing antibodies against specific human tissue antigens.

Type III (immune complex) reactions develop when the drug acts as an antigen, producing an immune complex vasculitis leading to serum sickness.

Type IV (cell-mediated) reactions occur when the drug antigen comes in contact with T cells, producing acute allergic dermatitis.

Nonimmunologic drug reaction, the more common type, results from overdose, cumulative toxicity, drug interactions, and metabolic changes.

Occurrence: Fairly common.

Age: Any age group.

Ethnicity: Not significant.

Gender: Occurs equally in males and females.

Contributing Factors: A family history of drug reactions; previous inoculation by the substance, and the individual's unique response to medication.

Signs and Symptoms: Parent complains, "my child has a rash." There may or may not be a history of itching. History should include a general medical history, a drug history, including dosage and duration of therapy, history of past drug reactions, and family history of drug allergies. Findings reveal a rash that may have the following characteristics:

Urticaria (type I): Pruritic, erythematous wheals or hives, varied in size and location. They change shape and location, and rarely last longer than 24 hours. Onset is minutes to days after exposure to the drug. Common drugs that precipitate a reaction via an immunologically mediated mechanism are acetylsalicylic acid, cephalosporins, griseofulvin, penicillins, sulfonamides, tetracyclines, and barbiturates. Nonimmunologic reactions that produce urticaria are reactions to alcohol, aspirin, codeine, estrogens, meperidine, and vancomycin.

Angioedema (type I): Large, deep areas of swelling; manifested by abdominal colic, hoarseness, stridor, and urticaria. Examples of responsible drugs are the above-mentioned ones that produce urticaria (type I).

Morbilliform eruptions: Symmetrically distributed, small macular or papular red spots, often confluent, starting at the head and neck and progressing downward. These reactions are not medication specific and are the most common of the reactions listed. Drugs most often associated with this eruption are barbiturates, carbamazepine, penicillins, phenothiazines, and streptomycins; less commonly associated are chloramphenicol, erythromycin, sulfonamides, and tetracylines.

Fixed drug eruptions: A solitary or a few sharply demarcated erythematous plaques, often tender and bulbous; often occur on the lips and genitalia. Common drugs are barbiturates, metronidazole, naproxen, nystatin, oral contraceptives, phenacetin, salicylates, sulfonamides, and tetracyclines.

Photosensitivity eruptions: Usually confined to the sun-exposed areas of the skin. They occur with the first exposure to the drug and are dose-related. Phototoxic reactions resemble a sunburn, whereas photoallergic reactions resemble eczema. Medications leading to a photosensitivity reaction are griseofulvin, nonsteroidal anti-inflammatory drugs, sulfonamides, and tetracylines.

Erythema multiforme minor: An acute, self-limited inflammatory disorder of the skin and one mucous membrane with distinctive target lesions. The most frequent causative agents are aminopenicillins, barbiturates, carbamazepine, sulfadiazine, sulfadoxine, and trimethoprim-sulfamethoxazole. Less commonly associated are cephalosporins, ibuprofen, rifampin, and vancomycin. Herpes simplex virus is often associated with erythema multiforme minor.

Stevens-Johnson syndrome (erythema multiforme major): Characterized by fever, headache, malaise, and severe involvement of the skin and at least two mucous membranes. Sulfonamides, barbiturates, aminopenicillins, and trimethoprim-sulfamethoxazole are examples of drugs that can cause this reaction. *Mycoplasma pneumoniae* may be associated with this syndrome.

Toxic epidermal necrolysis: Characterized by sudden onset of generalized, tender erythema, with areas of flaccid blistering, widespread denudation, and severe mucosal erosions. Nikolsky's sign, a sloughing of the skin when lateral pressure is applied, is usually present. Drugs that have been implicated are sulfonamides, barbiturates, aminopenicillins, and trimethoprim-sulfamethoxazole.

Leukocytoclastic vasculitis: Patients present with palpable purpuric lesions involving the lower extremities and other codependent areas. They may also have hemorrhagic blisters, urticaria, ulcers, nodules, and digital necrosis. Widespread organic and musculoskeletal responses may be noted. Usually occurs 7–14 days after exposure. Common drugs noted are ketoconazole, nonsteroidal anti-inflammatory drugs, penicillin and aminopenicillin, sulfonamides, and tetracyclines.

Erythema nodosum: An inflammation of the subcutaneous fat. Appears as erythematous, tender, subcutaneous nodules on the anterior lower extremities. Oral contraceptives, penicillins, sulfonamides, and tetracyclines have been implicated.

Unique eruptions: Caused by certain drugs. Some drugs, such as the tetracyclines, often permanently stain the teeth if given to children under age 6 or to pregnant women. Patients taking steroids may present with acnelike lesions, striae, and delayed wound healing. Phenytoin reactions consist of erythematous eruptions that become purpuric over time. Patients may present with fever, edema of the face, and tender, generalized lymphadenopathy. The reaction usually occurs 1–3 weeks after initial administration of the drug.

Diagnostic Tests: None.

Differential Diagnosis: Viral exanthems are indistinguishable from morbilliform eruptions, except by biopsy. A careful history is necessary.

Treatment: Discontinue the suspected drug immediately. For those with photosensitivity reactions, discontinue the drug and avoid UV lights. For pruritic lesions, may give diphenhydramine, 12.5–25 mg tid, or hydroxyzine (Atarax), 10–25 mg tid; prednisone, 1–2 mg/kg per day, is often given. Premeasured steroidal packaging, such as methylprednisolone (Medrol) 4 mg, 21-day dosepack or Sterapred/5 mg unipack, may be used to prevent recurrent or prolonged symptoms.

Follow-up: May use a telephone contact in 24 hours to assess therapeutic response.

Sequelae: Toxic epidermal necrolysis patients are at significant risk for pneumonia, pulmonary embolism, and fluid electrolyte disturbance. Thirty percent of patients with these complications die. Steroid use can put the patient at risk for yeast, fungal, and viral infections and can precipitate contact dermatitis.

Prevention/Prophylaxis: Taking a careful history of known allergies and taking into consideration a prior history of a reaction when prescribing medications.

Referral: None for minor reactions. Refer to a primary physician for any major drug reactions for definitive treatment.

Education: Instruct patient and/or caregiver about the dangers related to continued or recurrent use of the offending agent. If the patient is currently having a photosensitivity reaction, instruct the patient to avoid UV light, including riding in a car on a sunny day (UV light passes through glass).

Impetigo

Impetigo is a superficial skin infection caused by a gram-positive bacteria and characterized by pustular lesions that rupture early and form honey-colored crusts. Impetigo has several local folk names, such as "Indian fire."

Etiology: Most common agent is the gram-positive organism *Staphylucoccus aureus.*

Occurrence: Common.

Age: All age groups.

Ethnicity: Not significant.

Gender: Occurs equally in males and females.

Contributing Factors: Minor skin trauma, such as an insect bite, that allows penetration by the causative organism.

Signs and Symptoms: Patients present with concerns about their "sores." Parents may have treated child at home with OTC preparations without success. They often provide a history of an insect bite or other sore that the child has scratched; but they child may have no memory of trauma. There may be a history of contact with other children who have had similar lesions, such as other children in the family, daycare centers, or schools.

Physical findings include the presence of pustules with honey-colored crusts. The lesions may be on any body part, but are most common on the face. There may be a single lesion or multiple lesions. Usually there is more than one lesion because of the delay in seeking services.

Diagnostic Tests: Culture and sensitivity testing of the drainage from the lesion would be confirmatory, but this is not usually done.

Differential Diagnosis

Ecthyma, caused by Group A streptococci, is differentiated by the depth of the infection. When the crust is removed, rather than the shallow erosion as seen in impetigo, there is ulcer formation.

Herpes simplex also forms crusts, but upon questioning, the patient will report noticing a clear vesicle prior to crust formation.

Treatment

Topical

Mupirocin 2% (Bactroban), applied to the affected area three times daily; or gentamicin sulfate (Garamycin Ointment), applied to the lesions three or four times daily for 7–10 days.

Systemic

Cefadroxil (Duracef, Ultracef), infants and children, 25–50 mg/kg per day in divided doses q 12 hours for 10 days.

Cephalexin (Keflex), infants and children, 25–50 mg/kg per day in divided doses q 12 hours.

Cefaclor (Ceclor), infants and children, 20–40 mg/kg per day in divided doses q 8 hours for 10 days.

Follow-up: Reassess in 3–5 days for clinical response.

Sequelae: Usually none; however, a scar may result, especially in darker skinned persons.

Prevention/Prophylaxis: Not scratching insect bites and not using washcloths or other personal items that belong to an infected child.

Referral: None.

Education: Teach importance of good handwashing techniques, keeping fingernails short, and isolating the child's personal items (e.g., washcloth, drinking glass, linens) from others until lesions are healed.

Pediculosis (Lice)

Pediculosis is the infestation of hairy body areas by lice. Common areas of infestation include the head, axillae, and pubic area.

Etiology: Human-to-human contact with *Pediculus humanus capitis* (head louse) or *Phthirus pubis* (pubic or crab louse).

Occurrence: Common.

Age: Pediculosis is endemic among school-age children (*Pediculus humanus capitis*) and sexually active adolescents and young adults (*Phthirus pubis*).

Ethnicity: Not significant.

Gender: Occurs equally in males and females.

Contributing Factors: Using infested combs and clothing (caps), hanging garments together in school lockers, and engaging in sexual activity all contribute to becoming infested.

Signs and Symptoms: Child presents with complaint of "itchy" scalp, or the presence of the adult louse or eggs in other hairy areas of the body, such as the pubic area and axillae. Children are most often referred by the school nurse. Findings reveal itchy, red, excoriated areas. The offending louse may be seen on the hair shafts; the eggs (nits), which are small, white, translucent, and 2–3 mm in diameter, may be seen adherent to the hair shafts. Both the lice and the nits may be found in the seams of clothing.

Diagnostic Tests: Visualization of the adult lice and/or nits on the hair shafts.

Differential Diagnosis: None.

Treatment: Topical application of lindane 1% (Kwell) shampoo or lotion; permethrin 1% (Nix) or pyrethrin (A-200, Rid, R & C) shampoo; or malathion 0.5% (Ovid).

Head: Shampoo should be applied, left on for 5 minutes, and then rinsed thoroughly, followed by combing with a fine-tooth comb to remove the nits. This procedure may be repeated in 7 days.

Body: Lotion should be applied, left on for 4 hours, and then rinsed.

Pubis: Lotion should be applied, left on for 24 hours, and then rinsed. Procedure may be repeated in 4–5 days. Lindane is not indicated for infants or pregnant patients. Treat all family members and/or sexual partners. Wash all linens and clothing, iron the seams, and wash all the combs and brushes.

Follow-up: Return in 1 week for evaluation of treatment efficacy.

Sequelae: None.

Prevention/Prophylaxis: Not using combs, brushes, and clothing belonging to another person; and not hanging coats and jackets with the coats and jackets of others. In school, the child should be instructed to put coat in a plastic bag, rather than hanging it on a hook.

Referral: None.

Education: Instruct parents about proper application of medication. Educate parents and children about not using combs and other personal items belonging to others.

Pityriasis Rosea

Pityriasis rosea is an acute, self-limiting inflammatory pruritic dermatitis characterized by oval, slightly elevated, scaling patches and papules that are mainly located on the trunk. Days to several weeks before the generalized eruption, the patient will notice a single lesion, called a herald patch.

Etiology: Unknown.

Occurrence: Increased incidence in the winter months; occurs less commonly in summer months.

Age: Occurs in school-age children and adolescents.

Ethnicity: Not significant.

Gender: Occurs equally in males and females.

Contributing Factors: The possibility of a preceding viral respiratory infection has been suggested, but has not been proved.

Signs and Symptoms: The child often presents with complaints of itchy rash. May give a history of a single lesion (herald patch), 2–10 cm in diameter, several weeks before the generalized rash, which was thought to be ringworm.

Inspection reveals a pattern of rash distribution that, in whites, is mainly on the trunk; in African-Americans, the lesions appear mainly on the extremities.

The clinical presentation of tannish pink or salmon-colored, oval, minimally elevated, scaling patches, papules, and plaques typically follow cleavage, giving rise to the characteristic "Christmas tree" configuration. Pruritus may be mild to moderate.

Diagnostic Tests: None. When "atypical lesions" are noted, a serological test for syphilis should be done.

Differential Diagnosis

In *tinea corporis*, there are usually a few lesions. If in doubt, complete a KOH prep.

In *lichen planus*, the lesions are characteristically purple.

Secondary syphilis is the most important diagnosis to be considered. If there is no herald patch, or there are lesions on the palms of the hands and soles of the feet, or the person appears ill, do a serological test for syphilis.

Treatment: Moisturizing creams may be given for the dry skin and antihistamines, if needed, for the itching: diphenhydramine, 25–50 mg qid or hydroxyzine (Atarax) 10–25 mg qid. UV light therapy (UVB) may accelerate resolution. (Exposure to sunlight may help.)

Follow-up: None; the rash usually disappears in 2 weeks to 2 months.

Sequelae: None.

Prevention/Prophylaxis: None.

Referral: None.

Education: Reassure the patient that the lesions will disappear without specific treatment.

Scabies

Scabies, a pruritic maculopapular rash, results from epidermal infestation by the itch mite. Incubation period of 1 month.

Etiology: Human-to-human contact with the mite *Sarcoptes scabiei*.

Occurrence: Common.

Age: Occurs in any age, but is endemic among school-age children.

Ethnicity: Not significant.

Gender: Occurs equally in males and females.

Contributing Factors: Contact with other infected family members and pets.

Signs and Symptoms: Child presents with an itchy rash. Elicit a history of related illness in other family members and association with pets within the last month. The itching may keep the child awake.

Inspection reveals the classic distribution of burrows on the sides and webs of fingers, flexor surface of wrist, elbow, axillae, girdle area, and feet. The burrows are white and thread-like, with a black dot at the end of the burrow. The inflammatory papules are small and excoriated.

Diagnostic Tests: Skin scrapings of the lesions (using a no. 15 blade) from either the burrow or the papule, mounted on a slide with saline, may reveal the adult mite or eggs.

Differential Diagnosis

May be confused with *neurotoxic excoriations* if only excoriated areas are observed.

May be confused with *eczematous dermatitis* if infestation is widespread. Scrapings would be diagnostic.

Treatment: Treatment should include the identified child as well as all the family members. All linen and clothing should be washed in hot water and dried on hot cycle. The therapeutic agent (permethrin 5% [Elimite] cream) is applied to the entire body at bedtime and washed away in the morning. Oral antihistamines may be given for intense itching: diphenhydramine, 12.5–25 mg tid; or hydroxyzine, 10–25 mg tid.

Follow-up: Patients should return in 1 week. Some require a second treatment. Do not treat more than two times.

Sequelae: Secondary infection arising from the excoriated lesions.

Prevention/Prophylaxis: Treatment of family members and washing of clothing and linens is needed; scabies is very contagious, and treatment of the environment is critical to stop the spread.

Referral: None.

Education: Educate parents regarding the proper application of the therapeutic agent. Instruct parents to wash items such as clothing, bed linens, and favorite toys and stuffed animals. To prevent reinfection, care should be taken to treat the environment, including rugs, blankets, sofa, and chairs.

Seborrheic Dermatitis

Seborrheic dermatitis, also called cradle cap, is a chronic, superficial inflammatory process involving the areas where there are sebaceous glands, particularly in the scalp, the eyebrows, and face. It may also be seen in the groin and on the chest. Pruritus is variable. The mildest form is dandruff.

Etiology: It has been suggested that it is an inflammatory reaction to *Pityrosporum* (a yeast).

Occurrence: Common.

Age: Occurs in all pediatric age groups. If seen in infancy, it is usually outgrown by 6–8 months.

Ethnicity: Not significant.

Gender: Occurs equally in males and females.

Contributing Factors: Possible hormonal stimulation of sebum has been suggested by the incidence in infants and after puberty.

Signs and Symptoms: Parent may bring child in because of "cradle cap"; adolescents may present with the complaint of itchy scalp or facial scaling. Inspection reveals lesions with indistinct margins, mild-to-moderate erythema, and yellowish, greasy scaling. The lesions are bilateral and symmetrically distributed.

Diagnostic Tests: None.

Differential Diagnosis

In *atopic dermatitis*, the presence of lesions on the arms is a distinguishing characteristic.

Psoriasis may be distinguished by the involvement of the elbows and knees.

Treatment: Daily shampoo with mild soap or antiseborrheic shampoo containing 2% ketoconazole or selenium sulfide 2.5% (Selsun Rx 2.5% Selenium Sulfide Lotion, Exsel Shampoo). Use of OTC antiseborrheic shampoos. Low-potency topical steroid (hydrocortisone 1%) applied three times per day to facial lesions, if present. The patient may use ketoconazole ointment on the scalp if shampoos do not seem to be effective.

Follow-up: Reassess in 1–2 weeks for progress.

Sequelae: None.

Prevention/Prophylaxis: None.

Referral: None.

Education: Reassure parents of infants that the seborrheic dermatitis will resolve by ages 6–8 months. Instruct parents as to proper application of ointments as well as shampooing techniques.

Tinea

Tinea is a fungal infection of the epidermis found on a number of anatomical sites:

Tinea capitis: Scalp.
Tinea corporis (tinea circinata, ringworm): Glabrous skin.
Tinea cruris (jock itch): Groin, genitalia, pubic area.
Tinea pedis (athlete's foot): Feet.

The organisms depend on keratin for nutrition and thus do not invade deeper dermal layers. Tinea capitis, tinea pedis, and tinea corporis are contagious.

Etiology: The infection originates from contact with a pet or an infected person. The specific causative organisms are:

Tinea capitis: *Trichophyton tonsurans, Microsporum canis.*
Tinea versicolor: *Pityrosporum orbiculare.*
Tinea corporis: *Trichophyton rubrum, M. canis.*
Tinea pedis: *Trichophyton mentagrophytes.*

Occurrence: Common.

Age: Occurs across all pediatric age groups. Tinea capitis occurs most frequently in prepubertal children.

Ethnicity: Forty percent of asymptomatic inner-city children carry *Trichophyton tonsurans.* Most cases are seen in crowded inner cities, particularly among African-Americans (e.g., 12% of black females have tinea capitis) and Latinos.

Gender: Tinea capitis and tinea pedis are more common among males than females.

Contributing Factors: Susceptibility increases with exposure to infected animals; living in hot, humid areas; minor skin trauma that allows for penetration of the organism; tight hair braiding; and the use of hair pomades.

Signs and Symptoms: Child presents with a history of the presence of patchy, scaly lesions on a variety of anatomical sites. The findings are:

Tinea capitis: Noninflammatory; small, erythematous papules; hairs are gray, lusterless and broken off; inflammatory, pustular folliculitis to kerion formation. Erythematous, papular eruptions on scalp, possibly accompanied by itching and fever. In the black-dot type, the brittle hair breaks off and is left in the infected follicle, giving the appearance of a black dot; there is minimal hair loss or inflammation. Kerion is a boggy, erythematous nodule with perifollicular pustules. The presence of enlarged cervical lymph nodes is often noted.

Tinea corporis: An elevated, scaling border with central clearing is noted.

Tinea cruris: There are well-demarcated borders with erythematous papulovesicles and central clearing.

Tinea pedis: Chronic type involves fissuring, scaling, and macerations; hyperkeratonic type has moccasin distribution on soles of feet; vesicular, scaling. Acute type involves ulceration, maceration, oozing, and denudation.

Tinea versicolor: Changes in pigmentation (hypopigmentation and/or hyperpigmentation) are noted, as well as macules and scaly patches, especially on the trunk, neck, and shoulders.

Diagnostic Tests: Fluorescence of lesions using the Wood's light is useful for suspected infections of the scalp, but not for infections of the skin. KOH prep of scrapings or follicles is positive for the presence of fungal elements: spores and hyphae. Mycological cultures will aid in the differentiation between *Candida* infection and tinea.

Differential Diagnosis

Tinea Capitis

In *trichotillomania*, there would be irregular patches of alopecia containing stubble of broken hairs.

Alopecia areata has well-circumscribed, round patches of hair loss with smooth scalp. KOH prep would be confirmatory for tinea.

Tinea Cruris

In *intertrigio*, KOH prep is negative.

In *Candida infection*, KOH prep is negative and *Candida* also affects the scrotum.

Tinea Corporis

In *impetigo*, the vesicles, pustules, and crusts would be distinguishing features.

Tinea Pedis

In *hyperhidrosis*, KOH prep is negative.

Treatment

Tinea Capitis

Griseofulvin, 11 mg/kg per day; ultramicronized griseofulvin (Grispeg), 10 mg/kg per day with a fatty meal for 6 weeks. *Note*: Griseofulvin may inactivate birth control pills. Patients resistant to griseofulvin should be given itraconazole, 5 mg/kg per day for 4–6 weeks; or terbinafine, 10 mg/kg per day for 4 weeks. For severe inflammatory kerion, prednisone (1 mg/kg per day) for 5–7 days and erythromycin (30–50 mg/kg per day) may be given for 10 days.

Tinea Corporis

Topical imidazole (Lotrimin, Micatin), ciclopirox (Loprox), or an allylamine agent may be given twice daily for 14 days; or oral griseofulvin, 15–20 mg/kg per day for 4–8 weeks.

Tinea Cruris

Topical antifungals may be administered. In recalcitrant cases, give oral griseofulvin or ketoconazole.

Tinea Pedis

Administer topical antifungals.

Tinea Versicolor

Primary: Selenium sulfide (2.5% lotion or shampoo; leave on 10–15 minutes, and then shower off; use daily for 1 week); ketoconazole shampoo or cream 1–2 times per day for 1 week; oral ketoconazole 400-mg single dose; itraconazole 200-mg daily for 5 days.

Secondary: Selenium sulfide (2.5%) shampoo or lotion; benzoyl peroxide soaps; propylene glycol (50%) solution; oral ketoconazole 400-mg single dose.

Follow-up: Reevaluate at 2-week and monthly intervals for treatment efficacy. Monitor complete blood count monthly in children receiving long-term griseofulvin for leukocytosis. Also obtain liver function studies before starting drug and at 4 weeks. If serum glutamic oxaloacetic transaminase (SGOT) and serum glutamic pyruvic transaminase (SGPT) are elevated, stop drug.

Sequelae: Hair loss may be a permanent feature in kerion or may take 6 months to return. Bacterial and yeast overgrowth may be seen in tinea pedis.

Prevention/Prophylaxis

Tinea capitis: Not sharing combs, brushes, or headgear with others; evaluation and treatment of infected family members; washing linens; vacuuming and mopping floor with strong disinfectant, and not using oil on hair or scalp.

Tinea corporis: Keeping intertriginous areas dry, using absorbent powders, and avoiding tight clothing.

Tinea pedis: Maintaining good foot hygiene, wearing light footwear, and either throwing away or washing infected shoes.

Referral: Refer to a physician in cases of chronic infection or lack of response to treatment.

Education: Instruct patients regarding good foot hygiene; drying of feet; not sharing combs, brushes, or headgear; and inspection and treatment of infected animals. Teach medication administration, dosage, and side effects. Medication may be opened and sprinkled on ice cream.

Verucca

Verucca is a proliferation of epidermal cells resulting in a warty growth. There are three common types:

Verruca vulgaris: Firm, discrete gray or brownish gray papules with a diameter up to 1.0 cm; surface may be flat and smooth, but may become rough and fissured. These are found primarily on the hands and feet, but may occur anywhere on the body.

Verruca plantaris (plantar wart): Thick, firm, and flat, sometimes painful, lesions on soles of feet and sometimes palmar surfaces.

Verruca acuminata (condyloma acuminatum): Filiform, papular lesions in the perineal and genital areas.

Etiology: Infection with the human papillomavirus.

Occurrence: Common.

Age: All age groups.

Ethnicity: Not significant.

Gender: Occurs equally in males and females.

Contributing Factors: Chemotherapy and steroids may contribute to verruca vulgaris; verruca acuminata is sexually transmitted.

Signs and Symptoms: Patient presents with a complaint of a wart. Further history depends on the site of the wart. In genital warts, there is a history of sexual activity; in the common wart, there is a history of chemotherapy or steroid use. There may be multiple or single lesions.

Diagnostic Tests: None.

Differential Diagnosis: None.

Treatment

Verruca Vulgaris
May disappear in 6–9 months. However, the following may be effective: (1) application of 40% salicylic acid plasters, cut to fit the wart and left on for 5 days (reapply every 5 days; sometimes effective in 2–4 weeks); or (2) cryosurgery with liquid nitrogen.

Verruca Plantaris
Usually excision is the treatment of choice.

Verruca Acuminata
Apply topical 25% podophyllin in alcohol, and wash off in 4 hours. Retreat in 7–10 days if necessary. If the wart is not on the mucosa, it may be treated as a common wart and cryosurgically removed. Newer medications for home use are not recommended for children.

Follow-up: The patient should return to the clinic in 2 weeks for evaluation of treatment. If the area becomes very red or sore, or shows signs of infection, the patient should contact the office. If verruca acuminata is diagnosed, sexual abuse should be suspected.

Sequelae: Recurrences are often reported in 20–30% of treated cases.

Prevention/Prophylaxis: For verruca plantaris: cleaning the inside of shoes with alcohol, using shower shoes in public showers (e.g., after gym classes), and using clean towels and bath mats.

Referral: Refer patient to primary physician for cryosurgery.

Education: Instruct patients not to pick at lesions.

REFERENCES

General

Berhman, R, and Kleigman, R: Nelson's Essentials of Pediatrics. WB Saunders, Philadelphia, 1990.

Doenges, M, and Moorhouse, M: Nurse's Pocket Guide: Nursing Diagnoses with Interventions, ed 5. FA Davis, Philadelphia, 1995.

Green, M: Pediatric Diagnosis: Interpretation of Symptoms and Signs in Infants, Children and Adolescents, ed 5. WB Saunders, Philadelphia, 1992.

Hay, W, et al: Current Pediatric Diagnosis & Treatment, ed 12. Appleton & Lange, Norwalk, Conn, 1995.

Lookingbill, D, and Marks, J: Principles of Dermatology. WB Saunders, Philadelphia, 1993.

Steele, R: Clinical Handbook of Pediatric Infectious Diseases. Parthenon Publishing, New York, 1994.

Assessment

DeGowin, R: DeGowin & DeGowin's Diagnostic Examination. McGraw-Hill, New York, 1994.

Engle, J: Pocket Guide to Pediatric Assessment, ed 2. St. Louis, Mosby, 1992.

Flowers, F, and Hacker, S: Diligent diagnosis: Cutaneous manifestations of endocrine and gastrointestinal diseases. Mod Med 28, 1994.

Steele, R: Clinical Handbook of Pediatric Infectious Diseases. Parthenon Publishing, New York, 1994.

Swartz, M: Textbook of Physical Diagnosis: History and Examination, ed 2. WB Saunders, Philadelphia, 1994.

Alopecia

Baden, HP, et al: Loose anagen hair as a cause of hereditary hair loss in children. Arch Dermatol 128:1349, 1992.

Clore, ER, and Corey, A: Hair loss in children and adolescents. J Pediatr Health Care 5:245, 1991.

Healey, P, and Jacobson, E: Common Medical Diagnoses: An Algorithmic Approach, ed 2. WB Saunders, Philadelphia, 1994.

Vitulano, LA, et al: Behavioral treatment of children and adolescents with trichotillomania. J Am Acad Child Adolesc Psychiatry 31:139, 1992.

Atopic Dermatitis

Dahl, RE, et al: Sleep disturbances in children with atopic dermatitis. Arch Pediatr Adolesc Med 149:856, 1995.

Hogan, P, and Weston, W: An itch that won't go away. Contemp Pediatr 9:100, 1992.

Romeo, S: Atopic dermatitis: The itch that rashes. Pediatr Nurs 21:157, 1994.

Dermatitis

Fisher, A: Cosmetic dermatitis in childhood. Cutis 55:15, 1995.

Drug Eruptions

Bernstein, J: Nonimmunologic adverse drug reactions. Postgrad Med 98:159, 1995.

Bernstein, J: Allergic drug reactions: How to minimize the risks. Postgrad Med 98:159, 1995.

Krenek, G, and Rosen, T: Cutaneous drug eruptions: Patterns to help you identify the cause, control the problem. Consultant 35:1329, 1995.

Mandes, S: Serious and life-threatening drug eruptions. Am Fam Phys 51:1865, 1995.

Scabies

Wolf, R, et al: Scabies: The diagnosis of atypical cases. Cutis 55:370, 1995.

Seborrheic Dermatitis

Hurwitz, S: Skin lesions in the first year of life. Contemp Pediatr 9:110, 1993.
Janniger, CK, and Schwartz, RA: Seborrheic dermatitis. Am Fam Phys 52:149, 1995.
Peter, RU, and Richarz-Barthauer, U: Successful treatment and prophylaxis of scalp seborrhoeic dermatitis and dandruff with 2% ketoconazole shampoo: Results of a multicentre, double-blind placebo-controlled trial. Br J Dermatol 132:441, 1995.

Tinea

Anderson, N: Cutaneous dermatophytic infections: Special report: Mycology, January 14–17. In Cunha, B (ed): Health Care Information Projects. McGraw-Hill, New York, 1995.
Arndt, K: Manual of Dermatological Therapeutics. Little, Brown & Company, Boston, 1990.
Elewski, B: Superficial fungal infections of the skin: Diagnostic techniques. Special report: Mycology, January 9–13. In Cunha, B (ed): Health Care Information Projects. McGraw-Hill, New York, 1995.
Johnson, R: *Pityrosporum ovale* infestations. Special report: Mycology, January 29–34. In Cunha, B (ed): Health Care Information Projects. McGraw-Hill, New York, 1995.
Odom, R: Noninvasive fungal infections of the skin: Topical or systemic therapy? Special report: Mycology, January 18–23. In Cunha, B (ed): Health Care Information Projects. McGraw-Hill, New York, 1995.
Schwartz, R, and Janniger, C: Tinea capitis. Cutis 55:29, 1995.
Stevenson, L, and Brooke, D: Tinea capitis. J Pediatr Health Care 8:189, 1994.
Weston, W, and Lane, A: Color Textbook of Pediatric Dermatology. Mosby-Year Book, St. Louis, 1991.

Verruca

Kimble-Haas, S: Primary care treatment approach to nongenital verruca. Nurs Pract 21(10):29, 1996.
Miller, DM, and Brodell, RT: Human papilloma infection: Treatment options for warts. Am Fam Phys 53:135, 1996.
Vitulano, LA, et al: Behavioral treatment of children and adolescents with trichotillomania. J Acad Child Adolesc Psychiatry 31:139, 1992.

CHAPTER 7

HEAD, NECK, AND

FACE ASSESSMENT

Inspection, palpation, and percussion are the techniques used for assessing the head, neck, and face. Inspection begins as the patient enters the examining room, where the nurse practitioner (NP) observes for symmetry, distribution of hair, placement of eyes and ears, presence of apparent abnormalities, and the presence of edema or suspicious swellings. Palpation reveals the less obvious abnormalities. Percussion of the sinus area may be done in older children.

HEAD/NECK

In general, the head is larger than the chest until age 6, when the head reaches 90% adult size. The bones in the skull and in the face grow at varying rates. Inquire about alcohol use during pregnancy, about adverse birth events, and the shape of the head at birth.

Observations of the head denoting deviations from normal are frontal bossing, as seen in prematurity, rickets, and congenital syphilis. Fontanelles can indicate dehydration, intracranial defects, and malnutrition. In cases of rickets and mental retardation, there is flattening of the skull.

If tonic neck reflexes last longer than 3 months, suspect brain damage; head lag after 4 months suggests either mental or motor retardation. Nuchal rigidity indicates meningeal irritation.

FACE

Initial facial observations reveal the ability of the facial muscles to move. Does the baby smile? What does the face look like when the baby cries? "Allergic shin-

92

ers" may reveal chronic allergies. In addition, there are characteristic facies seen in Down's syndrome and fetal alcohol syndrome (FAS). In Down's syndrome, there is a small, brachycephalic head with a flat nasal bridge; a large, protruding tongue; small ears; upslanted palpebral fissures; and epicanthic folds. Facies in FAS may present with a small head with short palpebral fissures, short nose, and a long, smooth philtrum.

EYE

An examination of the eye begins with observation. Ptosis, or drooping of the upper lid, is seen in myasthenia gravis, damage to cranial nerve III, and damage to the sympathetic nerve, as seen in Horner's syndrome. An upward palpebral slant is normal, but if combined with epicanthal folds and hypertelorism, suspect Down's syndrome. Sunken eyes may indicate malnutrition, dehydration, or severe illness. Any interruption in the red reflex suggests an opacity in the cornea or lens, whereas an absent reflex occurs in cases of congenital cataracts or retinal disorders.

Visual acuity in the infant is determined on the basis of the perception of light. If there is an absence of blinking or absence of the pupillary reflex by 3 weeks after birth, the infant is probably blind, and a prompt referral should be made.

Visual acuity of 20/20 is developed by ages 6–7. The National Society for Prevention of Blindness has issued the following criteria for referral: (1) age 3 years, visual acuity 20/50 or less either eye; (2) age 4 years, visual acuity 20/40 or less either eye; or (3) if the difference in the two eyes is one line or more. The Snellen test may be used with children; the Child Recognition and Near Point Test (picture recognition), which tests from a distance of 13 inches, may also be used.

Color blindness or color sensitivity, a recessive X-linked trait, affects 8% of white males and 4% of African-American males. The incidence in females is 0.4%. Therefore, test males between ages 4 and 8 years for color blindness, using the Ishihara plates.

EARS

Low placement or deviated alignment of the ears suggests mental retardation or genitourinary malformations. There are cultural variations in ear wax: in whites and African-Americans, the wax is wet, sticky, and honey-colored; in Asians and Native Americans, it is dry and flaky. Children are at greater risk for the development of inner ear infections because of factors related to the maturity of the structures; a shorter, wider, and more horizontal eustachian tube; and increased lymphoid tissue in the lumen.

NOSE

The nose, which is located midline, should be symmetrical. Observe for displacement and deformities. Assessment of the patency of the nares in the early

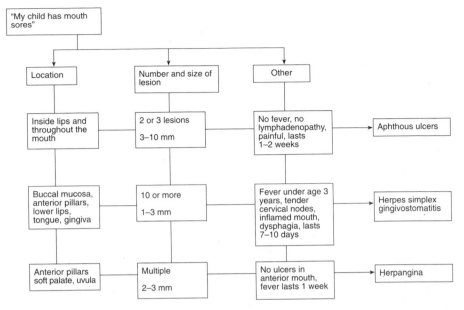

FIGURE 7–1 Evaluation of oral lesions.

newborn period is important because newborns are obligate nose-breathers. Inability to pass a catheter through the nares indicates choanal atresia, which requires immediate referral and intervention. Nasal flaring indicates respiratory distress. Development of the nose is complete by ages 16–18 years. On internal examination, observe for a deviated septum and the presence of drainage or polyps.

MOUTH/THROAT

Inspect the lips, buccal mucosa, tongue, teeth, palate, and oropharynx. Evaluate the sucking reflex in infants; during this process, the hard and soft palate may be evaluated. The presence of Epstein's pearls on the gums is normal, as is the presence of the "sucking" tubercule on the upper lip. Salivation begins at age 3 months; the child will continue to drool until he or she learns to swallow (Fig. 7–1).

Tooth eruption, which begins at approximately 6 months, should be complete by 30 months. In older children, evaluate for the presence of dental caries. There is a lower incidence of caries among African-Americans compared to whites, apparently because of their harder and denser tooth enamel.

Other cultural variations to consider include bifid uvula: cleft lip and cleft palate are most common among Asians and Native Americans and least common among African-Americans. Torus palatinus is most common among Native Americans, Eskimos, and Asians.

Using the penlight, inspect the tonsils. The color should be the same as that of the oral mucosa. Grade the tonsils on a scale of +1 to +4. With acute infection, you can expect an enlargement of +2, +3, or +4. Children often have tonsillar enlargements of +1 or +2 because of normal enlargement of the lymphoid tissue.

Concussion

A concussion is a brief period of unconsciousness, lasting seconds or minutes, occurring immediately after trauma and followed by normal arousal. A concussion grading scale is used by coaches to determine a player's eligibility for continued play:

Grade I concussion: No loss of consciousness occurs, or there is a brief state of confusion; amnesia lasts less than 30 minutes. Player may return to the game when fully recovered but must be carefully observed.

Grade II concussion: Loss of consciousness lasts less than 5 minutes; amnesia lasts more than 30 minutes but less than 24 hours. Player may return in 1 week if asymptomatic. After a second grade II episode, player may return if asymptomatic for 1 month. After a third grade II episode, player must end the season.

Grade III concussion: Loss of consciousness lasts more than 5 minutes; amnesia lasts longer than 24 hours. Player may return in 1 month if asymptomatic for 1 week. After the second grade III episode, player must end the season.

Etiology: A shearing lesion of white matter as the brain is shaken within the cranium, causing failure of axion conduction.

Occurrence: Common.

Age: All age groups.

Ethnicity: Not significant.

Gender: Occurs equally in males and females.

Contributing Factors: Falls and sports injuries are all contributing factors.

Signs and Symptoms: Child comes to clinic with history of an impact head injury. History should include description of the event. Evaluate the episode using the concussion scale as a guide. Perform a physical examination including a neurological examination. Usually the examination will be negative for any abnormal findings.

Diagnostic Tests: None.

Differential Diagnosis: Increased intracranial pressure (ICP) would be manifested by increasing irritability, lethargy, vomiting, and altered mental status.

Treatment: Observe level of consciousness and degree of amnesia. A computed tomographic (CT) scan may be indicated when there is prolonged unconsciousness.

Follow-up: Patient should return to clinic in 1 week for assessment of resolution of symptoms.

Sequelae: Retrograde or antegrade amnesia may occur. Retrograde amnesia is the inability to remember events immediately prior to the trauma. Antegrade amnesia is the inability to form new memories. The period of amnesia is related to the degree of the trauma. Focal or generalized brain swelling may occur if contusion or laceration has occurred. The athlete who returns to play while still experiencing symptoms and sustains a second head injury is at increased risk for experiencing a loss of autoregulation of cerebral blood flow, leading to increased ICP. This "second-impact" syndrome is associated with a high mortality rate.

Prevention/Prophylaxis: Increased safety measures to reduce risk of head injury, such as seat belts, car seats, gates at top of stairs, safe school yard equipment, and safety equipment for sports.

Referral: If parent is not capable of observing the child, then refer for admission to the hospital for observation.

Education: Teach parents how to observe for alertness, orientation, neurological functioning, increase in headaches, or vomiting. Teach parents how to test extraocular motions, pupillary reactions, and gait every 2–4 hours for 24 hours. Teach environmental safety, such as use of car seats, seat belts, and gates at top of stairs, as well as the importance of wearing protective head gear when participating in sports such as skateboarding and bicycling.

Craniosynostosis

Craniosynostosis, or premature closure of suture lines of the skull (usually involving sagittal, coronal, and lambdoid), may be associated with other disorders, such as Aperts' disease, Crouzon's disease, or metabolic disease (e.g., hyperthyroidism). Despite fusion of the skull bones, normal brain growth continues; any resultant disability (e.g., craniostenosis) depends on the duration of the process and the ability of the other sutures to compensate for brain growth. The clinical picture depends on which suture is affected.

Etiology: It is unknown what interferes with normal cranial growth.

Occurrence: Uncommon.

Age: Infancy.

Ethnicity: Not significant.

Gender: Occurs equally in males and females.

Contributing Factors: Metabolic disorders, such as hyperthyroidism and hypercalcemia, increase the incidence of craniosynostosis.

Signs and Symptoms: Abnormal or unusual shape of the head (craniostenosis) may be first noticed during a well-baby visit. Inspection reveals an elongation of the head anterior to posterior (most common because the sagittal suture is most often affected), an increase in cranial diameter from left to right (when the coronal sutures are affected), and fontanelles smaller than expected for age. Palpation reveals a suture ridge.

Diagnostic Tests: Skull x-rays to confirm physical findings. Thyroid panel may reveal hyperthyroidism, and serum calcium may be elevated.

Differential Diagnosis: Children with Down's syndrome have brachycephaly.

Treatment: Surgical intervention is done to reopen the suture line(s) that have prematurely closed. Often, a Teflon-type barrier is applied to keep suture line from prematurely closing again. Surgery is performed within the first 6 months of life to preserve normal skull shape and prevent compression and brain damage.

Follow-up: Monitor for appropriate growth and development and achievement of developmental milestones.

Sequelae: None, unless many or all of the sutures are involved and the brain is compromised.

Prevention/Prophylaxis: None.

Referral: Refer immediately to a pediatric neurologist for confirmation and surgical intervention, if needed.

Education: Reassure parents that they were not responsible for the defect.

Head Trauma

Head trauma, an injury of accidental or intentional origin to the head, causes the brain to move within the cranium. The injury may cause damage at the site of the trauma (coup), on the opposite side of the site of trauma (contrecoup), or in some cases, bilaterally. Head injury is the leading cause of morbidity and mortality in pediatric trauma patients. Head injuries are classified as mild, moderate, or severe (Table 7–1).

Common head trauma injuries occurring in children include cerebral edema, skull fractures, and acute subdural or epidural hematomas. Cerebral edema is a focal bruising or shearing of brain tissue. A skull fracture is a crack or fracture in the skull. It may be depressed or nondepressed. All patients with depressed fractures should be referred immediately. Acute subdural or epidural hematoma, which is associated with significant brain contusion, results in a collection of blood below the dura.

Etiology: Head trauma may be the result of a fall, a vehicular accident, or a sports-related injury. Severe head trauma in very young children is often

TABLE 7–1 CLINICAL CLASSIFICATION OF HEAD-INJURED PATIENTS

Mild	No loss of consciousness or amnesia. Alert and oriented. Asymptomatic or with only slight headache and dizziness.
Moderate	Possible findings: history of loss of consciousness, amnesia; posttraumatic seizures, vomiting, more than slight headache, listlessness, lethargy.
Severe	Possible findings: disoriented, unable to follow commands, decreasing level of consciousness, focal neurologic signs, penetrating skull injury or depressed skull fracture.

Source: Rosenthal, BW, and Begman, I: Intracranial injury after moderate head trauma in children. J Pediatr 115:346, 1989.

caused by abuse. Typically, the causes of head trauma vary by age group: young children fall, school-age children have pedestrian or bicycle accidents, and adolescents are victims of assault or motor vehicle accidents.

Occurrence: Annually, about 250,000 children per year sustain head trauma. Of those, about 150,000 sustain injury to the brain tissue, with 20% resulting in permanent neurological damage. Mortality range is 6–35%.

Age: All ages.

Ethnicity: Not significant.

Gender: Boys have a slightly higher incidence of traumatic injuries.

Contributing Factors

- Lack of safety helmets or precautions, such as child restraints in cars.
- Child abuse.
- Poor parental supervision.
- Drug or alcohol use, which can alter one's perceptions.
- Risk-taking behaviors, which can increase the incidence of injuries.
- Unsafe home and school environments.

Signs and Symptoms: Child is brought to the clinic or emergency room with a history of a fall or other type of closed head trauma. Obtain a detailed history related to the injury—where it occurred; length of time since the injury; if a fall, the distance and type of surface; whether safety equipment was worn; whether the child lost consciousness; whether the child could remember events before, during, and after the accident; and whether there has been vomiting, headache, or complaints of diplopia (Fig. 7–2).

A complete physical examination with a focus on the neurological examination is essential.

- Note vital signs; alterations may include irregular breathing, hypertension, and bradycardia.
- Assess pupil size, equality, reaction to light; perform a funduscopic examination.

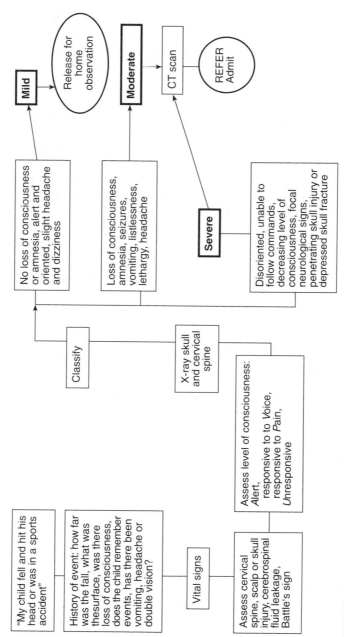

FIGURE 7-2 Evaluation of head injury.

- Examine the face for signs of associated facial injuries, such as mandibular fracture.
- Note the presence or absence of cerebrospinal fluid in the ears.

Assess the level of consciousness using the AVPU system. Is the child: Alert, responsive to Voice, responsive to Pain, or Unresponsive? The Glasgow Coma Scale (Table 7–2) is particularly beneficial in assessing children over 3. The Pediatric Trauma Scale is also useful (Table 7–3).

When a head injury has been sustained, there may be a history of a preceding event, such as a fall or an automobile accident. There may be accompanying injuries and apparent bruising.

If there is cerebral edema, there may be changes in strength and sensation, altered senses, altered level of consciousness, and increased ICP.

With a skull fracture, there will be swelling or depression of the skull, "raccoon eyes," altered level of consciousness, altered or normal neurological examination, and altered reaction to stimuli.

If a subdural or epidural hematoma is present, there may be altered level of consciousness, vomiting, lethargy, irritability, sluggish pupillary response, and seizures.

Vital signs will be altered and may include irregular breathing, hypertension, and bradycardia.

TABLE 7–2   GLASGOW COMA SCALE

Activity	Response	Score
Opens eyes	Spontaneously	4
	To sound	3
	To pain	2
	No response	1
Motor response	Obeys commands	6
	Localizes painful stimulus	5
	Responds to pain with:	
	Normal flexion	4
	Abnormal flexion	3
	Extension	2
	No response	1
Verbal response	Oriented	5
	Confused	4
	Inappropriate	3
	Incomprehensible	2
	No response	1
	Maximum score	**15**

Scoring: 13–15 = mild impairment; 9–12 = moderate impairment; 3–8 = severe impairment.
Adapted from Burns, C, et al: A Handbook for Nurse Practitioners. WB Saunders, Philadelphia, 1996.

TABLE 7–3 PEDIATRIC TRAUMA SCALE

Score	+2	+1	−1
Weight	>44 lb	22–44 lb	<22 lb
Airway	Normal	Oral/nasal airway	Intubated
BP	>90 mmHg	50–90 mmHg	<50 mmHg
LOC	Awake	Drowsy, but *no* history of LOC	Unresponsive
Open wound	—	Minor	Major or penetrating
Fracture	—	Minor	Open or multiple

Score of
<2 = 100% mortality
<6 = Increased risk for preventable mortality or morbidity
<8 = Immediate transfer

BP = blood pressure; LOC = loss of consciousness.

Diagnostic Tests: Skull series will reveal a fracture. Magnetic resonance imaging (MRI) or CT scan with and without contrast can show fractures, increased ICP, or bleeding.

H and H (hemoglobin and hematocrit) can show bleeding if values are decreased.
Electroencephalogram (EEG) will show seizure activity, if present.
A drug screen, if positive, will indicate the type and amount of drug use.
ICP levels will be increased in cases of severe injury.
Assess weight, blood pressure, open wounds, fracture, and level of consciousness.
Evaluate severity of situation with the Glasgow Coma Scale (see Table 7–2).
Consider CT scan, MRI, EEG, and x-ray of the neck (two views).
Evaluate severity using the Pediatric Trauma Scale (see Table 7–3).

Differential Diagnosis

Drug/alcohol intoxication, indicated by positive tests.
Meningitis, manifested by elevated white blood count (WBC), fever, and positive culture of fluid obtained via lumbar puncture.
Shaken baby syndrome, evidenced by the presence of retinal hemorrhage.
Child abuse.

Treatment: The airway should be maintained. Children should be hyperventilated to reduce ICP. Circulation should be evaluated and maintained. Hyperthermia should be avoided. Prompt consultation with neurosurgeon should be done. If trauma is mild, observe behavior for 24 hours for signs of neurological impairment, nausea, or vomiting.

Observe ears and nose for clear fluid, a sign of cerebrospinal fluid (CSF) leakage and basilar skull fracture. Evidence of intracranial hemorrhage may necessitate surgical intervention. Analgesia can be given for headache.

Follow-up: Follow-up interval depends on the injury sustained. Initially at 2 weeks post-trauma, the child should be seen by a neurologist and should maintain a regular schedule of visits with a health-care provider.

Sequelae: Death or permanent brain damage is possible. Although some children do recover, even mild head traumas may have cumulative effects.

Prevention/Prophylaxis: Maintenance of a safe environment at home and school. Safety measures for children, including safety helmets, car seats, and restraints. Adult supervision. Awareness of possible abuse or the potential for abuse.

Referral: A pediatric neurologist should be consulted for all cases of head trauma. Social services or child protective services should be called when abuse is suspected.

Education: Safety measures, including the use of helmets for bike riding, rollerblading, and skateboarding, should be stressed. Convey the importance of proper side rails on cribs and proper use of car seats and restraints. Assess house and schoolyard for the presence of hazardous equipment and surfaces. Warning signs of late sequelae, such as seizures, should be taught to parents.

Macrocephaly

Macrocephaly is an abnormal head size more than two standard deviations greater than the mean for age and sex. It may be due to hydrocephalus (enlargement of the ventricles), macrocrania (increased skull thickness), or megalencephaly (increased size of the brain). Macrocrania and megalencephaly are rare conditions.

Etiology: The cause of hydrocephalus is increased production, blockage of the flow, or impaired absorption of CSF, resulting in an increase in the size of the ventricles.

Occurrence: Uncommon.

Age: Hydrocephalus occurs in infancy.

Ethnicity: Not significant.

Gender: Occurs equally in males and females.

Contributing Factors: Choroid plexus papillomas (2–4% of childhood intracranial tumors) produce hydrocephalus without obstruction; intrauterine infections (toxoplasmosis); genetic factors are related.

Signs and Symptoms: Usually there are no specific signs noted by parents in the early infant period. Later, the child may be brought to the clinic because of vomiting, a problem with gait, or a headache. Findings may include impairment of upward gaze, "setting-sun sign," growth failure, enlarged head circumference (as compared to national standards), small anterior fontanelle, or a prematurely closed anterior fontanelle. Transillumination may show subdural effusion or presence of large cysts.

Diagnostic Tests: Skull films are not very reliable. CT, MRI, or if anterior fontanelle is open, ultrasound studies will help identify structural causes and determine whether the disorder is operable.

Differential Diagnosis: Tumors would be evident on the imaging studies.

Treatment: Continue monitoring growth and development; measure head circumference at each clinic visit until age 18 months, noting the size of the anterior fontanelle and comparing data with national standards for age. Surgical intervention for the placement of a shunt, which bypasses the obstruction and diverts the CSF to other sites, is done when macrocephaly is secondary to hydrocephalus.

Follow-up: Regular childhood visits.

Sequelae: Acute manifestations of increased ICP. If child has a shunt, watch for infection and "outgrowing" of the shunt.

Prevention/Prophylaxis: Prenatal care that includes assessment of rubella titer, treatment for maternal syphilis, avoidance of alcohol, and exposure to radiation during the prenatal period.

Referral: Referral to a pediatric neurologist for definitive diagnosis and care plan.

Education: Support for the parents as they deal with having a child with a chronic disability is very important. In cases involving children who have had this condition for some time, assist the parents in obtaining occasional respite care for their children.

Microcephaly

Microcephaly, an abnormal head size two standard deviations less than the mean for age, sex, height, and weight, may be congenital or acquired. In this disorder, the skull remains small because the brain does not grow. Primary microcephaly may be inherited through a familial autosomal dominant or recessive trait.

Etiology: Among the causes are transplacental transfer of toxins (alcohol, maternal phenylketonuria [PKU]), chromosomal disorders (trisomy 13, 18, or 21), and metabolic disorders (hypoglycemia, PKU).

Occurrence: Uncommon.

Age: Infancy.

Ethnicity: Not significant.

Gender: Occurs equally in males and females.

Contributing Factors: Maternal radiation during the first and second trimesters, maternal and perinatal infections, and genetics may be factors.

Signs and Symptoms: Parents may not notice the subtle changes in head size, but may bring the child to clinic because of seizures or developmental delay. Up to 6 months of age, chest circumference exceeds head circumference. There may be a backward slope to the forehead with narrowing of the bitemporal diameter. Progressive lack of growth in head circumference with advancing age may occur; fontanelles may close early.

Diagnostic Tests: Regular skull films are of little value; CT or MRI scans reveal intracranial calcifications, malformations, or atrophic patterns of brain growth. If history warrants, obtain antibody titers for toxoplasmosis, cytomegalovirus, rubella, herpes simplex virus, and syphilis.

Differential Diagnosis

Craniosynostosis, defined as premature closure of the skull suture lines, is differentiated by CT or MRI and demonstrates that the brain is growing normally.

In *Rett's syndrome,* normal mental ability and head circumference exist until 6 months. Between 5 and 30 months, there is a decline in language and development of mental retardation; between ages 2 and 4 years, head circumference decreases and there is loss of purposeful hand skills.

Treatment: Supportive, directed at management of neurological and sensory deficits that may occur.

Follow-up: Regular monitoring of growth and development.

Sequelae: Mental retardation due to diminished brain growth.

Prevention/Prophylaxis: Good prenatal care that treats maternal infections promptly can decrease the incidence of microcephaly. Protection of the maternal pelvis from radiation during the first and second trimesters is essential to avoid affecting the fetus' skull.

Referral: Immediate referral to a pediatric neurologist for definitive diagnosis and plan of care.

Education: Provide genetic counseling for parents of children with significant microcephaly.

Cervical Lymphadenitis

Cervical lymphadenitis is an acute, unilateral cervical adenitis accompanied by local pain, fever, and tenderness. Any node may be involved, but the cervical node is the most common. The size of the node ranges from that of a walnut to an egg; it is firm, tender, and associated with local erythema. The condition is sequela to infections of the ear, nose, and throat.

Etiology: Most common infective agents are Group A β-hemolytic *Streptococcus* (70%), *Staphylococcus* (20%), and viruses (10%).

Occurrence: Common.

Age: All pediatric age groups.

Ethnicity: Not significant.

Gender: Occurs equally in males and females.

Contributing Factors: Breaks in the mucous membrane that occur during teeth eruption, allowing inoculation by mycobacteria; exposure to cats plus a minor skin lesion allowing entrance of the causative organism.

Signs and Symptoms: Child is brought to the clinic with the complaint of "swollen glands" and fever. History should include which nodes are involved and past medical history, particularly any past infections. Palpation reveals a large, swollen, taut, firm, and/or tender mass in any lymph node, usually cervical or inguinal (Fig. 7–3). Record the measurements of the node(s) for future comparison. Observe the neck for protective torticollis. Examine each tooth for the presence of a periapical abscess.

Diagnostic Tests: Complete blood count (CBC)—a WBC greater than 20,000/mm³ with a shift to left is often seen. Obtain a throat culture to identify a specific organism, a screen to determine the presence of streptococcal infection, and a culture aspirate of the node to identify a specific organism. Obtain a tuberculin (TB) skin test, as early tuberculosis of the cervical nodes may be confused with lymphadenitis.

Differential Diagnosis

Thyroglossal duct cyst: This is often mistaken for submandibular lymph node, but the cyst moves upward in the neck when the patient protrudes the tongue.
Cystic hygroma: This finding may be associated with a large tongue.
Mumps: Disease affects the parotid gland(s), usually bilaterally and crossing the angle of the jaw.
Ranula: This is a bluish retention cyst of the sublingual gland on one side of the frenulum under the tongue.
Brachial cleft cyst: This cyst occurs along the anterior border of the sternocleidomastoid muscle. Although rarely seen, drainage is clear and mucoid, when present.

Treatment

Nonpharmacological
Apply cold compresses or an ice bag to relieve symptoms.

Pharmacological
During the first few days, give analgesics for pain. If a periapical abscess is suspected, begin prophylactic penicillin V, 40 or 60 mg/kg q 6 hours for 10 days, to prevent facial cellulitis, and refer patient to a dentist. Other regimens include the following:

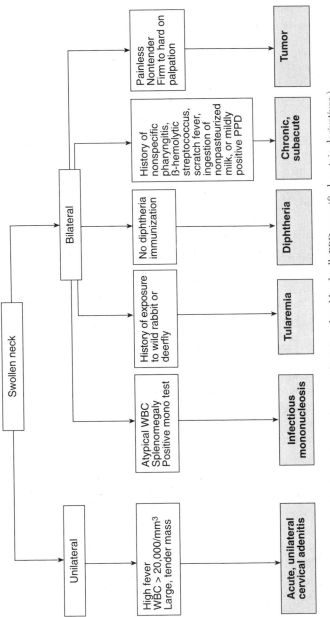

FIGURE 7–3   Differential diagnosis of neck masses. (WBC = white blood cell; PPD = purified protein derivatives.)

Cefadroxil (Duricef, Ultracef), Infant and Children, 25–50 mg/kg per day in divided doses q 12 hours, or once daily, if tolerated, for 7–10 days
or
Dicloxacillin, 15 or 20 mg/kg in divided doses q 6 hours for 10 days
or
Erythromycin, 250 mg q 6 hours for 10 days [Eryped, 30–50 mg/kg per day in four divided doses for 10 days]
or
Amoxicillin/clavulanate (Augmentin), 40 mg/kg per day in divided doses q 8 hours for 10 days

Follow-up: Patient should return to clinic daily. There is usually a good response after 48 hours of treatment.

Sequelae: If untreated, illness may progress to suppuration of the node, a poststreptococcal glomerulonephritis, and bacteremia.

Prevention/Prophylaxis: Adequate treatment of streptococcal infections.

Referral: Refer patient to primary care physician in cases of acute bilateral adenitis; if periapical abscess is suspected, refer to a dentist. Refer to primary-care physician if no improvement in 24 hours, for aspiration of node for identification of infective agent; if there is no marked improvement after the 10 days of antibiotics, refer for incision and drainage. Refer to primary care physician for admission to the hospital if child is less than 6 months old, or is toxic, dehydrated, dysphagic, or dyspneic.

Education: Stress the importance of completing the therapeutic regimen to avoid complications. Use good handwashing technique to lessen cross-contamination if there is drainage from the node.

Torticollis (Wry Neck)

Torticollis is a contracture of the sternocleidomastoid muscle secondary to muscle or bone pathology. Clinically there is a shortened muscle, a rotation of the head toward the opposite side, and a tilting of the head toward the involved side.

Etiology: In infancy, torticollis occurs as a result of an injury during delivery, congenital deformities of the cervical spine, spinal cord or cerebellar tumors, syringomyelia, rheumatoid arthritis, or shortening of the muscle. In older children, it may occur as a sequela of an upper respiratory infection.

Occurrence: Unknown.

Age: Any pediatric age group.

Ethnicity: Not significant.

Gender: Occurs equally in males and females.

Contributing Factors: In older children, infectious agents are implicated as contributing to the problem.

Signs and Symptoms: Parent brings child to the clinic with a complaint such as, "My child isn't holding his head right."
　　Inspection reveals a muscular deformity characterized by chin rotation to the side opposite the affected muscle contracture. On palpation, there may be a mass in the midportion of the muscle.

Diagnostic Tests: Obtain cervical spinal x-rays; in infants, there is a 20% incidence of concomitant hip dysplasia, and therefore hip x-rays should be done.

Differential Diagnosis: Tumors and cervical spine defects will be visible on the radiographic films.

Treatment: Usually resolves after passive stretching (congenital), but may require the use of traction or a cervical collar (acquired).

Follow-up: In infancy, follow the regular well-baby visits. Monitor the status of the muscle after the stretching exercises are implemented. In the acquired form, reevaluate in 7–10 days.

Sequelae: If untreated, the child may have unsightly asymmetry of the face and cranial vertebrae.

Prevention/Prophylaxis: None.

Referral: If the cause is congenital and treatment is not effective within the first year, obtain surgical consultation and intervention to release the contracture. In the acquired form, obtain an immediate referral for consultation and possible surgical intervention.

Education: Instruct parents in methods of passive exercise. Reassure parents that they are not at fault for either the congenital or acquired forms of the condition.

Aphthous Stomatitis

Aphthous stomatitis is the painful recurrence of ulcerations of the buccal mucosa and lips also known as canker sores.

Etiology: Unknown; may be an autoimmune or allergic response.

Occurrence: Common.

Age: Any pediatric age group (peak onset, 10–19 years).

Ethnicity: Not significant.

Gender: Occurs equally in males and females.

Contributing Factors: Chocolate, nuts, and tomatoes have been suggested as offending agents. Hereditary factors have been implicated, as has increased stress.

Signs and Symptoms: Patient complains of painful sores in mouth. Inspection reveals two to five painful, pin-sized vesicles covered with a yellowish gray membrane inside lips and mouth. If the membrane is removed, there will be a raw area. There is no fever and no lymphadenopathy.

Diagnostic Tests: None.

Differential Diagnosis

Herpangina is an acute viral infection accompanied by fever. Oral lesions are papulovesicular with a zone of erythema and ulcers ranging from grayish yellow to white. Ulcers appear on the soft palate and tonsillar pillars, not on the buccal mucosa or gingivae.

Herpetic stomatitis causes small, irregular vesicles that leave ulcers when they rupture. These ulcers are characteristically red at the edge with a gray center. The patient is febrile and has enlarged cervical lymph nodes.

Treatment: Supportive; apply topical antacids to lesions four times per day or steroidal mouthwash (0.1%). Recommend a bland diet, avoiding salty food, to reduce pain during eating. (*Note:* Do not use smallpox vaccine, antibiotics, chemical cautery, and products containing *Lactobacillus*.)

Follow-up: None, if lesions heal.

Sequelae: None.

Prevention/Prophylaxis: Avoid food that may trigger the reaction.

Referral: None.

Education: None.

Glossitis

Glossitis is an inflammation of the tongue characterized by painless, circular or elliptical, smooth areas devoid of papillae and surrounded by a narrow ring of hyperkeratosis; pattern may change daily. This is also known as "geographic tongue" or benign migratory glossitis.

Etiology: Unknown.

Occurrence: Common.

Age: Usually prior to age 6 years.

Ethnicity: Not significant.

Gender: Occurs equally in males and females.

Contributing Factors: Unknown.

Signs and Symptoms: Parent complains that the child's tongue "looks funny." Inspection reveals characteristic lesions.

Diagnostic Tests: None.

Differential Diagnosis

Fissured tongue (scrotal tongue): Characterized by numerous irregular fissures on dorsum. Occurs in 1% of persons and is usually a dominant trait. May be seen in persons who chew on their protruded tongues (e.g., those with trisomy 21).

Coated tongue (furry tongue): Occurs as a result of impaired mastication and when the patient is on a liquid or soft diet.

Treatment: None.

Follow-up: None.

Sequelae: None.

Prevention/Prophylaxis: None.

Referral: None.

Education: Reassure parents that the condition is benign and will resolve in several months.

Herpes Simplex Stomatitis

Herpes simplex stomatitis is a viral infection of the oral mucosa and oropharynx.

Etiology: Herpes simplex virus, type 1.

Occurrence: Common.

Age: Any age, but predominantly in children aged 1–3.

Ethnicity: Not significant.

Gender: Occurs equally in males and females.

Contributing Factors: Immune deficiencies and increased stress are suggested factors.

Signs and Symptoms: Children may complain of a burning sensation in the mouth 26–48 hours before lesions appear. In infants, there is a history of irritability, drooling, and feeding problems. Inspection reveals multiple, grouped lesions on erythematous base on tongue and the buccal and gingival mucosa, along with friable, red gums; lesions may extend to the pharynx. There may be swollen cervical nodes and fever.

Diagnostic Tests: None.

Differential Diagnosis

Aphthous stomatitis: Painful ulcers are present throughout the mouth; there is no fever or adenopathy.

Vincent's angina: Crater-like ulcers are present on the gingival margins, covered with a whitish gray membrane. Gums are tender and bleed easily. Patient may have submaxillary adenopathy.

Herpangina: This is an acute illness in which the patient is febrile. Oral lesions are papulovesicular lesions. The lesions are on the palate and tonsillar pillars, not on the buccal mucosa.

Thrush: This is characterized by white, raised patches on the oral mucosa, lips, tongue, and pharynx that are difficult to remove; usually there is no fever or adenopathy.

Treatment: Supportive: condition usually lasts for 7–14 days. Suggest a bland diet and increased liquids for sore mouth. Do not prescribe steroids because they may cause spread of the infection. For severe cases, may give acyclovir suspension 200 mg/5 mL, 10 mg/kg per dose, qid for 7 days.

Follow-up: None, if lesions heal.

Sequelae: Immunosuppressed patients may have severe chronic disease and esophageal involvement. Some patients have episodic recurrences; recurrent lesions (fever blisters) are usually perinasal or perioral, at the mucocutaneous junction, with a tingling sensation in the prodromal phase. The vesicles and subsequent crusts resemble impetigo.

Prevention/Prophylaxis: None.

Referral: None.

Education: Instruct parents and children not to share drinking glasses or toothbrushes.

Thrush

Thrush is an infection of the oral mucosa with the yeast *Candida albicans.*

Etiology: Hand-to-mouth contact with the causative organism, *C. albicans.*

Occurrence: Common.

Age: Any pediatric age group, but predominantly in infants.

Ethnicity: Not significant.

Gender: Occurs equally in males and females.

Contributing Factors: Factors include long-term antibiotic use and immune disorders.

Signs and Symptoms: Parent complains that child is a "problem feeder" and may report having noted lesions. Child may refuse to eat because mouth is painful.

Inspection of the mouth reveals adherent, painful, white, curdlike plaques with mucosal ulceration. Assess the diaper area for evidence of a candidal diaper rash.

Diagnostic Tests: None.

Differential Diagnosis

Herpetic lesions are small, irregular vesicles that leave ulcers when they rupture. The lesions are characteristically red at the edge with a gray center.

Aphthous ulcers (canker sores) are pin-sized vesicles that leave grayish yellow ulcers covered with a similarly colored membrane. If the membrane is removed, there will be a raw area.

Treatment

Infants

Nystatin, oral suspension, 1,000,000 units, 1–2 mL onto lesions four times per day for 1 week.

Older Children

Nystatin, oral suspension, 200,000–500,000 units four times per day as a mouthwash.

Fluconazole (Diflucan, 10 mg/mL), 6 mg/kg first day, then 3 mg/kg for 6 more days.

Clotrimazole troches 10 mg four times per day.

For refractory lesions, gentian violet 0.5–1.0% to paint the lesions (messy and colorful, but often effective).

Follow-up: Reevaluate in 1 week for efficacy of treatment.

Sequelae: Left untreated, condition may develop into disseminated candidiasis.

Prevention/Prophylaxis: Wash all toys, synthetic nipples, pacifiers, and if child is breastfed, mother's nipples to prevent reinfection. Stop antibiotics and steroids if possible.

Referral: None.

Education: Instruct parents about washing toys, nipples, and pacifiers.

Chalazion

A chalazion is a granulomatous inflammation of the meibomian glands.

Etiology: Unknown.

Occurrence: Common.

Age: All age groups.

Ethnicity: Not significant.

Gender: Occurs equally in males and females.

Contributing Factors: Retention of the secretions of the meibomian glands.

Signs and Symptoms: Child comes to clinic with the complaint of a "red, scratchy eyelid." Inspection reveals edema of the lid, swelling, and irritation. Swelling may be seen in the tarsus of the lid, generally appearing subconjunctivally as a red or gray mass.

Diagnostic Tests: None.

Differential Diagnosis: None.

Treatment: Warm compresses to the eyelid four to five times per day. Often resolves spontaneously after application of compresses. Local incision may be required if chalazion is refractory to treatment. Application of an antibiotic ointment four to five times per day to the eyelid. Continue the antibiotic for several days after the lesion has subsided. Sulfacetamide sodium (Sodium Sulamyd) ophthalmic ointment 10%, 0.5–1.0 cm in conjunctival sac four times daily for 7 days.

Follow-up: None.

Sequelae: None.

Prevention/Prophylaxis: None.

Referral: Refer to primary care physician for incision and drainage if necessary.

Education: Instruct parent or caregiver in the application of the "ribbon" of antibiotic ointment from the tube.

Conjunctivitis

Conjunctivitis is an inflammation and/or infection of the conjunctivae with a rupture of small vessels, causing bleeding into the sclera.

Etiology: Common causative agents are bacterial (*Staphylococcus, Streptococcus pneumoniae, Haemophilus influenzae, Neisseria gonorrhoeae, Chlamydia*); viral (adenoviruses 3, 4, or 7 [30–40%]); allergic processes; and chemicals or other irritants.

Occurrence: Common.

Age: All age groups.

Ethnicity: Not significant.

Gender: Occurs equally in males and females.

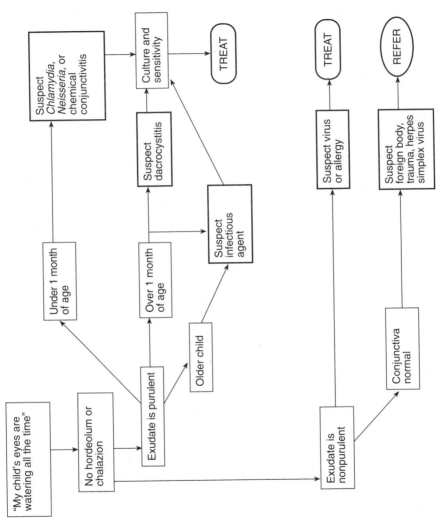

FIGURE 7–4 Conjunctivitis.

Contributing Factors: Silver nitrate administered at time of delivery, allergies, and colds have been implicated.

Signs and Symptoms: Child presents to clinic with complaint of "pink eye"; older children describe an itchy, scratchy sensation. Caregivers will give history of sticky eyelids on awakening, swelling of lid, and photophobia (Fig. 7–4).

Physical findings vary depending on the underlying cause: (1) watery discharge (viral or allergic); and (2) purulent discharge (usually bacterial; if associated with otitis media, suggestive of *H. influenzae* as causative agent). Other distinguishing characteristics are erythema of conjunctivae; preauricular adenopathy (viral agents); cobblestone papillae beneath upper lid; stringy, thick, mucoid discharge (vernal conjunctivitis); and primary skin lesion of single or grouped vesicles or crusted ulcers (primary herpes infection). Vision is normal (Fig. 7–5).

Diagnostic Tests: Culture the discharge on all infants under 1 month to determine the specific organism.

Differential Diagnosis

Keratitis: Severe pain and corneal swelling.
Endophthalmitis: Acute onset, pain, and loss of vision.
Anterior uveitis: Irregular pupils, pain, and poor vision.
Kawasaki syndrome: Usually no drainage; acute illness accompanied by erythematous rash.
Stevens-Johnson syndrome: Follows a viral illness or drug reaction; mucosal lesions in the mouth are characterized by three areas of color (target lesions).

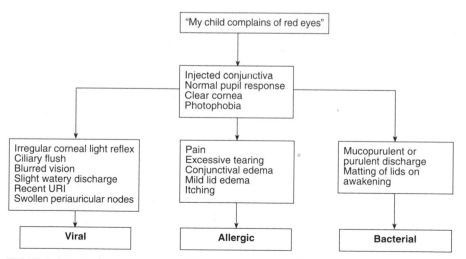

FIGURE 7–5 Evaluating red eyes. (URI = upper respiratory infection.)

Measles: Erythematous maculopapular rash, coryza, and Koplik spots.

Juvenile rheumatoid arthritis: Usually a fever, rash, and arthralgia.

Vitamin A deficiency: Usually the presence of a malabsorption syndrome, as seen in persons with cystic fibrosis or those who are on fad diets.

Treatment

Bacterial

Trimethoprim sulfate 0.1% plus polymyxin B sulfate 10,000 units/mL (Polytrim Ophthalmic Solution), 1 drop two to four times per day (children over 2 months)

or

Sulfacetamide sodium ophthalmic ointment or solution (Sulamyd), 1%, five times daily for 7–10 days

or

Tobramycin 0.3% plus dexamethasone 0.1% (Tobradex Ophthalmic Ointment or Solution), 2 drops two to four times per day and

Application of cool compresses.

Viral

Self-limiting (usually associated with upper respiratory infection).

Application of cool compresses.

To prevent secondary infection, sulfacetamide solution 1% five times daily.

Allergic

Apply cold compresses and treat underlying problem.

Prescribe Acular 0.5% (ketorolac tromethamine) solution, 1 g per day.

Chemical

Flush eye with a copious amount of tepid water or normal saline.

Follow-up: Child should return to clinic in 2–3 days if there is no improvement; parent should call back immediately if condition becomes worse, child complains of pain, or child initially gets better and then gets worse.

Sequelae: A secondary bacterial infection may develop. If untreated, the long-term effects may be blepharitis, corneal ulcers (bacterial infection), sloughing of the cornea, or corneal ulcer (chemical irritation).

Prevention/Prophylaxis: Proper handwashing techniques and proper disposal of compresses. Instruct parents to avoid cross-contamination by keeping child's washcloth and towels separate from those of other family members.

Referral: Consult with ophthalmologist for prompt referral for corneal ulcer, chemical conjunctivitis, complaints of pain, photophobia, and any irregularities in pupil size, as well as for infants under age 1 month.

Education: Instruct parents in proper eye care:

Wipe eyes gently from inner canthus to avoid spreading infection to the other eye. Clean eye before instilling medication.

To instill ointment or drops, pull down inner canthus of lower eyelid toward center of eye; apply a thin ribbon of ointment or drops to the "pocket." Rubbing of eyes can cause the infection to spread to the other eye. Instruct parents to teach child not to rub his or her eyes.

Eye Injuries

Eye injuries include any trauma, accidental or nonaccidental, to the eye or its structures.

Etiology: Foreign body, lacerations, abrasions, burns, fractures, contusions, child abuse (shaken-baby syndrone).

Occurrence: Fairly common.

Age: All age groups.

Ethnicity: Not significant.

Gender: Occurs equally in males and females.

Contributing Factors: Lack of knowledge about safety when using hammers, firearms, or chemicals, and exposure to ultraviolet light.

Signs and Symptoms: Child is brought to the clinic with a complaint such as, "I have something in my eye." Obtain a history of the event, the activity engaged in, where the activity took place, time elapsed before seeking health care, any home remedy used, and the presence of pain or bleeding.

Foreign body: Evert the upper lid; inspection will usually reveal the foreign body in the furrow immediately behind the margin of the upper lid.

Corneal foreign body: Refer immediately to primary care physician or ophthalmologist.

Intraocular foreign body: Refer immediately to ophthalmologist.

Injuries to the eyelids (ecchymosis and lacerations): Refer to primary care physician or ophthalmologist.

Corneal injuries: Refer to primary care physician or ophthalmologist.

Burns: Refer to primary care physician or ophthalmologist.

Diagnostic Tests: Vision testing. If the patient cannot take the Snellen test, obtain gross vision by having the patient count upheld fingers. Radiographic studies are done to determine the presence of any fracture of the orbit.

Differential Diagnosis: None.

Treatment

Conjunctival foreign body: After visualizing the foreign body, gently remove with a moist cotton applicator.

Corneal and intraocular foreign bodies: should be referred immediately to the primary care physician or ophthalmologist.

Follow-up: For minor injuries, patient should return in 24 hours; those with major injuries should return to the clinic after the period of hospitalization.

Sequelae: If not treated promptly and appropriately, there could be loss of vision or loss of the entire eye.

Prevention/Prophylaxis: Wear safety goggles when working with tools or hazardous chemicals, or when exposed to ultraviolet light. Do not allow children to play with firearms, fireworks, or other harmful items.

Referral: After initial assessment, refer all ocular injuries to the primary care physician or ophthalmologist.

Education: Teach (1) the safety rules related to tools and hazardous substances, (2) the dangers and safety measures related to ultraviolet rays, and (3) firearm safety.

Hordeolum

Hordeolum is an abscess of the sebaceous glands of the lid margin. External hordeolum is commonly called a "sty." Internal hordeolum is an acute infection of the meibomian glands.

Etiology: The infective agent is a staphylococcal organism, usually *Staphylococcus aureus.*

Occurrence: Common.

Age: All age groups.

Ethnicity: Not significant.

Gender: Occurs equally in males and females.

Contributing Factors: Hand-to-eye contact with the infective agent.

Signs and Symptoms: Parent complains, "My child has a sty." Obtain history of duration of illness, other persons at home with the problem, and what they have done at home in an attempt to cure the sty. Findings include localized tenderness, redness, and swelling.

Diagnostic Tests: None.

Differential Diagnosis: None.

Treatment

Nonpharmacological
Apply warm, moist compresses to the eyelid four times per day.

Pharmacological
Apply an antibiotic ointment to the eyelid four to five times per day. Continue the antibiotic for several days after the lesion has subsided.

Sulfacetamide sodium ophthalmic ointment 10%, 0.5–1.0 cm in conjunctival sac four times per day for 7 days.

Follow-up: None.

Sequelae: None.

Prevention/Prophylaxis: Good handwashing techniques. Purchase new eye makeup, throwing out the old makeup as well as the old applicators. Keep child's wash cloth and towels separate from those of other family members. Dispose warm compresses properly to prevent reinfection.

Referral: None, unless treatment is ineffective or the lesion needs to be incised and drained.

Education: Instruct parent and/or patient in good handwashing techniques and to take care not to cross-contaminate the eyes. Older children and adolescents should not wear eye makeup until the infection has cleared.

Nasolacrimal Duct Obstruction

This condition is defined as obstruction of the nasolacrimal duct with or without an infectious process. There may also be a concomitant infection of the lacrimal sac, termed dacrocystitis.

Etiology: Failure of nasolacrimal duct to canalize completely.

Occurrence: Common.

Age: Infancy.

Ethnicity: Not significant.

Gender: Occurs equally in males and females.

Contributing Factors: Failure of tears to drain or stasis of tears in the tear sac predisposes infants to infection, usually with *Staphylococcus aureus.*

Signs and Symptoms: Child presents with a history of persistent tearing and mucoid discharge in the inner corner of the eye; may have matting of the eyelashes during sleep. Inspection reveals watering of the eye(s), with tears spilling over onto the cheek. If dacrocystitis is present, there will be swelling and erythema medial and inferior to the inner canthus, and purulent material may be expressed from the duct opening.

Diagnostic Tests: None; may do culture of exudate to assess for infective organisms.

Differential Diagnosis: Excessive lacrimation is an early sign of congenital glaucoma, as are photophobia and a cloudy cornea.

Treatment: Gently massage the lacrimal sac, expressing exudate toward the nose to clear the passage. Instill antibiotic ointment or drops, as indicated.

Follow-up: Evaluate monthly; if no improvement by 6 months of age, refer patient to the ophthalmologist.

Sequelae: May be secondary inflammation due to the obstruction.

Prevention/Prophylaxis: None, except for proper eye care to prevent secondary infection.

Referral: If no improvement in 6 months, refer patient to ophthalmologist for surgical intervention.

Education: Instruct parents in lacrimal massage and in the proper manner of instillation of medications.

Nystagmus

The involuntary ocular movements are classified as follows:

Pendular (undulatory): Equal in each direction of gaze.

Jerking (rhythmic): Slow component followed by quick, corrective component.

Congenital: Jerky movements, present in all directions of gaze, usually decrease when eyes converge.

Latent: Occurring when one eye is covered.

Etiology: Varies by classification: poor vision (pendular), congenital (jerky), inner ear disease, secondary to central nervous system (CNS) disease (jerky).

Occurrence: Fairly uncommon (less than 2%).

Age: All age groups.

Ethnicity: Not significant.

Gender: Occurs equally in males and females.

Contributing Factors: Physiologic disease, CNS disease, drug and/or alcohol toxicity.

Signs and Symptoms: Child presents with a history of spontaneous, involuntary movements of one or both eyes. Family history, drug and chemical history, illnesses, and duration of symptoms are all avenues of investigation.

Inspection reveals rapid eye movements. Notations of the plane and the rate of movement assist in the classification: equal in all directions, pendular; quicker movements in one direction, jerky.

Diagnostic Tests: A funduscopic examination may reveal cataracts, retrolental fibroplasia, decreased visual acuity, and weakness of the ocular muscles.

A neurological examination is indicated because premature infants with persistent or horizontal nystagmus are predisposed to intracranial hemorrhage. Horizontal nystagmus is often associated with a brain tumor.

Problems related to cranial nerve VIII (vestibular branch of auditory nerve) may also be a source of nystagmus. The rotational test is done (if nystagmus does not occur after rotation, there is labyrinth damage). The caloric test is then done to determine which labyrinth is affected. Screening for vestibular abnormalities may be done using the past pointing test in which the arm moves to the side of the disorder. In the Romberg test, child will fall toward the side of the vestibular lesion.

Differential Diagnosis: None. Nystagmus is a symptom of an underlying disorder. Clarification of the type of nystagmus provides some diagnostic clues for identifying the cause. End-point nystagmus, which occurs when the child looks out of the far corner of the eye, is not true nystagmus.

Treatment: To treat nystagmus, the underlying cause must be treated.

Follow-up: Follow-up is done with respect to the underlying cause and in concert with the consulting physician.

Sequelae: Later outcomes include extreme vertigo, oscillopsia, and permanent nystagmus. Permanent disability and even death can occur if underlying causes are not found and treated.

Prevention/Prophylaxis: None.

Referral: Immediate referral to a primary care physician, ophthalmologist, and neurologist.

Education: Explain possible causative factors to parents and the need for referral to a specialist.

Strabismus

Strabismus, or abnormal ocular alignment, is nonparallelism of the visual axes in the various fields of gaze. It is usual in infants up to age 6 months, may be transitory in infants aged 6–18 months, and is abnormal after age 18 months. Nonparalytic strabismus is characterized by a constant angle of deviation in all fields. Strabismus may be classified as follows:

Esotropia (convergent strabismus): Eye turns medially.
Exotropia (divergent strabismus): Eye turns laterally.
Hypertrophia: upward deviation of the eye.
Hypotrophia: downward deviation of the eye.
Esophoria: tendency of eyes to converge.
Exophoria: tendency of eyes to diverge.

Etiology: In paralytic strabismus, a motor imbalance caused by paresis of an extraocular muscle causes the condition. In nonparalytic strabismus, muscle weakness, visual defects, intracranial hemorrhage, lead poisoning, and infection have been implicated.

Occurrence: Occurs in 2–3% of children.

Age: Occurrences past age 6 months require further investigation.

Ethnicity: Not significant.

Gender: Occurs equally in males and females.

Contributing Factors: There is often a family pattern of strabismus. Febrile illness, head injury, fatigue, or stress may precipitate concomitant (nonparalytic) strabismus.

Signs and Symptoms: In infants and young children, strabismus is usually identified at the time of the well-baby visit. Parents of an older child may bring the child to the clinic because an abnormal look to the eyes is apparent. The onset and duration should be investigated. Examination of the eye reveals ocular deviation.

Diagnostic Tests: Visual accuracy tests can identify any defect causing the problem.

Hirshburg test (corneal light reflection test): When a light is shined into the eyes, the light should fall nearly in the center of each pupil. Lateral displacement indicates esotropia; nasal displacement indicates extropia.

Alternate cover test: The movement of the covered eye is observed when the cover is removed. If the eye remains in the deviated position, atropia is present; if it returns to center, it is normal.

Cardinal positions of gaze: There will be limited movement in one direction of gaze if strabismus is present. Testing each eye separately assists in determining the presence of true paralysis of an extraocular muscle.

Differential Diagnosis: Sudden onset indicates intracranial hemorrhage, encephalitis, lead poisoning, or intraorbital tumors. Hypoglycemic patients may have transient strabismus.

Treatment: Surgical intervention is done to correct strabismus due to muscular problems. In cases of strabismus due to other physical problems, underlying causes should be treated.

Follow-up: Follow-up depends on the cause and treatment. Care should be provided in conjunction with the referring physician.

Sequelae: Monocular strabismus may develop in persons with amblyopia.

Prevention/Prophylaxis: Prompt identification and treatment of underlying cause will prevent further complications.

Referral: Refer to ophthalmologist any child over age 6 months with presenting history and physical examination indicating the presence of strabismus. Refer to ophthalmologist any child under age 6 months if strabismus is fixed or constant.

Education: None.

The Common Cold

The common cold, a viral infection of the upper respiratory tract, is limited to the nasopharynx and nasal mucosa. A cold is a highly communicable disease, extremely common in the pediatric population; it is the second most commonly diagnosed illness seen in the primary health-care setting.

Etiology: Viruses of many different types (approximately 100), with rhinovirus being responsible for about one third of all colds, cause the common cold or upper respiratory infection. Parainfluenza virus, respiratory syncytial virus, and coronavirus are the other most common viral agents that cause colds.

Occurrence: Fall, winter, and early spring, or during a community outbreak. In children, winter still remains the most likely time during which the majority of colds are seen.

Age: Preschoolers get colds more frequently (between three and nine per year) than any other age group of children.

Ethnicity: Not significant.

Gender: Occurs equally in males and females.

Contributing Factors: Exposure to second-hand smoke, smoking, environmental pollutants, crowded areas, and day-care settings increases the incidence of colds.

Signs and Symptoms: The child and/or parent may report that rhinorrhea, nasal stuffiness, and a thin, watery discharge from the nose have been present for 1–4 days. Mouth breathing and frequent sneezing will also be reported. For infants, the temperature ranges from normal to 102°F, whereas older children rarely are febrile. A decreased appetite, poor feeding, and a mildly upset stomach will also be reported. The child appears ill and fussy. Postnasal drip and swollen, erythematous nasal mucosa are noted. Auscultation reveals some referred nasal sounds, with occasional coarse breath sounds in the upper lobes.

Diagnostic Tests: None are indicated; however, if a CBC is performed, there may be slight leukopenia followed by leukocytosis.

Differential Diagnosis

Pertussis, measles, and diphtheria in the early stages are differentiated by their clinical courses, which quickly become more serious. Auscultation in these diseases reveals findings that suggest lower respiratory infections.

Sinusitis, which causes a persistent fever and an accompanying cough and headache, are differentiated by symptoms.

Allergic rhinitis is differentiated by history, seasonality of the disease, and other allergic symptoms.

Cocaine use, which can produce chronic congestion and watery rhinorrhea, is differentiated by a drug screen.

Treatment: Symptomatic treatment is the most appropriate regimen for the common cold or upper respiratory infections. Comfort measures such as elevating the head of the bed, using saline nasal spray up to four times a day, and taking acetaminophen for fever are all effective modes of treatment. Increasing the child's fluid intake helps to liquefy secretions. A cool-mist humidifier is also helpful for infants and toddlers, but it must be cleaned daily.

Oral antihistamines have not been shown to cause a significant reduction in the symptoms or discomfort of a cold.

Follow-up: Regular childhood visits, unless the cold fails to resolve within 2 weeks or there is a worsening of symptoms.

Sequelae: No serious sequelae have been documented.

Prevention/Prophylaxis: Although many have suggested administering vitamin C for colds, most studies have shown that it has no impact on the incidence or severity of colds. Some risk does exist, however, with taking vitamin C in high doses, as vitaminosis has been frequently documented. Good nutrition, avoidance of crowds when a community outbreak has been noted, adequate rest, and good hygiene are the best ways to decrease the spread of colds.

Referral: Referral is rarely needed, but if the cold does not resolve within 1–2 weeks or the symptoms worsen, the patient should be referred to a pediatrician.

Education: Parents and children should be taught that this self-limiting disease has few, if any, serious consequences. Although parents often request antibiotics at the health-care visit, antibiotics are of little value in the treatment of a cold. Parents should also be made aware that if their child has school-age siblings, has a large family, or attends a day-care center, he or she is more likely to get colds.

Nasal secretions, which contain the virus, can be on the skin, clothing, or toys; thus handwashing can decrease the spread of the cold. The importance of handwashing should be stressed to both the child and the caregiver because the disease spreads by hand-to-mouth contact.

Croup

Croup or laryngotracheobronchitis, an acute viral respiratory illness of short course (3–7 days), generally follows an upper respiratory infection. It is characterized by a barky cough, variable respiratory distress, and biphasic or inspiratory stridor.

Etiology: Parainfluenza, respiratory syncytial virus (RSV), adenovirus, and influenza A are all thought to be the causative agents.

Occurrence: Usually during the fall and winter.

Age: Children ages 6 months to 5 years.

Ethnicity: Not significant.

Gender: Not significant.

Contributing Factors: Exposure to affected persons.

Signs and Symptoms: Parent usually reports that the child had a mild cold or rhinitis and was awakened by a "barking cough." The child appeared frightened and at times unable to catch his or her breath. Chest retractions and nasal flaring are usually seen. There may or may not be a fever. Between episodes of cough, the child will appear well. Inspection shows the child to have occasional nasal flaring during the coughing episode. The child may seem irritable and restless. Substernal retractions are noted. Palpation may reveal displacement of the cardiac apical beat toward an area of atelectasis. Percussion reveals dullness, which may indicate consolidation or atelectasis of the lung. Auscultation will reveal tachycardia, bronchial breathing, and rales.

Diagnostic Tests: Laboratory tests are usually not helpful or indicated. An x-ray of the neck may show subglottic narrowing (the Staple sign) but is not indicated in most cases. If the child shows signs of clinical deterioration, an RSV titer, arterial blood gases (ABGs), and CBC should be done. The RSV titer, if positive, may indicate that the coughing is not related to croup, but rather RSV infection.

A CBC or urinalysis should be obtained to determine dehydration. ABGs should be monitored to see whether PCO_2 is greater than 45 or PO_2 less than 70. These results would indicate the need for supplemental O_2 and aggressive therapy.

Differential Diagnosis

Foreign body aspiration: Can affect all ages; differentiated by a sudden onset, no fever, normal WBC count, and no growth in blood culture; can affect all ages.

Epiglottitis: Affects children aged 1–8 years; onset over several hours; patient usually febrile; blood culture positive for *H. influenza*, swollen epiglottis apparent on x-ray.

Peritonsillar abscess: Febrile process; affects children ages 1 and older; blood culture positive; tonsils swollen and covered with exudate.

Treatment: The risk of obstruction increases when intubation is attempted, so care should be taken. A tracheostomy set-up should be available in the room. The treatment of choice for croup is as follows: (1) cool-mist humidifiers, with or without additional oxygen; (2) racemic epinephrine, 0.25 mg in 2.5 mL normal saline nebulization, every 2 hours for the hospitalized patient; and (3) steroid, either intravenously (IV) or orally (PO) (methylprednisolone [Solu-Medrol] IV 1 mg/kg q 6 hours or dexamethasone PO q 6 hours).

A child may be treated as an outpatient if there are no signs of dehydration or if PCO_2 and PO_2 are normal. If PCO_2 is greater than 45 or PO_2 less than 70, the child should be hospitalized. Do not use any sedation or respiratory-depressing agents on the child. It is also important to calm the parents.

Follow-up: Reexamine patient in 2–3 days to ensure that there are no signs of infection.

Sequelae: Rarely will the disease progress to the point where intubation or tracheostomy are necessary. For the most part, children recover completely, without any permanent respiratory system damage. Occasionally, bronchitis develops after an episode of croup. When this is suspected, appropriate antibiotic therapy should be instituted.

Prevention/Prophylaxis: Children should avoid close contact with other children who exhibit signs and symptoms of croup or bronchitis. Prompt attention to and treatment of respiratory problems can improve outcomes for infants with croup.

Referral: If the disease does not respond to treatment within 1–2 days or if there is a worsening of symptoms, a pediatrician should be consulted.

Education: Parents should be taught how to treat a recurrence of a croup attack; they should either go outside to expose the child to cold air or go into the bathroom, turn on the hot water, and mist the room. They should also be taught to inform the health-care provider of the episode, but if the child is in acute distress, to bring the child to the emergency room immediately.

Epiglottitis

Epiglottitis is an acute and potentially fatal respiratory infection. Inflammation of supraglottic structures can very rapidly cause acute airway obstruction. It is a true pediatric emergency, and a physician should be present at all times during the patient's treatment.

Etiology: *H. influenzae* type B (almost always).

Occurrence: Generally in late fall or early winter.

Age: Primarily ages 3–7 years; however, *H. influenzae* epiglottitis may occur at any age, including infancy and older childhood.

Ethnicity: Ethnicity is not significant.

Gender: Male to female ratio is 3 : 2.

Contributing Factors: Sore throat is a possible factor.

Signs and Symptoms: The parent usually reports a quick onset of fever, sore throat, and difficulty swallowing and breathing. For the most part, no other family members are ill. Auscultation reveals inspiratory and expiratory stridor. The pediatric NP can observe nasal flaring and retractions. The pharynx is inflamed and there is an increased amount of saliva, sometimes resulting in drooling. Some rhonchi may be heard on auscultation. If the disease progresses, increasing cyanosis, air hunger, and progression to coma may occur. A cherry-red epiglottis may be visualized, but the NP should take care not to induce a laryngospasm when examining the throat. The child may be observed to sit leaning forward, with a hyperextended neck ("sniffing-dog" position).

Diagnostic Tests

CBC (expect highly elevated WBC).
Blood cultures (usually positive for *H. influenzae* type B).
X-rays of the lateral neck show "thumbprint sign."
"Cherry red sign" is noted—swollen, enlarged, cherry-red epiglottis.

Differential Diagnosis

Croup syndrome is generally diagnosed by a barking cough and is usually a nonprogressive disease.

Bacterial tracheitis has symptoms that develop more slowly and nearly always follows a viral infection. There is an accompanying brassy cough.

Pertussis is accompanied by a characteristic spasmodic, whooping cough.

Foreign bodies are differentiated by x-ray or direct inspection of the trachea and larynx.

Retropharyngeal abscess progresses more slowly, and palpation of the posterior wall reveals a fluctuant mass.

Treatment: Swift and careful management should be instituted in consultation with a physician. The primary goal is to maintain an adequate airway. It is imperative to plan treatment in advance. A patent airway should be maintained, and supplies to accommodate immediate intubation should be present with the patient at all times. Skilled personnel prepared to perform airway stabilization and ventilation support (anesthesiologist and otolaryngologist) should be present. Child should be kept calm, preferably in parent's arms. Staff must accompany child to radiology department.

Nasotracheal intubation or elective tracheotomy is the procedure of choice after diagnosis. Generally, children are intubated for 2–3 days.

IV antibiotic therapy—ampicillin (100–200 mg/kg IV divided into four doses) and chloramphenicol (25 mg/kg once daily for neonates; 50–100 mg/kg divided q 6 hours in children)—often is the initial choice until results of sensitivities are available.

Follow-up: One week after discharge from the hospital the child should return to the primary-care office.

Sequelae: Laryngeal obstruction, pneumonia, or cervical lymphadenitis may result from epiglottitis. If the disease progresses untreated, it will lead to asphyxia and death.

Prevention/Prophylaxis: Conjugated *H. influenzae* type B vaccine can be given.

Referral: Refer if epiglottitis is suspected. Hospitalize child *immediately* and refer to anesthesiologist and otolaryngologist.

Education: Parents should be kept informed as to the condition of the child. They should be educated regarding the possible treatment modalities, including intubation and tracheostomy.

Epistaxis

Epistaxis is blood loss from the nose arising from the Kiesselbach area.

Etiology: Commonly occurs as a result of trauma (picking nose) and excessive dryness of the mucous membrane. Less common causes are vascular malformation, hypertension, nasopharyngeal angiofibroma (adolescent males), and allergic rhinitis.

Occurrence: Common.

Age: Occurs in any age group.

Ethnicity: Not significant.

Gender: Occurs equally in males and females.

Contributing Factors: Vigorous nose blowing, allergies, chronic bleeding disorder (von Willebrand's disease, thrombocytopenia), family history of bleeding disorder, other spontaneous blood loss, and aspirin usage.

Signs and Symptoms: Child presents with a history of spontaneous nosebleed. The frequency may range from daily to monthly. Obtain a detailed history of the present nosebleed (e.g., trauma, extended use of nasal sprays containing phenylephrine, type of home heating system, nasal insertion of a foreign body, duration of nosebleed). Obtain a family history of bleeding disorders or illnesses such as rheumatic fever and sickle cell disease. Ask about color of stools (tarry stools indicate that the bleeding did not occur recently). Upon examination, the anterior portion of the nasal septum will have a red, raw surface with crusts. Observe for the presence of a foreign body or polyps. Evaluate the Kiesselbach area for telangiectasia, hemangiomas, or varicosities (structural defects). Observe the color and character of the nasal mucosa to determine allergic rhinitis (Fig. 7–6).

Diagnostic Tests: Obtain a hematocrit at baseline and 6–12 hours after the nosebleed to determine whether the bleeding is related to anemia. (*Note:* if there is a family history of bleeding disorder, easy bleeding, other spontaneous loss of blood, a nosebleed lasting more than 30 minutes, onset of nosebleed before age 2 years, or a drop in hematocrit after a nosebleed, obtain a hematologic workup.

Differential Diagnosis

Allergic rhinitis: Rubbing, picking, and itching of the nose due to boggy, inflamed mucosa predisposes patients to nosebleeds.

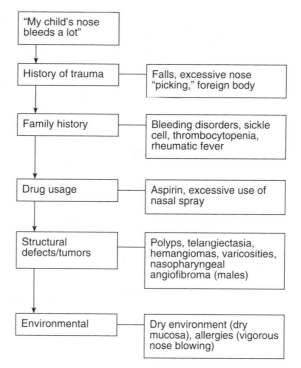

FIGURE 7–6 Evaluation of epistaxis.

Chronic bleeding disorders: If the patient has history of easy bleeding after lacerations or surgical procedures, together with family history of bleeding tendencies, an in-depth evaluation is indicated.

Treatment: If the child is having an active nosebleed, he or she should sit with head down, pinch nose at site for 10 minutes, and then reapply pressure if bleeding is not stopped. (*Note:* Use of cauteries is contraindicated because of their destruction of the septal tissue.) If identified, remove any foreign bodies. If simple anemia is present, treat with an iron supplement, 3 mg/kg per day before breakfast for 2 months.

Follow-up: Patient should return in 6–12 hours for a follow-up hematocrit. If anemic and placed on iron therapy, reevaluate hematocrit level in 2 months.

Sequelae: Mild anemia; less than 5% of children have a bleeding disorder.

Prevention/Prophylaxis: Parent or patient should apply petroleum jelly daily until 5 days elapse without a nosebleed occurring, and then weekly for 1 month; avoid giving aspirin; discourage vigorous blowing or picking of the nose; and increase humidity in patient's room in dry climates.

Referral: In cases of recalcitrant nosebleeds or a suspected bleeding disorder, refer to a primary care physician or otolaryngologist. To induce vasoconstriction, apply a pledget soaked with 0.25% phenylephrine nose drops; 1% lidocaine with 1 : 1000 epinephrine inserted into the nose is usually effective. The most potent vasoconstricting agent is 1% cocaine, but this is rarely used.

Education: Instruct parents in home techniques to stop bleeding. Caution parents about the causes of nosebleeds, such as insertion of foreign bodies and rubbing or picking the nose. Instruct parents as to measures to increase humidity in the home (e.g., using a vaporizer, simmering water on the stove). Parents should avoid giving the child aspirin. Reassure parents that the amount of blood loss always appears to be greater than what is actually lost; a normal hematocrit is very comforting to parents.

Foreign Bodies in the Nose

A foreign body inserted into the nose can obstruct the nasal passage.

Etiology: The most common objects inserted are buttons, beans, nuts, and marbles.

Occurrence: Common.

Age: Usually children aged 3–6 years.

Ethnicity: Not significant.

Gender: Occurs equally in males and females.

Contributing Factors: The natural curiosity of the 3- to 6-year-old child, and improper storage of objects most likely to be inserted.

Signs and Symptoms: Child presents to the clinic with a history of known insertion of a foreign object (parent or caregiver saw the activity), the "nose smells," or abnormal sounds are heard on respiration. Often the first indication is a unilateral, purulent, foul-smelling rhinitis, with occlusion of the nasal passage. Inspection reveals presence of a foreign body.

Diagnostic Tests: None.

Differential Diagnosis: None.

Treatment: Removal of the object. If child is cooperative, the pediatric NP may attempt to remove the object by having the child vigorously blow nose while leaning over a basin to reduce risk of aspiration, and irrigating the contralateral nasal passage with normal saline solution. The overflow of the solution into the closed passage will often bring the object out. If you can observe any space around the object, insert a #8 balloon catheter past the object, inflate the catheter balloon, and gently remove the catheter, thus extracting the object. Treat inflammation and/or infection with amoxicillin, 40 mg/kg per day in three divided doses for 10 days.

Follow-up: None for simple removal with no evidence of infection. If infection is present, patient should return in 10 days for evaluation of therapeutic response.

Sequelae: None.

Prevention/Prophylaxis: Instruct the child not to insert anything into bodily orifices.

Referral: Refer to primary care physician or otolaryngologist if object is not easily removed or child is unable to cooperate.

Education: Instruct parents as to the proper storage of offending objects.

Hearing Loss

Normal hearing ranges from 0 (threshold of hearing) to a 120-decibel (dB) hearing loss (HL), which is the threshold for pain. The following are HL values for children:

Normal threshold for hearing: 0–5 dB Hz
Minimal HL: Up to 25 dB Hz
Mild HL: 25–40 dB Hz
Moderate HL: 40–55 dB Hz
Moderately severe HL: 55–70 dB Hz
Severe HL: 70–90 dB Hz
Profound HL: Greater than 90 dB Hz

The two mechanisms are:

Conductive: Caused by a problem in the external or middle ear.
Sensorineural: Caused by a problem medial to the stapes, inner ear, auditory nerve, or brain.

Any HL lasting up to 72 hours is classified as acute; any HL lasting more than 72 hours is classified as chronic.

Etiology: Conduction abnormality due to middle ear disease, congenital infections such as rubella, perinatal complications such as kernicterus, or genetic deafness (dominant or recessive).

Occurrence: Common: 1 in 1000 full-term infants at birth and 1–3% of all premature infants. Between 33% and 50% of cases have a genetic basis. Sensorineural loss is more common if HL becomes more severe.

Age: All age groups.

Ethnicity: Not significant.

Gender: Occurs equally in males and females.

Contributing Factors: Recurrent otitis media.

Signs and Symptoms: Parent may bring child to the clinic at age 12–18 months with the complaint, "He is not talking like my other children"; or the HL may be discovered at a regular well-baby visit, or as a result of testing because of otitis media. The child may complain that the ear is painful or feels full. History should include queries as to family history of HL; noise exposure associated with work or recreation; and past medical history, including medications, head trauma, history of flying or diving, recurrent otitis media. If the hearing loss is acute, a prior viral infection or episodes of otitis media may be the cause.

Typical auditory symptoms found in conductive loss include otalgia and otorrhea, which are compatible with the findings of either otitis externa or otitis media. The sensation of aural fullness is associated with otitis media and eustachian tube dysfunction. Fluctuation in hearing intensity is noted with otitis media, eustachian tube dysfunction, and genetic forms of HL. Tinnitus and vertigo are noted less frequently; hyperacusis is not noted in conductive loss.

In sensorineural HL, otalgia and otorrhea are absent; sensation of aural fullness and hearing fluctuation are mildly present. Sound sensations, however, are overly loud and uncomfortable; the sensation of different pitches of the same tone (hypercusis and dipacusis) is strongly evident in sensorineural HL.

Examination of the ear, external canal, and tympanic membrane (TM) may reveal cerumen in the canal, otitis externa, or otitis media. Pneumatic otoscopy may be helpful in establishing the diagnosis of tympanic immobility. Perforation of the TM may be noted.

Diagnostic Tests: Diagnostic testing should begin in the newborn nursery and at each well-baby visit. The majority of these tests require a licensed audiologist.

Behavioral observational audiometry should be done at all visits during the regular physical examinations from birth to age 3 years. The bell is rung, and the observer watches for the reaction from the infant. By age 4 months, the child should turn the head toward the sound.

Office tympanograms can assist in determining the presence of effusion and eustachian tube dysfunction. Office audiometry can provide basic screening, identify a need for referral, and enhance effective treatment.

The Rinne test and the Weber test, which use a 512-cycle tuning fork, can be performed on older children; they are not reliable in young children. The Rinne test, which evaluates air and bone conduction, is positive when air conduction of sound elicited from a 512-Hz tuning fork is twice as long as bone conduction. The Weber test for unilateral HL is very sensitive, because sound localizes to the ear with the conductive HL.

Differential Diagnosis: Examine the ear for underlying cause, such as otitis media with effusion or otitis externa with swelling that occludes the ear canal.

Treatment: Remove the impacted cerumen, if indicated. Treat the otitis media. Fit the child for hearing aids. Cochlear implants benefit some children.

Follow-up: Return to clinic in 10 days for evaluation of otitis and for hearing reassessment.

Sequelae: Acute HL due to head trauma or ototoxic drugs is irreversible. Progressive HL occurs if HL is not detected and treated early (e.g., if cause is recreational or work-related, such as in situations with continuous exposure to loud sounds). Loss of communication occurs as a result of HL.

Prevention/Prophylaxis: Genetic counseling, improved prenatal care, prompt treatment of otitis media, wearing ear plugs if HL is work-related.

Referral: Refer any suspicion of a sensorineural loss to an audiologist. Refer to primary care physician and otolaryngologist for definitive diagnosis, testing (audiologist), and treatment. Refer parents to a parent-centered program for the hearing impaired and to a support group.

Education: Teach parents what behaviors to watch for to assess HL, such as the child turning a radio or TV very loud or speaking in a very loud voice, or the child's failure to hear when being spoken to in a normal tone of voice.

Otitis Externa

Otitis externa is an inflammation of the skin lining of the ear canals accompanied by swelling, pain, and itching; there is no HL until the canal is occluded. There are four categories:

Localized: An infected nodule is noted on the skin; it may be a furuncle or a boil.

Generalized: Infection involves the entire ear canal.

Acute: Tenderness is noted on traction of the pinna and/or pain on pressure over the tragus; patient may have regional lymphadenopathy.

Chronic: Ear canal is dry, pruritic, not tender; cerumen is absent, and there may be some erythema of the skin.

Etiology: Conversion of the pH from acid to alkaline in the ear canal, trauma to the canal, contact dermatitis, or irritation from chronic drainage from a perforated TM. Localized, usual agent is *Staphylococcus aureus;* generalized, *Pseudomonas aeruginosa;* chronic, usually caused by a fungus.

Occurrence: Common, seen more often during the summer months.

Age: All age groups.

Ethnicity: Not significant.

Gender: Occurs equally in males and females.

Contributing Factors: Contributing factors include use of hair sprays and dyes, accumulation of wax in the canal, and increased wetness or moisture in the canal.

Signs and Symptoms: The child is brought to the clinic with the complaint of "pain in the ear." History should include the duration of the condition, location and quality of the pain, activities preceding the onset, and home treatment already given. Type of inflammation is categorized as follows:

Localized: Infection is localized, perhaps with purulent, bloody drainage.

Generalized: There may be a foul-smelling discharge and swelling of the canal.

Acute: Canal is red and edematous. There is tenderness on traction of the pinna and/or pain on pressure over the tragus. Regional lymphadenopathy is present if disease has progressed.

Chronic: Dry canal; skin may be slightly red and edematous, with no ear wax.

Diagnostic Tests: Obtain a culture of the ear drainage for identification of the organism.

Differential Diagnosis

Cellulitis: Usually involves the total auricle.

Foreign body: None found on inspection of the canal in otitis externa.

Tympanic membrane rupture with drainage: Not found on inspection of the canal and tympanic membrane with otitis externa.

Treatment: Clean exudate from the canal. When instilling ear drops, have the patient lie down with ear upward for 5 minutes, or keep the head bent with the ear upward for 5 minutes. Give acetaminophen for pain. Cortisporin Otic Solution Sterile (polymyxin B, neomycin, hydrocortisone), four drops in the affected ear, four times daily, for 7 days; Cortic ear drops (chloroxylenol, pramoxine hydrochloride, hydrocortisone), four drops in the affected ear, four times daily, for 7 days; or Domeboro otic solution, four to six drops in the affected ear, four times daily, for 7 days. Give systemic antibiotics only if there is fever or lymphadenopathy.

Follow-up: Patient should return to clinic in 7–10 days for reevaluation and therapeutic response.

Sequelae: Allergic reaction to the neomycin in the ear drops.

Prevention/Prophylaxis: Parent and/or patient should be instructed to (1) keep objects such as hairpins and swabs out of the ear canal; (2) wear ear plugs when swimming to keep water out of the canal; and (3) instill alcohol drops in the ears before and after swimming.

Referral: None, except for recalcitrant cases.

Education: Teach children not to pick at their ears, especially with sharp objects. Teach that the ear is self-cleaning, and that poking the ear with swabs just pushes the wax farther down the canal. Teach children to use ear plugs before swimming.

Otitis Media

Acute otitis media is an inflammation of the middle ear characterized by pain, a bulging eardrum, or a perforated eardrum with drainage of purulent material. *Otitis media with effusion* is fluid in the middle ear without signs and symptoms of infection. Otitis media is considered chronic or persistent if there are six episodes by the age of 6 years, five episodes in 1 year, or three episodes in 6 months.

Etiology: Bacterial infections (*Streptococcus pneumoniae, H. influenzae, Moraxella catarrhalis* are the most common pathogens), viral infections (influenza A, RSV, coxsackievirus, adenovirus, and parainfluenza virus are the most common), immune reactivity, and allergic rhinitis.

Occurrence: Common.

Age: Any pediatric age group, but most common from 6–36 months and from 4–6 years; incidence decreases after 6 years of age. Chronic otitis media is more common in children whose first episode occurred before 1 year of age.

Ethnicity: Otitis media is more prevalent among Native Americans and Alaskan and Canadian Eskimos; it occurs in African-Americans less than in whites. Effusion is more likely to occur in white children under age 2.

Gender: Males are at greater risk than females.

Contributing Factors: Risk is increased in premature infants, children with Down's syndrome, and babies fed in the supine position. Children who attend day-care centers, have parents who smoke, and who have a family history of otitis media are also at greater risk.

Signs and Symptoms: The child with acute or recurrent otitis media presents with a complaint of "tugging at ears," ear pain, fever, irritability, and sleep disturbances. Not all children have ear pain; nausea, vomiting, diarrhea, and upper left quadrant abdominal pain may also be evident. In otitis media with effusion, the child is usually asymptomatic (Fig. 7–7).

Acute otitis media: Assess the color, transparency/opacity, vascularity, and mobility of the TM with both positive and negative pressures. Mobility of the TM will be diminished or absent. The TM may be red (note whether the child is crying; the degree of redness mirrors the degree of crying) and bulging, showing loss of landmarks. In 50% of cases, the TM will be yellow, indicating pus behind the drum. Retraction of the TM suggests eustachian tube dysfunction.

Otitis media with effusion: The ear drum, which may be retracted or convex, is opaque with mobility diminished. Landmarks are blurred. May see the air-fluid level or the presence of air bubbles with an amber or bluish fluid.

Diagnostic Tests: Use tympanometry to confirm the presence of fluid in the middle ear. Persistent middle ear dysfunction is prognostic for the increased

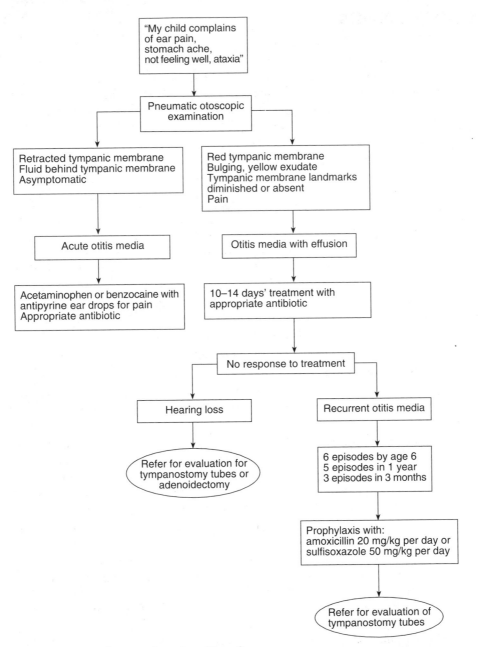

FIGURE 7–7 Evaluating and treating otitis media.

risk of recurrence. Children who have had otitis media with effusion for 3 months should undergo hearing tests.

Differential Diagnosis: *Toothache* (examine mouth and tap each tooth to elicit tenderness), *foreign body in the ear* (found on examination), *furuncle in the canal* (found on examination), and *temporomandibular joint dysfunction.*

Treatment

Antibiotics

- *Acute otitis media* (10–14 days of treatment): Amoxicillin (Amoxil), 20 mg/kg in three divided doses q 8 hours. Effective against *Streptococcus, Escherichia coli, Proteus mirabilis,* and *Bacteroides fragilis,* but no β-lactamase coverage.
- Amoxicillin/clavulanate potassium (Augmentin), 40 mg/kg per day based on amoxicillin component, in three divided doses, q 8 hours. Effective against *H. influenzae, M. catarrhalis, Streptococcus pneumoniae, Streptococcus pyogenes, Staphylococcus aureus, E. coli, P. mirabilis,* and *B. fragilis,* and gives β-lactamase coverage.
- Cefaclor (Ceclor), 40 mg/kg per day in three divided doses, q 8 hours. Effective against *M. catarrhalis, Streptococcus pneumoniae, Streptococcus pyogenes, E. coli, P. mirabilis,* and β-lactamase coverage, and gives partial coverage for *H. influenzae* and *Staphylococcus aureus.*
- Cefixime (Suprax), 8 mg/kg per day single dose for children under 50 kg and less than 12 years old. For children over 50 kg and over age 12, give adult dosage, 400 mg. Effective against *H. influenzae, M. catarrhalis, Streptococcus pneumoniae, Streptococcus pyogenes, E. coli,* and *P. mirabilis,* and gives β-lactamase coverage.
- Cefpodoxime proxetil (Vantin), 10 mg/kg per day in two divided doses. Effective against *H. influenzae, M. catarrhalis, Streptococcus pneumoniae, Streptococcus pyogenes,* and *P. mirabilis,* and gives β-lactamase coverage.
- Cefprozil (Cefzil), 15 mg/kg q 12 hours. Effective against *H. influenzae, M. catarrhalis, Streptococcus pneumoniae, Streptococcus pyogenes, P. mirabilis,* and *E. coli,* and gives β-lactamase coverage.
- Cefuroxime axetil (Ceftin), 30 mg/kg divided twice daily for children under age 13; 250–500 mg bid if over age 13. Effective against *H. influenzae, M. catarrhalis, Streptococcus pneumoniae, Streptococcus pyogenes, P. mirabilis, Staphylococcus aureus,* and *E. coli,* and gives β-lactamase coverage.
- Erythromycin ethylsuccinate and sulfisoxazole acetyl (Pediazole), 50 mg/kg per day in four divided doses based on the erythromycin component, every 6 hours. Effective against *H. influenzae, M. catarrhalis, Streptococcus pneumoniae, Streptococcus pyogenes,* and *Staphylococcus aureus,* and gives β-lactamase coverage.
- Loracarbef (Lorabid), 30 mg/kg per day in two divided doses q 12 hours. Effective against *H. influenzae, M. catarrhalis, Streptococcus pneumo-*

niae, Streptococcus pyogenes, Staphylococcus aureus, E. coli, and *P. mirabilis,* and gives β-lactamase coverage.

- Trimethoprim (TMP)/fulfamethoxozole (SMX) (Bactrim, Septra), 8 mg TMP/40 mg SMX daily in two divided doses. Effective against *H. influenzae, M. catarrhalis, Streptococcus pneumoniae,* most strains of *Streptococcus pyogenes, E. coli, Staphylococcus aureus,* and *P. mirabilis,* and gives β-lactamase coverage.

Analgesics

Acetaminophen may be given for discomfort. Relief for ear pain may be obtained through the use of ear drops containing antipyrine and benzocaine (Auralgan).

Recurrent otitis media (three episodes in 6 months or four episodes in 12 months): Consider antibiotic prophylaxis during high-risk seasons (winter and spring): amoxicillin (Amoxil), 20 mg/kg per day; or sulfisoxazole (Gantrisin), 50 mg/kg per day.

Otitis media with effusion: Consider a trial of antibiotics (discussed previously). Usually resolves spontaneously in 3–4 months. The Clinical Practice Guidelines do not recommend corticosteroids, antihistamines, or decongestants for the treatment of otitis media with effusion.

Follow-up: Have the child return in 48–72 hours if there is no improvement. Child should return to clinic in 10 days to evaluate therapeutic response. (*Note:* fluid may remain behind the eardrum for 3–4 months before fully absorbed.) Reevaluate children on prophylaxis at 2- to 3-month intervals for asymptomatic effusion.

Sequelae: Mastoiditis, labyrinthitis, petrositis, facial paralysis, and intracranial complications are all possible sequelae of otitis media and otitis media with effusion. Delayed language-skill development may be associated with recurrent or chronic otitis media.

Prevention/Prophylaxis: Parents should be taught to prevent otitis media by taking steps to avoid contributing factors: for example, feeding infant in an upright position, keeping child away from day care and sick playmates (or using small day-care facilities), and avoiding passive smoke. Mothers should breast-feed children during infancy. Prescribe prophylaxis as noted under therapy.

Referral: If HL occurs, prophylaxis fails to prevent recurrence, or child is allergic to penicillins or sulfa drugs, refer to an otolaryngologist for tympanostomy tube evaluation and insertion. Children who fail to respond to medical treatment for otitis media with effusion in 3–4 months should be referred to an otolaryngologist for evaluation for tympanostomy tube insertion, and evaluation of adenoids. Tonsillectomy is not recommended as a treatment option for otitis media with effusion.

Education: Instruct parents in ways to prevent ear infections: avoiding exposure of the child to passive smoke, not propping bottle, keeping child away from sick children, and watching child's swimming habits (child should not dive and should not submerge his or her head in water greater than 2 feet deep). Child may be more comfortable with chest and head elevated at bedtime. Parents should make sure the child takes all the medication, even if there seems to be improvement.

Pharyngitis/Tonsillitis

Pharyngitis is an inflammation of the pharynx; the term tonsillitis is used when the tonsils are involved.

Etiology: In children less than age 2, the agent is a virus (e.g., adenovirus, enteroviruses, Epstein-Barr virus, coxsackievirus A); over age 5, the agent is Group A streptococcus; and in adolescents, the agents are *Clostridium haemolyticum, Mycoplasma* (10% of adolescents), and gonococcus.

Occurrence: Common; peak incidence is in late fall, winter, and spring.

Age: All age groups.

Ethnicity: Not significant.

Gender: Occurs equally in males and females.

Signs and Symptoms: Infants usually present with a low-grade fever with serous or serous-mucoid rhinitis; toddlers with a low-grade fever, irritability, anorexia, and cervical adenitis; and adolescents with a low-grade fever and sore throat. (*Note:* In Group A β-hemolytic streptococcus, look for acute onset of sore throat, dysphagia, fever, malaise, vomiting, headache, abdominal pain, cough, and rhinorrhea.)

Findings in bacterial infections include erythematous pharynx, edematous uvula, enlarged tonsils with discrete yellow exudate, petechial stippling with moderate redness of the soft palate, and tender submandibular nodes. If the agent is a strain of streptococcus, there may be a red and finely punctate rash (sandpapery with Pastia's sign) starting on the trunk and spreading peripherally to cover the entire body, characteristic of scarlet fever.

Viral pharyngitis produces vesicular or ulcerative lesions, and rash. There are six types of viral presentations:

Infectious mononucleosis: Exudative tonsillitis, cervical adenopathy, fever, palpable spleen, presence of 20% atypical lymphocytes or positive mononucleosis test.

Herpangina: Herpangina ulcer found on anterior tonsillar pillars and sometimes on the palate and uvula.

Lymphonodular pharyngitis: Small, yellow-white nodules in the same distribution as in herpangina.

Hand, foot, and mouth disease: Ulcers on tongue and oral mucosa; vesicles on palms, soles, and interdigital areas.

Pharyngoconjunctival fever: Exudative tonsillitis, fever, and conjunctivitis.

Rubeola: Small white specks (Koplik spots) on examination of the buccal mucosa.

Diagnostic Tests

CBC with differential to assess infectious process.

Throat swab for rapid streptococcus test, culture, and sensitivity.

Mononucleosis spot test for possible infectious mononucleosis.

Throat culture for gonococcus if child abuse is suspected or sexual history indicates participation in orogenital sex.

Throat cultures for children on prophylactic penicillin (e.g., those with sickle cell anemia) because of negative throat swabs.

Differential Diagnosis

Retropharyngeal abscess: Asymmetrical swelling of tonsils, tonsillar fossae, and soft palate; uvula shifted to opposite side.

Peritonsillar abscess: Difficulty swallowing, hyperextension of the head, and possibly a forward bulge in the posterior pharyngeal wall.

Treatment

Nonpharmacological

Viral: Give supportive care; force fluids and gargles.

Bacterial: Force fluids.

Pharmacological

Analgesics for fever and discomfort, as well as the following antibiotics:

- Penicillin V (phenoxymethyl penicillin): Acid-resistant penicillin (Pen V K), supplied as tablets, oral suspension, and drops, 15–30 mg/kg per day, q 6–8 hours. If patient is allergic to penicillin, erythromycin (macrolide antimicrobial) 30–50 mg/kg per day, divided q 8 hours.
- *Second-generation cephalosporins:*
  - Cefaclor (Ceclor) 20–40 mg/kg per day, divided q 8 hours (*note:* may cross-react with penicillin).
  - Cefuroxime axetil (Ceftin, 125–250 mg bid for children under 13; 250–500 mg bid for children over age 13.
  or
  - *Amoxicillin plus clavulanate* (Augmentin; β-lactam antibiotic with a β-lactamase inhibitor): Amoxicillin, 20–40 mg/kg per day, plus clavulanate, 5–10 mg/kg per day, divided q 8 hours.
  Oral suspension: Amoxicillin 125 mg plus clavulanate 31.25 mg/5 mL; or amoxicillin 250 mg plus clavulanate 62.5 mg/5 mL.
  Tablets: Amoxicillin 250 mg/clavulanate 125 mg, or amoxicillin 500 mg/clavulanate 125 mg. (*note:* may cause diarrhea, urticaria)

Child can return to school after 24 hours on antibiotics.

Follow-up: Patient should return in 1 week for assessment of therapeutic response. If caused by streptococcus, repeat throat screen at that time.

Sequelae: Complications include otitis media and peritonsillar abscess; if causative agent is streptococcus, acute rheumatic fever and acute glomerulonephritis (1–4 weeks postinfection) may ensue.

Prevention/Prophylaxis: Prompt and complete treatment of infection. If streptococcus is the offending organism, screen and treat other symptomatic family members. Although there is a carrier stage, which is noncontagious and self-limiting, there is no specific test or treatment during this period.

Referral: Consult or refer for suspected peritonsillar abscess. Patients in whom infections continue to develop despite the use of prophylactic penicillin should be referred to an otolaryngologist for possible tonsillectomy.

Education: Stress the importance of increasing fluid intake and of prohibiting the sharing of drinking glasses and eating utensils.

Rhinitis

Rhinitis is an inflammation of the nasal mucosa characterized by congestion and increased nasal secretions. There are two groups of patients: those without associated nasal eosinophilia, who often experience increased symptoms related to changes in temperature and environmental pollutants; and those with associated nasal eosinophilia, who have no history of atopy and have negative skin tests. The latter is less common in children. Symptoms of allergic rhinitis are more severe in the morning.

Etiology: Alterations in nasal mucosa related to immune-mediated conditions, infection, overuse of topical decongestants, irritants, nasal polyps, and ciliary defects have all been suggested as probable causes.

Occurrence: Occurs in 10% of children.

Age: After ages 4–5.

Ethnicity: Not significant.

Gender: Occurs equally in males and females.

Contributing Factors: Pollens, dust, and molds contribute to the allergic response, as well as smoke and chemical irritants.

Signs and Symptoms: Child is brought to clinic with the complaint of a "runny" nose. History should include onset, severity, type of nasal secretion, and the identification, if possible, of precipitating factors. Past and current medical history, including medications, should be obtained. Note the pattern of onset, season of the year, and time of day. Ask about family history of allergies and other allergic manifestations. Past history may include a history of recurrent epistaxis.

Inspection reveals a boggy, edematous nasal mucosa with a large amount of clear drainage. Pale mucous membranes with swollen turbinates are observed obstructing the nasal passage. Eyes may be watery, and the sclera and conjunctiva may be red. Purulent secretions indicate secondary infection. There are usually dark shadows under the eyes ("allergic shiners") and a transverse crease over the bridge of the nose (from the "allergic salute"). Other findings you might find on physical examination include a high, arched palate; a geographic tongue; and mouth breathing.

Diagnostic Tests: Nasal smears demonstrate eosinophils. Allergy testing or radioallergosorbent testing (RAST) shows the specific allergen.

Differential Diagnosis

Purulent rhinorrhea suggests sinusitis; can be confirmed by changes on radiographic films.
Congenital abnormalities are usually observed during the neonatal period.
Foreign bodies are usually unilateral, with a bloody, purulent discharge.
Nasal polyps are uncommon in childhood.
Nonallergic rhinitis with eosinophilic syndrome has a negative family history of atopy, negative skin tests, and adult onset.
Vasomotor rhinitis is similar to nonallergic rhinitis, having autonomic nervous system imbalance as a suggested cause.

Treatment

Nonpharmacological
Environmental control should be exercised, thereby avoiding or limiting contact with irritants.

Pharmacological
- *Antihistamines:* Use of sustained-release antihistamines is not recommended for children under age 7. Use the smallest dose that relieves symptoms. If the first drug used is not effective, switch drug classes.
  - *Alkylamines:* (1) Chlorpheniramine maleate (Chlor-Trimeton), 0.35 mg/kg per day in four divided doses; (2) brompheniramine maleate (Dimetane), 0.5 mg/kg per day in three to four divided doses for children under age 6; for children over age 6, 4 mg q 4–6 hours.
  - *Ethanolamines:* (1) Carbinoxamine maleate (Clistin), 4–8 mg q 6–8 hours; (2) clemastine fumarate (Tavist-1 Tablets), 1.34–2.68 mg (one to two tablets) q 12 hours; (3) diphenhydramine hydrochloride (Benadryl), 4–6 mg/kg per day q 6–8 hours; (4) loratadine (Claritin), 10 mg/10 mL (over age 6; 2/3 tsp per day; 10-mg chewable tablet daily for children over age 12); (5) Cetirizine (Zyrtec), 10 mg once daily for children over age 12.
  - *Other:* Terfenadine (Seldane), 60 mg q 12 hours
  - *Nasal sprays:* (1) cromolyn nasal sprays, in a metered nasal spray, one to two sprays twice daily; (2) topical nasal steroids, for use in resistant cases of allergic rhinitis or rhinitis medicamentosa (prescribe for 1–3

weeks); (3) beclomethasone (Vancenase, Beconase), one to two sprays bid; (4) flunisolide (Nasalide); mometasone (Nasonex), two sprays qid for children 12 years and over.

- *Decongestants:* Administer when antihistamine therapy is inadequate.
  - Pseudoephedrine hydrochloride, 4 mg/kg per day in four divided doses

Follow-up: Patient should return in 1 week for assessment of therapeutic response.

Sequelae: Overuse of nasal decongestants can cause rhinitis medicamentosa, characterized by dry, sore nasal mucosa.

Prevention/Prophylaxis: To identify precipitating factors, have the family perform an environmental survey of heating system, presence of pets, carpeting, exposures to noxious substances, etc. Have the family avoid or limit the child's exposure to these factors.

Referral: Refer to primary care physician or an allergist for allergy testing.

Education: Instruct the family in methods of reducing allergens in the home: changing pillows, covering mattress and pillows with plastic, eliminating rugs in the bedroom, daily damp mopping of floors, and avoiding contact with pets and other precipitating factors. Instruct patient in the proper method of using nasal sprays.

Sinusitis

Sinusitis is an acute inflammation of the paranasal sinuses, most commonly the ethmoid and maxillary sinus.

Etiology: The infective agents most commonly identified include *Streptococcus pneumoniae, H. influenzae, Moraxella catarrhalis,* and β-hemolytic streptococcus; viruses have been isolated in 10% of cases.

Occurrence: Common.

Age: Occurs in the ethmoid sinus after age 6 months, the maxillary sinus after age 1, and the frontal sinuses after age 10.

Ethnicity: Not significant.

Gender: Occurs equally in males and females.

Contributing Factors: Edematous obstruction of the nasal ostia, decreased ciliary action in the paranasal sinuses, and increased mucus production promote the development of retention of secretions leading to sinusitis.

Local factors that contribute are allergic rhinitis, upper respiratory infection, overuse of topical decongestants, nasal polyps, tumors, foreign bodies, swimming and diving, dental extractions, and cigarette smoke.

Signs and Symptoms: The parent and child present with a complaint such as, "The cold won't go away, and the nasal drainage is green." The detailed history of the present illness should include time of onset, duration of symptoms, and change in symptomatology. Usually the pediatric NP will find that the present illness has existed for 7–10 days as a "cold," with nasal discharge, postnasal drip, and a daytime cough. Often there has been a low-grade fever. Older children may complain of a headache or a sense of fullness in the head.

Findings may include halitosis (if a morning visit), painless periorbital swelling, and tenderness when the facial areas are palpated or percussed (older children). Location of the pain indicates specific sinus: ethmoid, retroorbital, maxillary, upper malar or zygomatic, frontal, or over the eyebrows. In children over age 10, transillumination of the maxillary and frontal sinuses will reveal clouding. Examination of the nares reveals injected mucosa with purulent drainage. Test nasal patency by compressing one side of the nostril and having the child blow through the nose. Examination of the throat reveals an exudate in the area of the tonsillar pillars. An examination of the chest may reveal wheezing in children with reactive airway disease.

Diagnostic Tests: Radiographic studies are not done routinely, but are indicated if there is facial swelling with an unknown cause, acute sinusitis not responsive within 48 hours, or chronic or recurrent sinusitis of at least 3 months' duration. A Waters view (occipitomental) for the maxillary sinus is usually sufficient. Other views are the Caldwell view (anteroposterior) for the frontal and ethmoid maxillary, and the submental-vertex and lateral views for the sphenoidal. Positive findings in children over age 1 will show opacities of the involved sinus, air/fluid levels, or a mucosal thickening of greater than 5 mm. Such findings may also be present in children with colds or nasal allergies. Limited CT is a diagnostic alternative.

If there are complications or the patient is immunocompromised, consider a sinus aspiration for diagnostic purposes.

In chronic sinusitis, evaluate for allergies, immune defects, and cystic fibrosis.

Differential Diagnosis

Viral upper respiratory infection resolves spontaneously.

Group A streptococcal infection is differentiated by a positive streptococcus test.

Cystic fibrosis may be ruled out by a negative sweat test.

Foreign body in the nose may be ruled out by tests of nasal patency, as well as radiographic studies. Dental infections may be ruled out by an inspection of the mouth and by tapping each tooth to evaluate tenderness.

Treatment

Nonpharmacological

Parents may restore moisture to the air by running a vaporizer; they may also place warm washcloths on the child's face.

Pharmacological

- *Analgesics* for pain.
- *Salt water nose drops* (1/4 tsp salt to 6 ounces boiled water).
- *Antibiotics* (*note:* amoxicillin is the drug of choice):
  - Amoxicillin (Amoxil), 40 mg/kg per day in three divided doses for 10 days

  or

  - Amoxicillin and potassium clavulanate (Augmentin), 40 mg/kg per day in three divided doses for 10 days

  or

  - Cefaclor (Ceclor), 20–40 mg/kg per day in three divided doses for 10 days

  or

  - Cefixime (Suprax), 8 mg/kg per day for 10 days
  (not to exceed 1g/day) *or*
  - TMP-SMX (Septra), 8 mg/kg TMP, 40 mg/kg SMX daily in two divided doses for 10 days

  or

  - Cefpodoxime proretil (Vantin) 10 mg/kg per day in two divided doses

  or

  - Cefprozil (Cefzil) 15 mg/kg q 12 hours for 10 days
- The efficacy of *decongestants* has not been established.
- Do not use *antihistamines* unless the child has allergies because they slow the movement of secretions.

Follow-up: Patient should return to clinic in 48 hours if there is no improvement with therapy; otherwise, in 2 weeks for evaluation of therapeutic response.

Sequelae: Chronic or recurrent sinusitis may develop in some patients. The most frequent cause is allergic rhinitis, but this sequela may also be caused by structural defects, such as a deviated septum, a nasal polyp, or a foreign body, or by diving into water feet first. Orbital cellulitis may occur if infection spreads into the orbit through the sinus wall.

Prevention/Prophylaxis: Prevention of spread of upper respiratory infection by proper handwashing. The use of steam or saline reduces secretions and improves mucociliary clearance, thus producing a mild decongestant effect. Patient should avoid swimming and diving during the treatment period, avoid exposure to smoke-filled rooms, and stop smoking.

Referral: Patients with chronic or recurrent sinusitis not caused by diving or allergies should be referred to an otolaryngologist. Refer patient to a primary physician or otolaryngologist if development of an orbital cellulitis is suspected.

Education: Instruct the parents to run a vaporizer to add moisture to the air. Application of a warm, wet washcloth over the face may relieve some of the discomfort. Child is not to swim or dive during the duration of treatment. If the child smokes, emphasize the importance of smoking cessation.

REFERENCES

General

Berhman, R, and Kleigman, R: Nelson's Essentials of Pediatrics. WB Saunders, Philadelphia, 1990.
Berman, S: Pediatric Decision Making. BC Decker, Philadelphia, 1991.
Doenges, M, and Moorhouse, M: Nurse's Pocket Guide: Nursing Diagnoses with Interventions, ed 5. FA Davis, Philadelphia, 1995.
Green, M: Pediatric Diagnosis: Interpretation of Symptoms & Signs in Infants, Children, and Adolescents. WB Saunders, Philadelphia, 1992.
Hay, W, et al: Current Pediatric Diagnosis & Treatment, ed 12. Appleton & Lange, Norwalk, Conn, 1995.
Hoekelman, RA: Primary Pediatric Care, ed 2. Mosby–Year Book, St. Louis, 1992.
Jarvis, C: Physical Examination and Health Assessment. WB Saunders, Philadelphia, 1992.

Assessment

US Public Health Service: Vision screening in children. Am Fam Phys 50:587, 1994.

Concussion

Bronstein, R: On-field management of football injuries. J Musculoskel Med 12:14, 1995.
Colorado Medical Society Sports Medicine Committee: Guidelines for the Management of Concussion in Sports (Revised). Colorado Medical Society, Denver, 1991.
Genuardi, F, and King, W: Inappropriate discharge instructions for youth athletes hospitalized for concussion. Pediatrics 95:216, 1995.
Fick, D: Management of concussion in collision sports: Guidelines for the sidelines. Postgrad Med 97:53, 1995.

Head Trauma

Goldstein, B, and Powers, K: Head trauma in children. Pediatr Rev 15:213, 1994.
Hahn, M: Pediatric head trauma. Adv Nurse Pract 3(9):35, 1995.
Inaba, A, and Seward, P: An approach to pediatric trauma. Emerg Med Clin North Am 9:523, 1991.
Johnson, M, and Gerring, J: Head trauma and its sequelae. Pediatr Ann 21:362, 1992.
Sampson, J, et al: Initial management of pediatric trauma. Am Fam Phys 45:2621, 1992.
Techlenburg, F, and Wright, M: Minor head trauma in the pediatric patient. Pediatr Emerg Care 7:40, 1991.

Cervical Lymphadenitis

Park, Y: Evaluation of neck masses in children. Am Fam Phys 51:1904, 1995.

Aphthous Stomatitis

Peterson, M, and Baughman, R: Recurrent aphthous stomatitis: Primary care management. Nurse Pract 21(5):36, 1996.

Conjunctivitis

Ruppert, S: Differential diagnosis of pediatric conjunctivitis (red eye). Nurse Pract 21(7):12, 1996.

The Common Cold

Gerchufsky, M: Respiratory synctial virus. Adv Nurse Pract 1(13):29, 1996.
Urhach, A: What's behind that chronic cough? Contemp Pediatr 9:106, 1993.

Croup

Cressman, W, and Meyer, C: Diagnosis and management of croup and epiglottiditis. Pediatr Clin North Am 41:265, 1994.

Epiglottitis

Cressman, W, and Meyer, C: Diagnosis and management of croup and epiglottiditis. Pediatr Clin North Am 41:265, 1994.

Epistaxis

Goldman, JL, et al: Embolization as the definitive treatment of epistaxis in the pediatric patient. Ear Nose Throat J 74:490, 1995.

Murray, AB, and Milner, RA: Allergic rhinitis and recurrent epistaxis in children. Ann Allergy Asthma Immunol 74:30, 1995.

Hearing Loss

Buttross, S, et al: Early identification and management of hearing impairment. Am Fam Phys 51:1437, 1995.

Rukenstein, M: Hearing loss: A plan for individualized management. Postgrad Med 98:197, 1995.

Otitis Externa

Polk, S: Making sense of swimmer's ear: Treatment of otitis externa. Adv Nurse Pract 2(7):25, 1994.

Otitis Media

American Academy of Pediatrics Otitis Media Guideline Panel: Managing otitis media with effusion in young children. Pediatrics 94:766, 1994.

Claessen, JQ, et al: Persistence of middle ear dysfunction after recurrent otitis media. Clin Otolaryngol 19:35, 1994.

Eden, A, et al: The rise of acute otitis media. Patient Care 29:22, 1995.

Eden, A, et al: Otitis media with effusion: Sorting out the options. Patient Care 29:52, 1995.

Giebink, GS: Preventing otitis media. Ann Otolaryngol Rhinol Laryngol (suppl) 163(17):20, 1994.

Hanson, M: Acute otitis media in children. Nurse Pract 21(5):72, 1996.

Mandel, EM, et al: Efficacy of 20- versus 10-day antimicrobial treatment for acute otitis media. Pediatrics 96:5, 1995.

Stevenson, L, and Brooke, D: Managing otitis media with effusion in young children. J Pediatr Health Care 9:36, 1995.

Pharyngitis/Tonsillitis

Ajulo, SO: The significance of recurrent tonsillitis in sickle cell disease. Clin Otolaryngol 19:230, 1994.

Aujard, Y, et al: Comparative efficacy and safety of four-day cefuroxime axetil and ten-day penicillin treatment of group A beta-hemolytic streptococcus pharyngitis in children. Pediatr Infect Dis J 14:295, 1995.

Guggenbichler, JP: Cefetamet pivoxil in the treatment of pharyngitis/tonsillitis in children and adults. Drugs (suppl 3): 47:27, 1994.

Rhinitis

Jobst, S, et al: Assessment of the efficacy and safety of three dose levels of cetirizine given once daily in children with perennial allergic rhinitis. Allergy 49:598, 1994.

Smolensky, MH, et al: Twenty-four hour pattern in symptom intensity of viral and allergic rhinitis: Treatment implications. J Allergy Clin Immunol 95:1084, 1995.

Murray, AB, and Milner, RA: Allergic rhinitis and recurrent epistaxis in children. Ann Allerg Asthma Immunol 74:30, 1995.

Sinusitis

Corren, J: Making the clinical diagnosis of sinusitis: Clinical focus, symposium: Sinusitis in Primary Care. Patient Care 27:11, 1993.

Middletown, D: Acute sinusitis: When a child's cold persists. Fam Pract Recert 15(12):33, 1993.

Slavin, R: The pathophysiology of sinusitis: Clinical focus, symposium: Sinusitis in Primary Care. Patient Care 27:3, 1995.

Stafford, C: Successful medical management of sinusitis: Clinical focus, symposium: Sinusitis in Primary Care. Patient Care 27:18, 1993.

Stevenson, L, and Brooke, D: Clinical acute sinusitis. J Pediatr Health Care 9:136, 1995.

CHAPTER 8

CHEST ASSESSMENT

When the nurse practitioner (NP) assesses the chest, the cardiac and respiratory systems are of particular importance. To assess these systems properly, the NP needs to develop an organized method for evaluating the chest, know appropriate baseline functioning parameters (Table 8–1), and be able readily to recognize deviations from the norm. These skills will enable the NP to diagnose and treat problems when they are found (Fig. 8–1).

Chest assessment requires an examination of the lungs and heart, as well as observation of vital clues related to respiratory and cardiac efficiency. These clues may be found during other parts of the examination aside from that of the chest. Cardiac and respiratory problems may involve the skin (altered coloration, temperature, and turgor), finger tips (clubbing), overall height-weight ratio (too

TABLE 8–1 RANGE OF NORMAL VITAL SIGNS

Age	Pulse (beats/min)	Respirations (breaths/min)	Systolic Blood Pressure (mm Hg)
Newborn	125	64–70	
1 yr	120	35–40	
2 yr	110	31–35	96
4 yr	100	26–31	96
6 yr	100	23–36	96–98
8 yr	90	21–23	104
10 yr	90	21	110
12 yr	85–90	21	115
14 yr	80–85	21–22	118–120
16 yr	75–80	20	120–124

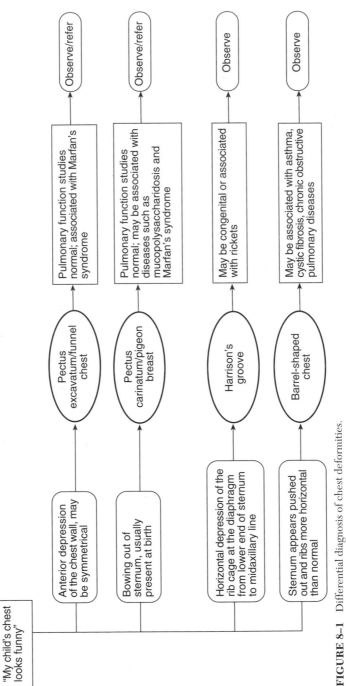

FIGURE 8–1 Differential diagnosis of chest deformities.

small for age), nutrition (problems associated with eating), and development (delayed or missed milestones).

Because respiratory problems are the leading cause of illness in children and one of the main reasons children present for health-care visits, this area should be well understood by the NP. Cardiac defects, both congenital and acquired, are also a major problem for children because the functions of the respiratory and cardiac systems are intimately associated—one system often depends on the other for proper functioning and the well-being of the child.

When examining the heart and lungs, the NP needs to modify the examination for the infant, child, and adolescent. Because of differences in physical size and developmental levels, each age group requires a unique and careful approach to produce accurate assessments.

Physical examination of a child's chest should always begin with a thorough family history of the respiratory or cardiac problems, prenatal and perinatal course, exposure to teratogens, medications taken either during the pregnancy or presently being taken by the child and the reasons for these, problems with eating, weight gain or loss, exercise pattern and tolerance, review of current concerns and symptoms, environment, and a review of systems. The nurse practitioner then needs to rely on observation skills. For both cardiac and respiratory problems, history and observation often provide the most vital clues needed for an accurate diagnosis.

Cardiac Assessment

In children, the major problems with cardiovascular function are due to congenital heart disease. Approximately 13 in 1000 live births result in a child with congenital heart disease. Approximately 90% of congenital heart disease cases result from a genetic predisposition that interacts with environmental triggers, such as drugs, a variety of viruses and bacterial infections, and chromosomal abnormalities. Acquired heart disease occurs much less frequently in this population and results from infection, environmental factors, autoimmune problems, and familial tendencies.

Congenital heart disease can be divided into three groups:

Obstructive lesions: Cause pressure overloads because of either an obstructive or a stenotic lesion. The most common of these anomalies are aortic stenosis (AS), coarctation of the aorta (COA), and pulmonary stenosis (PS).

Left-to-right shunt: Results in volume overload. Ventricular septal defect (VSD), atrial septal defect (ASD), and patent ductus arteriosus (PDA) are the most common anomalies in this group.

Cyanotic lesion: Produce central cyanosis. Anomalies include tetralogy of Fallot (TOF), transposition of the great arteries (TGA), and tricuspid atresia (TA).

These nine anomalies represent approximately 90% of all cardiac problems found in children.

Other problems that have cardiac origin or impact on the cardiac system should also be considered when assessing children. While not common, Kawasaki syndrome may have profound effects on the cardiac system, resulting in an aneurysm. Rheumatic fever can also affect the heart and cause irreparable damage. Syncope, alterations in blood pressure, and apnea of infancy also are intimately related to cardiac function. A thorough history can often differentiate these more acute problems from a congenital anomaly, which is chronic.

Therefore, the diagnosis of either a congenital or acquired heart disease, a cardiovascular disease, or other problems associated with the cardiovascular system is based on a thorough, comprehensive history, a physical examination, and diagnostic tests. While taking the history, question the parent about exposure to teratogens, medication use, or excessive weight gain during the pregnancy. The mother's age, if greater than 40 during the pregnancy, may also be a factor in the incidence of cardiac problems. The detection of genetic disorders, infections, and fetal distress during the prenatal or perinatal period should also be discussed thoroughly. Familial risk factors such as myocardial infarction, hypercholesterolemia, hypertension, obesity, siblings with congenital heart disease, genetic syndromes, or xanthomas should be questioned. Questions specifically related to the child also need to be asked, such as these:

Has your child ever had a change in skin color during feeding or crying?
Does your child tire easily during physical activities, and does your child seem to need more naps or rest times than other children?
Has anyone ever told you that your child has a heart murmur?
Does your child seem to assume a squatting position frequently?
Has your child ever had a "blue spell" during exercise?
How frequently does your child acquire respiratory infections, and how severe are the episodes?
How would you describe your child's exercise and diet?
Does your child ever complain of being dizzy or lightheaded, or has your child ever fainted?
What is it about your child's condition today that makes you think there may be something wrong with his or her heart?

Although there are other questions the NP may ask, these can provide vital clues to a cardiac problem.

Examination of the infant can be done while the infant is in the arms of the mother, and it should be done when the child is not crying so that sounds can be heard accurately. A thorough assessment of vital signs is essential. Pulse rate, if increased beyond normal, may indicate anxiety, fever, severe anemia, hyperthyroidism, or excitement. The rhythm of the pulse, if irregular, needs to be further evaluated. A bounding pulse may indicate PDA; a weak or absent pulse may represent an obstructive lesion, such as COA. If the child is afebrile, respiratory rates in excess of 40 breaths/min indicate tachypnea, which needs further investigation. This symptom is particularly indicative of a problem if the child is asleep. Blood pressure assessment should begin between ages 2 and 3 and should be done at each examination.

> In children between ages 2 and 10, the systolic pressure can be calculated by the use of the following equation:
>
> $$90 + (2 \times \text{age in years})$$

Pulse pressure differences (i.e., differences between systolic and diastolic pressure) are generally between 20 and 50 mm Hg throughout childhood. Differences of less than 20 mm Hg or more than 50 mm Hg may indicate excitement, fever, hypertension, or previous exercise (high) or aortic regurgitation, PDA, or other cardiac pathology (low).

The next step in a cardiac assessment is the physical examination. Because young children are not always cooperative during a cardiovascular examination, the NP needs to have a flexible approach. Observe physical development, the color of the skin, nail beds, and muscle tone before undressing the child. Mottling, excessive perspiration, or the presence of xanthomas can be signs of a cardiac problem. Next, palpate the brachial pulses and assess for rate, rhythm, and volume. An abnormally full pulse can indicate the possibility of PDA or aortic insufficiency, whereas a slow or shallow pulse may indicate an outflow obstruction (Fig. 8–2).

Undress the child, place the child in the recumbent position, and observe the chest for any abnormalities. A child who has exhibited respiratory distress secondary to heart failure should have an obvious left-sided chest prominence, increased respiratory rate, and subcostal retractions. Using the right hand, palpate the thorax, placing two fingers just left of the xiphoid process. The hand should be resting on the right ventricle. A faint impulse, will be felt but anything more forceful indicates an enlarged heart. Apical pulses should be palpated for any abnormalities. To determine whether there is a prominent pulmonary artery, palpate the second intercostal space at the left sternal border. A prominence in this artery might indicate an arterial or ventricular septal defect. Using the index finger, palpate the suprasternal notch, assessing for a thrill or abnormal pulsation. Working in the opposite direction, the NP can further determine whether there are any palpable thrills or sounds. Next, the NP should palpate the liver, which is normally not more than 1 cm below the costal margin. If hepatomegaly is present, the NP should suspect potential heart failure.

Auscultate with both the diaphragm and the bell of the stethoscope. Innocent murmurs are rarely heard in newborns and therefore should be thoroughly evaluated. Approximately 30% of children beyond the neonatal period are found to have an innocent murmur. Innocent murmurs are those that occur in the absence of significant heart disease or structural abnormality of the heart. They may be classified as follows:

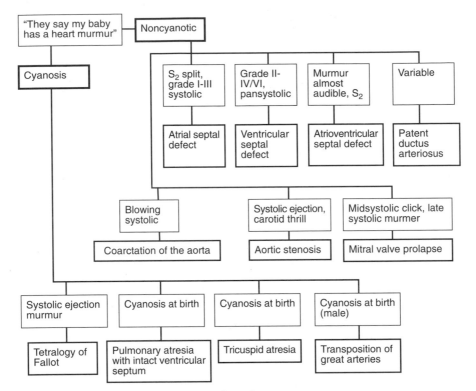

FIGURE 8–2   Noncyanotic versus cyanotic heart disease.

Still's murmur: A low-pitched, soft murmur occurring in the early to mid phase of systolic timing and best heard at the apex and left sternal border of the heart when the child is in a supine position.

Basal ejection murmur: A higher pitched, blowing sound best heard in the pulmonic area in the supine position.

Pulmonary outflow murmur: A short systolic murmur that is heard at the axillary region or back and disappears during infancy as the pulmonary arteries enlarge.

Venous hum: A continuous murmur, described as a humming sound. It is best heard in the infra and supraclavicular areas when the child is lying down, head turned to one side, or when the jugular vessels are occluded. The intensity of this murmur can range from grade III to grade VII (Table 8–2).

Loud, coarse systolic murmurs noted before the infant is discharged from the hospital usually suggest an obstructive heart problem. A high-pitched murmur, heard only in the left axillary area or back, suggests constriction of the aorta and *prompt* referral to a pediatric cardiologist should be made.

TABLE 8–2   GRADATION OF HEART MURMURS

Grade 1: Barely audible in quiet room by experienced examiner
Grade 2: Soft, but easily audible; limited radiation
Grade 3: Moderately loud; moderate to wide radiation
Grade 4: Loud; associated with palpable thrill
Grade 5: Audible with stethoscope chest piece in incomplete contact with skin
Grade 6: Audible with chest piece 1 cm away from skin

Palpation of brachial and femoral pulses is also a part of the complete cardiac examination. Absent or diminished femoral pulses, cool lower extremities, and decreased blood pressure in the lower extremities are all suggestive of COA. Blood pressure measurements should be done on upper and lower extremities, and significant deviance from the norm (see Table 8–1) should be followed up with an echocardiogram.

Finally, when examining the infant, the NP should make the infant cry to assess the skin and mucosal tissue for color changes. Circumoral cyanosis and purple discoloration of the inside of the infant's mouth suggest a serious problem resulting in central cyanosis, and prompt referral to a pediatric cardiologist should be made.

Heart sounds can provide the NP with other important clues related to a variety of heart problems. Although the first, second, and third heart sounds (S_1, S_2, and S_3) are normal for children, the fourth heart sound (S_4) is pathologic and requires immediate referral.

Examination of the older child also includes a careful observation of the chest, respiratory effort, skin turgor and color, physical development, assessment of pulses, and nail-root skin angle (looking for clubbing). Pulses will vary with size, age, and activity of the child. Persistent bradycardia, a pulse rate less than 60 beats/min, generally indicates an atrioventricular (AV) block; therefore, the child should have an electrocardiogram (ECG) and be referred to a cardiologist. In a child of this age, an organic problem should be suspected if there is a thrill and a grade IV–VI heart murmur.

When examining teen-agers, include them in the history taking as much as possible. Organic symptoms in a previously undetected cardiac disease are uncommon, but all complaints should merit careful evaluation. Chest pain is a fairly common complaint, often diagnostic of costochondritis, in teen-agers. Although chest pain rarely represents a cardiac problem, these complaints require careful evaluation. The evaluation should include a thorough physical examination, an ECG, appropriate laboratory studies to include a complete blood count, a lipid profile, arterial blood gas (ABG) studies, and a chest x-ray. Generally, in the teen-age population, the symptom of most concern is syncope, which may represent AS, a complete AV block, prolonged QT interval syndrome, hypertrophic myopathies, sick sinus syndrome, or pulmonary hypertension. Suspicion of these problems should be adequately evaluated and the patient referred to a cardiologist.

Cardiac assessment is a compilation of all the skills the NP brings to his or her practice:

Listening to obtain the most complete history.

Observing to provide a thorough picture of the child's overall appearance.

Palpating pulses to identify lifts, heaves or thrills, and organomegaly.

Auscultating for the heart rate and rhythm, components of the cardiac cycle, heart sounds and murmurs, bruits, or other adventitious sounds.

Developing an intuitive sense and being aware of one's own scope of practice when assessing the cardiac system.

Assessment of the respiratory system is another challenge for the NP; the next section describes this assessment. Note the interconnectedness of the cardiac and respiratory systems: They are, in effect, evaluated simultaneously during a chest assessment.

Respiratory System

Respiratory problems, which routinely occur in children, are by far the most common reason parents seek medical care for their child. Often, parents have used a number of over-the-counter medications before coming to the health-care setting. The types of medications or treatments used, and the results obtained, are vital pieces of information for the NP to elicit when taking the history. Although upper respiratory illnesses are less serious than lower respiratory problems, adequate assessment of both is essential. Assessment of the respiratory system begins with seeking information related to the history of the specific respiratory concerns, conducting a review of systems, and performing a systematic and meticulous physical examination of both the upper and lower respiratory system as well as the sinuses (see Chapter 7). When indicated, the assessment may include ordering appropriate laboratory examinations, such as a chest x-ray, blood tests (e.g., complete blood count [CBC], ABGs [Table 8–3]), blood cultures, and pulmonary function tests.

Examination of the upper respiratory system should include the nostrils, nasopharynx, throat, upper portion of the trachea, eustachian tubes, ears, and sinuses. The maxillary and ethmoidal sinuses develop and become clinically important as early as infancy, the sphenoidal sinuses about the third or fourth year of life, and the frontal sinuses between ages 6 and 10. When examining the lower respiratory system, the lungs are the primary area of examination.

Keep in mind that virtually all lower respiratory illnesses result from some form of airway obstruction: a foreign body, thickened mucosa or edema, spasms of the smooth muscles, or extrinsic compression. The younger the child, the more potentially hazardous the obstruction becomes; that is, because they are

TABLE 8–3 NORMAL ARTERIAL
BLOOD GAS VALUES

PaO_2	90–100 mm Hg
$PaCO_2$	38–42 mm Hg
Capillary PaO_2	Approximately half the arterial
Capillary $PaCO_2$	Same as arterial

physiologically smaller, the obstruction becomes life-threatening more quickly. In a child with a barking cough, the NP should realize that this type of cough is a function of the inspiratory effort being used to remove the upper airway obstruction and may be a sign of croup (Fig. 8–3). When expiratory efforts are hampered in some way, wheezing often results (Fig. 8–4). This is particularly true in asthma. When chronic overinflation of the lungs occurs, the NP will note that the chest circumference (anteroposterior diameter) increases, resulting in a barrel-chest appearance, which can help the NP properly diagnose a lower respiratory problem. When percussing the overinflated chest, the NP will note hyperresonance as opposed to a dull sound, which will be heard in cases where a mass has somehow increased the chest diameter.

Be sure to note the chest wall shape, not only for size discrepancies but for deformities (see Fig. 8–1). Pectus excavatum and pectus carnatum are usually cosmetic problems and rarely represent underlying pathologies. The color of the skin should also be examined. A cyanotic appearance may indicate poor oxygenation due to either a respiratory or a cardiac problem. The NP should note whether there is equal movement on both sides of the chest. Young children (under 6) usually use abdominal muscles more than adults. If this movement is minimal or absent, a respiratory problem should be suspected. The spine must be examined as well. Marked abnormalities such as scoliosis may impede the pulmonary function of the child by changing the shape and size of the thoracic cage. Scoliosis may become evident in the preteen years and progress rapidly, so careful examination of the spine is important.

The history of the illness should be obtained from the child (or parent) and should include the following questions:

What are the symptoms that brought you here today?

Have the breathing problems (e.g., cough, runny nose) gotten worse over the last few days or hours?

Do any family members or persons in school or day care (including babysitters' homes) have the same symptoms?

Have there been problems like this in the past?

What types of treatments have been used, and how effective have they been?

Are there any congenital problems that may be contributing to this problem?

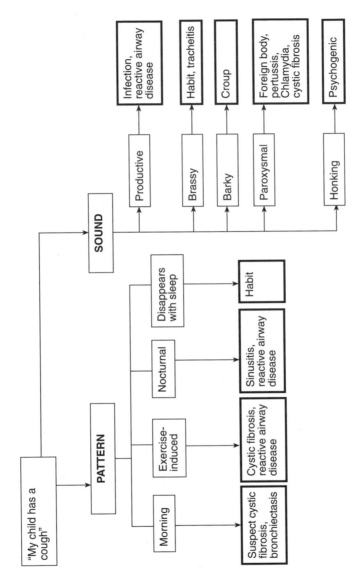

FIGURE 8–3   Differentiation of cough.

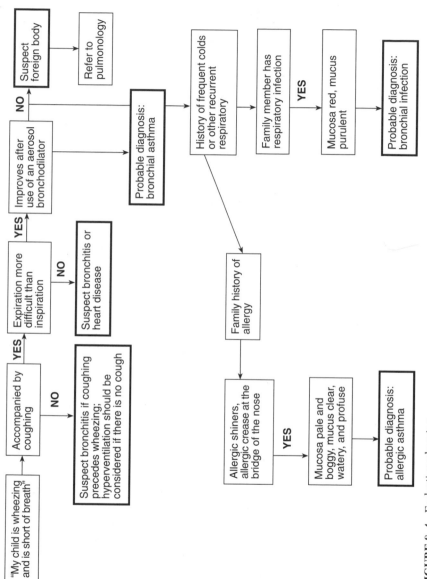

FIGURE 8–4 Evaluating wheezing.

Is there anything in the environment that may have triggered this problem?

These questions are a good starting point for the NP to gather the patient's history. The history should always include in-depth information on the family and child.

The NP then needs to perform a physical examination that begins with obtaining vital signs and observing the client. Examination is best accomplished with the younger child sitting in the parent's lap; the older child should sit on the examination table. Be sure to ensure privacy during the examination.

Tachypnea, retractions, and nasal flaring are key indicators of a serious respiratory problem, usually with the lower respiratory tract. Tests for rhinorrhea in the nose; the color, consistency, and odor of the mucus; the turbinates; and the child's ability to breathe through each nostril should be performed and findings noted. In young children, a malodorous discharge may suggest the presence of a foreign body in the nose. Care should be taken during examination of the child, and if necessary, removal of the object. If bleeding is reported to the NP, make note that the main reason children have nosebleeds is that they pick their noses, which may cause an abrasion inside one or both of the nostrils. Epistaxis in children under 2 that lasts longer than 20 minutes is an ominous sign, possibly indicating a bleeding disorder or a tumor. The throat, pharynx, and tonsils should then be examined. With the use of a light and tongue blade, carefully assess these areas. For the younger child, the parent may report a reluctance to eat or drink or that they suspect that the child's throat hurts. For the older child, be sure to ask if and when their throat hurts. Also ask what makes it feel better or worse. Commit the following to memory when examining the mouth: *If epiglottiditis is suspected, do not examine the mouth, and certainly do not use a tongue blade, because this may make the child unable to breathe.*

When auscultating the chest, rhonchi or referred nasal or breath sounds are commonly heard with upper respiratory problems such as pharyngitis, sinusitis, rhinitis, and tonsillitis, whereas crackles or rales are more commonly auscultated with a lower respiratory tract infection such as asthma, bronchitis, croup, tuberculosis, chest wall trauma, and respiratory syncytial virus (RSV). When determining the degree of the child's distress, several factors should be quickly evaluated, including anxiety level, respiratory rate and rhythm, the use of accessory muscles, color of skin and mucosa, breath sounds, and pulse oximetry. Remember the following rule of thumb when using oxygen saturation telemetry: If the child's reading remains greater than 92% O_2 saturation level, he or she is not necessarily in danger, but anything below that level compromises the child's oxygen level, thus requiring supplemental oxygen.

Efficient and thorough assessment of the respiratory system is essential in children, especially when they are under 2. Using a systematic approach and obtaining as much information during the history as possible before the examination are essential components of a complete respiratory examination.

Chest Wall Trauma

Chest wall trauma, which results in a variety of chest injuries, accounts for 25% of all traumatic deaths. Injuries associated with chest trauma include fractured ribs, pulmonary contusions, pneumothorax, hemothorax, sternal fractures, and widened mediastinum. Aortic rupture, which often accompanies widened mediastinum, is fatal in 80–90% of all cases. If three or more adjacent ribs are fractured, "flail chest" may develop. Flail chest impairs the bellows action of the chest, causes intense pain, and affects the child's ability to cough and clear secretions. If a pulmonary contusion occurs, there is a greater risk of impaired oxygenation and the pulmonary system is compromised. Pneumothorax can result from a blunt or penetrating chest trauma. Occasionally, a pneumothorax can develop spontaneously. Pneumothorax can be closed or open; open pneumothorax results from a penetrating chest injury.

Hemothorax, another injury resulting from chest trauma, is defined as a collection of blood in the pleural space, which results from laceration of the chest wall, heart, great vessels, or lung tissues. A hemothorax results in impaired ventilation, but the greatest danger associated with this problem is hypovolemic shock. A sternal fracture, characterized by pain, can result in additional problems, including cardiac arrhythmias, right ventricular impairment, cardiac tamponade, and ventricular aneurysms. A widened mediastinum may result in an aortic tear, which is potentially fatal.

Etiology: Chest wall trauma results from blunt or penetrating injuries. These injuries can be the result of a motor vehicle accident (MVA), seat belt injury, stabbing, shooting, crushing injuries, or other forms of trauma.

Occurrence: Although the incidence of chest wall trauma is not available, 25% of all deaths result from traumatic chest injuries.

Age: Any age.

Ethnicity: Not significant.

Gender: Slightly higher in males than females.

Contributing Factors: Risk-taking behaviors may contribute to the incidence of chest wall injuries. Abuse should also be considered when there is no evidence of accidental injury.

Signs and Symptoms: Generally a traumatic incident will be reported in which the chest has suffered a penetrating or blunt injury. There may be a report of respiratory difficulty, chest pain, or hemoptysis. The time and type of injury should be elicited, if possible, from either the patient or the person accompanying them.

Inspection commonly reveals shallow breathing and splinting of chest. Poor color (cyanotic or pale) and uneven chest expansion are also noted. In the case of an open pneumothorax, the pediatric NP may feel or hear air escaping from the chest. Bruising, swelling, and bleeding may also be observed.

Touching the patient often elicits a pain response. Swelling at each site of the injury is also noted. Diminished or unequal expansion of the chest, crepitus, or deformity over fracture sites is felt with rib fractures. Right jugular distention and peripheral edema occur with right-sided heart failure. Absent or rapid pulses may be felt.

When a pneumothorax is present, auscultation with the stethoscope often reveals decreased air exchange. Various cardiac and pulse arrhythmias may also be noted. Hypotension is present in a tension pneumothorax, whereas tachycardia is present in a hemothorax. Pulmonary rales are often heard; when cardiac tamponade has occurred, muffled sounds will be auscultated.

Diagnostic Tests

X-rays reveal fractures and also show when a pneumothorax is present.
ECGs define irregular cardiac functioning. ABGs demonstrate the need for supplemental oxygen.
A hemoglobin and hematocrit demonstrate the need for blood.

Differential Diagnosis: None.

Treatment: Refer patient immediately to a tertiary-care setting. The goals of treatment are to maintain satisfactory respiration, stabilize cardiac problems, and treat shock, bruises, contusions, and fractures as promptly as possible. Cover open chest wounds quickly, but allow one side of the dressing to remain slightly open. If the patient shows signs of deterioration, open the dressing completely to allow air to escape; then close dressing with only one side open. A thoracotomy is the required treatment for pneumothorax. Treatment for a hemothorax includes oxygenation, volume replacement, surgical intervention, and chest-tube insertion. Providing supplementary oxygen is also a priority. Because this treatment regimen is complicated and requires specialized care, the NP should refer the child to a physician in a tertiary-care or trauma setting.

Follow-up: All follow-up should be appropriate for the particular injury. Generally an appointment should be made for 2 weeks posthospitalization. Patients should be told to call the health-care provider if any changes occur before their appointment date.

Sequelae: Respiratory failure and death can be the result of even a simple blunt trauma injury. Pay careful attention to all aspects of the patient's condition. Lingering pain from a rib fracture may persist for several months.

Prevention/Prophylaxis: Safety measures can prevent these types of injuries. Seat belt injuries, however, do account for a measurable portion of blunt chest injuries in an MVA.

Referral: *All* cases of chest wall trauma should be immediately referred to a tertiary-care setting for supervision by a physician.

Education: The importance of safety measures such as seat belts and child restraints should be taught to all parents. The dangers of traumatic injuries should be stressed.

Costochondritis

Costochondritis is the unilateral inflammation of the costochrondral junctures, usually the left side, involving the fourth to sixth ribs. The pain radiates to the back and abdomen. There is either minimal or no swelling. Tietze's syndrome involves the second sternochrondral junction at the right sternoclavicular junction, is accompanied by painful swelling at the junctions, and is aggravated by respiratory movement.

Etiology: Unknown.

Occurrence: Common.

Age: School-age children, usually adolescents.

Ethnicity: Noncontributory.

Gender: Occurs equally in males and females.

Contributing Factors: Unknown.

Signs and Symptoms: Child presents with a history of chest pain that radiates to back and/or abdomen. The pain, which varies in intensity, is accentuated by palpation or movement. There is marked tenderness on palpation over the costochrondral junctions with minimal or no swelling. The pain is not increased by coughing or swallowing.

Diagnostic Tests: Chest x-ray to rule out problems related to pulmonary or diaphragmatic causes of chest pain. ECG to rule out problems related to cardiac causes of chest pain.

Differential Diagnosis

Pericarditis patients present with sharp, stabbing chest pain that increases with deep breathing, coughing, swallowing, or twisting of the thorax.

Pleurisy produces sharp pain that increases with deep breathing, coughing, and arm movements.

Slipped rib syndrome is characterized by sudden onset of pain. The eighth, ninth, or tenth rib is usually involved.

Precordial catch (Texidor twinge) causes sharp, shooting pain at the left sternal border or cardiac apex.

Muscle strain or spasm involves the muscles. There is a history of participation in strenuous sports.

Treatment: Analgesics for the discomfort.

Follow-up: None.

Sequelae: None.

Prevention/Prophylaxis: None.

Referral: None.

Education: Instruct parents that costochondritis is a self-limiting illness. Reassure the parents and child that the child is not having a heart attack.

Spontaneous Pneumothorax

Pneumothorax is the dissection of air from the alveolar spaces into the interstitial spaces of the lung.

Etiology: Unknown.

Occurrence: Pneumothorax occurs more commonly in children with asthma or cystic fibrosis. It may occur as a complication of infection, a tracheostomy, ventilatory support, or chest trauma.

Age: Spontaneous pneumothorax occurs in adolescents and young adults.

Ethnicity: Noncontributory.

Gender: Occurs more often in males than females.

Contributing Factors: Underlying obstructive or restrictive lung disease.

Signs and Symptoms: Child complains of respiratory distress. Observation reveals retraction and often a shift of the larynx, trachea, and heart toward the unaffected side. Auscultation reveals markedly decreased breath sounds on the affected side; percussion is tympanic.

Diagnostic Tests: Radiographic studies assess the severity of the pneumothorax and differentiate between pneumopericardium (air surrounding the heart) and pneumomediastinum (heart and mediastinum outlined with air).

Differential Diagnosis: Diaphragmatic hernia, lung cysts, congenital lobar emphysema, and cystic adenomatoid malformations may be distinguished by chest films.

Treatment

Small pneumothorax: Observation. Administration of 100% oxygen increases the nitrogen pressure gradient between the lung air and the blood, thus hastening resolution.

Large or symptomatic pneumothorax: Needle aspiration and insertion of chest tube drainage.

Follow-up: None.

Sequelae: Pneumopericardium and pneumomediastinum are life-threatening.

Prevention/Prophylaxis: None.

Referral: Refer to pediatrician or surgeon for immediate hospitalization and insertion of chest tube in symptomatic cases.

Education: None.

Congenital Cardiac Defects

Congenital cardiac defects, the most common group of congenital anomalies encountered in infants, are structural abnormalities of the heart. Although all congenital anomalies are present at birth, congenital cardiac defects are recognized any time from the early neonatal period up until later in childhood, and in some cases, not until adulthood. The severity and type of anomaly usually directly relates to how early it is discovered, with the most severe anomalies being identified at birth or within 48 hours of birth. This coincides with the time necessary for the change from fetal to neonatal circulation.

Congenital anomalies are classified into three categories:

Cyanotic lesions include TOF, TA, pulmonary atresia, and truncus arteriosus, and transposition of the great vessels.

Acyanotic lesions include PDA, ASD, VSD, truncus arteriosus, and AV canal defect.

Obstructive lesions include PS, AS, and COA.

Incidence: Congenital cardiac defects affect approximately 1% of the North American population. Of that 1%, the specific incidence of defects is estimated in the discussion that follows. VSD, the most common defect, occurs 25% of the time. Because of the frequency of this disorder, VSD will be treated as a separate protocol in this chapter. Other acyanotic defects are seen in the following frequencies: PDA, 12%; truncus arteriosus, 2%; AV canal defect, 2%; and ASD, 10%. Obstructive defects occur in the following frequency: COA, 6%; AS, 5%; PS, 10%; and endocardial cushion defect (ECD), 4%. Cyanotic defects with their incidence are as follows: transposition of the great arteries (TGA), 4%; TOF, 5–9%; and TA, 2%.

Etiology: Chromosomal abnormalities, familial association, a combination of genetic and environmental catalysts, and teratogens. Deficiency of fetal growth or failure of component parts to align or fuse in utero can also cause cardiac defects.

Gender: For the most part gender is not a factor, but COA and PDA occur in a male-to-female ratio of 2 : 1. In ASD the female-to-male ratio is 2 : 1.

Contributing Factors: Prematurity and increased altitude may increase the incidence of PDA. There is an increased incidence of ASD among children with Down's syndrome and Ellis-van Crevell syndrome. Other factors include maternal exposure to certain teratogens, use of addictive drugs including cigarettes, and exposure to certain viruses or illness during the prenatal period.

Signs and Symptoms: If congenital cardiac defects are evident at birth, there will usually be tachycardia and tachypnea or apnea. These signs may be accompanied by hypothermia and feeding or swallowing difficulties along with poor intake of fluids. The prenatal history may reveal exposure to rubella or other teratogens, use of medications, illness history, and bleeding during the prenatal period. There may be a positive family history of congenital heart disease. The parents may report repeated gastroesophageal reflux in younger children. Older children may have a history of exercise intolerance, fatigue, and episodes of squatting, as reported by a parent. Parents may also report that the child frequently sighs. The following is a list of the specific symptomatology for individual congenital cardiac defects:

TGA:	Cyanosis from birth
	Dyspnea
	Slow weight gain
	Feeding difficulties
TOF:	Cyanosis from birth
	Dyspnea with exercise
	Squatting, hypoxia
	Irritability
	Tachycardia followed by weakness and syncope
	Exercise intolerance
	TET spells
	Increased fatigability
	Hypercyanotic spells worsened by crying, defecation, or feeding (ages 2–3 months)
AS:	Mild exercise intolerance
	Chest pain and/or syncope with exertion
ASD:	Increased incidence of respiratory infections
	Slight physical underdevelopment
	Increased fatigue and exertional dyspnea
PDA:	Asymptomatic in newborns
	Diaphoresis during feeding
	Poor feeding
	Falling asleep during feedings
Truncus arteriosus:	Cyanosis
	Dyspnea on exertion
	Increased fatigability
	Occasional hypoxic spells
AS:	Fatigability
	Dyspnea
	Occasional angina
	Syncope

A cardiac thrill or heave is detected in ASD, VSD, PS, and ECD. In COA, pulse rate is decreased in the dorsalis pedis and in the femoral and popliteal areas; the brachial, radial, and carotid arteries have bounding pulses; and increased blood pressure is noted in the arms, together with a corresponding decreased blood pressure in the legs. In AS, there is a difference between the peripheral pulses (right arm greater than left arm); the skin and mucous membranes may appear cyanotic or pale; and there is a narrow pulse pressure. In TOF, hepatomegaly is present, along with an observable sternal lift due to right ventricular hypertrophy. Also there is clubbing of the fingers and toes; these digits will feel cooler to touch. In TGA, hepatomegaly is noted.

In AS, a systolic ejection click murmur transmits to the neck. In ASD, there is a wide, fixed split S_2, ejection systolic murmur, and a diastolic flow murmur that is best heard at the left lower sternal border. In ECD, there is an abnormally split S_2, and either a diastolic flow murmur at the apex of the heart or a pansystolic murmur. In PS, an abnormally split S_2, a systolic ejection click, and an ejection systolic murmur may be heard over the pulmonic area. In VSD, there is an accentuated S_2, with either a diastolic flow murmur at the apex or a pansystolic murmur heard. In COA, there may be an audible ejection systolic murmur heard over the intrascapular area of the back. In TGV, there is a sharp S_1 and a loud single or narrowing split S_2. In TOF, there is a loud or harsh systolic ejection murmur or a holosystolic murmur at the mid lower sternal border. In truncus arteriosus, there is a grade III–IV/VI harsh, pansystolic ejection murmur in the upper right sternal border. When AS is present and the problem is located at or in the valve itself, an opening snap is heard. When the lesion is severe, there is a pronounced S_2 split. In PS, there is a grade III–IV/VI harsh murmur in the mid to late ejection phase murmur at the upper left sternal border in the pulmonic region. In severe or pronounced cases, cardiomegaly or hepatomegaly may be revealed when percussion is performed on the abdomen.

Diagnostic Tests: A number of tests may assist the NP in diagnosing the various heart defects. In general, these should be performed by the cardiologist. Usually, if a defect is suspected, the NP may initiate differentiation of the defect by ordering an ECG and chest x-ray, followed by an echocardiogram. ABGs, hemoglobin, and hematocrit are also needed. The following are some other diagnostic tests that may also be performed along with the specific cardiac disorders:

ASD: Chest x-ray reveals cardiomegaly. Abnormal ECG shows a right axis deviation and paradoxical motion of the ventricular septal wall.

VSD: In a small shunt, x-ray reveals few findings. In larger defects, cardiomegaly is noted, the aorta is small to normal, and the pulmonary markings are increased. The ECG is normal in small defects; in larger ones, there is pronounced left ventricular hypertrophy. An echocardiogram reveals defects of 4 mm or greater, generally pinpointing their location.

PDA: If shunt is large, x-ray will reveal an enlarged heart; ECG shows left ventricular hypertrophy. Cardiac catheterization shows an increased oxygen saturation near the pulmonary artery.

For any cyanotic defect, the following tests along with an echocardiogram may be useful in diagnosing a problem. An x-ray will show a boot-shaped contour of the heart and increased vascular markings. The ECG will be normal at first and later will reveal prominent P waves, right axis deviation, or right ventricular hypertrophy. Cardiac catherization reveals the right-to-left shunt and the size of the defect.

Differential Diagnosis

For cyanotic heart defects, *acyanotic defects.*
For acyanotic defects, *cyanotic defects.*

Functional murmur.

For VSD, *peripheral pulmonic stenosis.*

Metabolic abnormalities, which can be differentiated by tests to exclude cardiac problems.

Polycythemia, not related to a congenital cardiac defect.

Heart failure during the first few days of life, which is related to metabolic disorders, thyroid diseases, hypomagnesemia, or hypocalcemia.

Treatment: When a CCD is suspected, referral to a pediatric cardiologist is required and should be accomplished as quickly as possible. The following are specific treatment regimens:

ASD: Elective surgery may be performed between ages 2 and 4.

VSD: Small defects generally close on their own; if large, the defect should be closed during the first year of age.

PDA: The ductus arteriosis usually closes spontaneously during the first 2 years of age. In the preterm infant in whom closure is needed, indomethacin (0.1–0.3 mg/kg) is given every 8–24 hours by mouth (PO) or parenterally every 12 hours with a maximum of three doses. Surgery is done only if the shunt is severe.

TGA: Prostaglandin E_1 (0.05–0.2 µg/kg per min) is given to delay closure of PDA. Morphine sulfate (0.1–0.2 µg/kg) is given to relax the right ventricle; supplemental oxygen is used. Surgery is necessary, but still considered risky. Closure is sometimes delayed when certain defects (e.g., TGA and COA) require surgery but the surgery needs to be postponed.

TOF: Instruct the parents to hold the child in the knee-chest position during hypoxic episodes. Surgery (Blalock-Taussig procedure) is done in infants aged newborn to 4 months; this procedure increases the oxygen saturation and the pulmonary outflow, but complete repair is done when the child is 10 kg, or by 9–12 months.

AS: Surgery, if performed during the neonatal period, has a high mortality rate. The parents and child need to be cautioned to avoid sports because of the high rate of sudden death associated with these activities.

COA: Surgery, either as an emergency during the neonatal period or electively between ages 2 and 4 years, should be performed. The stenotic area is excised, and the ends of the artery are then reanastamosed.

PS: Vulvoplasty is done in a catheterization facility.

Follow-up: When a defect is suspected during the neonatal period, the infant should be referred to the cardiologist for follow-up. Referral is usually done during the first weeks of life or, when the defect is thought to be life-threatening, immediately. Follow-up continues for life; although some problems necessitate monthly visits, others are followed up on a yearly basis. If surgery is done, the same follow-up holds true in that rarely does the surgery have to be repeated, although some procedures are done in stages. Routine check-ups should be maintained; immunizations should be given as scheduled, including vaccines for pneumonia and influenza.

Sequelae: With early identification, appropriate intervention can be achieved, allowing these children to lead normal lives. Some (e.g., those with severe defects or AS) may not be able to participate in certain sports activities. Occasionally, parents become overly protective, refusing to allow the child to partake fully in activities; an emotional tug of war between the child and parent can result in conflict. For some of the more severe anomalies, death can result either when a child is not treated early or as a result of the intervention (surgery).

Referral: All children with suspected congenital cardiac defects *must* be referred to a pediatric cardiologist immediately.

Education: Parents need to know what treatments (medication or surgery) are needed and the prognosis of the specific defect. The rationale for various treatment regimens should also be carefully explained to the parents. When necessary, psychological counseling may be recommended for the parents and child who are not coping with the diagnosis. Long-term outcomes of the disease should be reviewed at each visit to assess the child and parents' level of understanding.

Ventricular Septal Defect

VSD is a common anomaly defined as a hole or defect in the intraventricular septum of the heart, resulting in a right-to-left shunt. Blood crosses the defect during systole and flows out to the pulmonary artery, causing pulmonary overload. The hemodynamic effects depend on the size of the defect.

Etiology: In most cases, the cause of VSD is unknown; however, it may accompany a chromosomal abnormality.

Occurrence: VSD occurs in 1.5–2.5 in 1000 live births. There has been a marked increase in the occurrence of VSD during the last two decades. It occurs more frequently in premature or low-birth-weight infants.

Age: Usually detected between 2 and 6 weeks of age, but may be detected as early as day 1 of life.

Ethnicity: Not significant.

Gender: Occurs equally in males and females.

Contributing Factors: When any of the following are present, the risk of VSD increases: Down's syndrome, trisomy 13 and 18, maternal exposure to rubella, maternal alcohol problems resulting in fetal alcohol syndrome, and phenylketonuria (PKU).

Signs and Symptoms: Parents will report no symptoms if the defect is small. In the case of a large VSD with a significant shunt volume, there may be a report of tachypnea, fatigue, exercise intolerance, dyspnea on exertion or with feedings, a slow growth rate, or frequent upper respiratory infections (URIs). No cyanosis will be noted. The child may be smaller than expected or may experience difficulty feeding. Palpation with a small VSD may or may not reveal a thrill at the lower left sternal border. With a moderate VSD, there may be a louder left ventricular apical impulse with or without a thrill. In a large VSD, there will be a right ventricular lift and thrill. If the patient is in heart failure, there will also be hepatomegaly.

Percussion may reveal slight cardiomegaly, but in the very early days this will not be detected. In small VSDs, a normal S_1 and S_2 are heard with a holosystolic or long systolic, harsh, blowing murmur at the left and right sides of the sternum.

In a moderate VSD, a frequently heard wide split between S_1 and S_2 may or may not be accentuated. There is a harsh, holosystolic blowing murmur.

In a large VSD, S_1 may be accentuated, whereas S_2 is narrowly split. There may also be a thudding sound at the apex. There is usually a holosystolic, blowing murmur at the left sternal border.

Diagnostic Tests

Chest x-ray: Normal with small VSD. Heart may be slightly to moderately enlarged in a moderate or large VSD.

ECG: Normal in small VSD. A moderate or large VSD causes left ventricular hypertrophy, left axis deviation, and left atrial enlargement. If right ventricular hypertrophy is present, one should suspect pulmonary hypertension.

Differential Diagnosis

Atrial septal defect: Differentiated by an echocardiogram and the position and quality of the murmur

Congestive heart failure (CHF), which can accompany the VSD: Differentiated by an echocardiogram and the presence of elevated cardiac electrolytes; ECG usually essentially normal

Treatment: Spontaneous closure occurs in up to 50% of all cases with no intervention. However, if CHF due to VSD occurs, surgical intervention will be warranted. Large defects require vigorous treatment of respiratory problems.

Follow-up: Every 6 months, close monitoring with a pediatric cardiologist is important.

Sequelae: Generally, small VSDs have no significant sequelae. A large untreated defect that does not close, can lead to CHF.

Prevention/Prophylaxis: None—VSD is a congenital defect.

Referral: Patient should be referred to a pediatric cardiologist when the murmur is first detected. The NP along with the cardiologist can provide continued follow-up.

Education: Reassure parents that the majority of VSDs close spontaneously. Parents must schedule health visits regularly, both with primary health-care provider and the cardiologist. The parents should also be taught to identify signs that the condition is worsening, such as poor weight gain, feeding problems, and shortness of breath.

Hypertension

Hypertension occurs when blood pressure is above the 95th percentile for age. Because hypertension is a potentially serious problem, all children should have their blood pressure taken routinely, starting at age 3 years. Table 8–1 lists normal blood pressures.

Systolic blood pressure, which gradually increases with age, should be correlated with weight and height throughout adolescence. Hypertension may be either primary or secondary.

Etiology: Sixty percent of all cases of hypertension can be genetically linked. In primary hypertension, heredity, salt intake, diet, stress, and obesity may all contribute to primary hypertension. Secondary hypertension is most frequently found in children with renal disorders. Additionally, certain foods or substances (e.g., sodium, nicotine, caffeine, licorice), medications (e.g., oral contraceptives, sympathomimetics, monoamine oxidase inhibitors, corticosteroids), or toxic exposure to certain elements (e.g., lead) or drugs (e.g., amphetamines, cocaine) can also lead to hypertension.

Occurrence: In infants and young children, secondary hypertension is more common than primary. Hypertension (primary and secondary) occurs in about 5–7% of all children and 10–15% of the adult population.

Age: All age groups.

Ethnicity: Hypertension occurs more often in African-Americans than in any other group.

Gender: The prevalence of hypertension is slightly increased among males, but females are found to have hypertension with increasing frequency.

Contributing Factors: Heredity, obesity, and smoking are the leading contributors to the incidence of primary hypertension. Physical problems, particularly renal problems and congenital cardiac defects, and certain medications can also contribute.

Signs and Symptoms: Because hypertension is generally a silent disease, there are often no signs. Of greater importance is a known familial history of hypertension. Occasionally, the child will have frequent headaches, nosebleeds, visual difficulties, or shortness of breath. Also, there may be a history of renal problems and/or unexplained febrile episodes throughout childhood.

Inspection may reveal short stature; otherwise, there will not be any visible signs. Obesity may be obvious.

Palpation may reveal a significant difference in upper and lower extremity pulses, especially with COA. Edema may be present and kidney abnormalities may also be evident. The abdomen should be carefully assessed for masses and costovertebral angle tenderness. In neonates, respiratory distress, irritability or lethargy, vomiting, apnea, or seizures may also be observed.

The presence of café au lait spots or depigmented areas of skin may signify hypertension secondary to neurofibromatosis. Fundus examination may reveal arterial changes, exudate, or hemorrhages. Auscultation may reveal a murmur with hypertension secondary to COA. If renal artery stenosis is present, a bruit may be heard over the costovertebral angle.

Diagnostic Tests: The most useful tool is to take the child's blood pressure with the appropriate size cuff in two positions (sitting/standing/lying) and on both arms and at least one leg. If elevated on two or more occasions, other follow-up should be initiated.

A urinalysis should be done. Hematuria, proteinuria, leukocyturia, or an elevated blood urea nitrogen or plasma creatine could indicate renal disease. Hypokalemia, hypochloremia, or metabolic alkalosis may also reveal a kidney problem. ECGs and chest x-rays are often requested, but are generally normal until the late stages of hypertension.

Echocardiograms are useful in determining specific cardiac defects.

Differential Diagnosis

White coat hypertension: A rise in blood pressure that occurs only when the patient is in the health-care provider's office.

Renal diseases, cardiac abnormalities or *renovascular hypertension.*

Lead toxicity: May be indicated by a serum lead level greater than 10 but more likely greater than 50.

Drug toxicity, especially illicit drugs: Can be detected by urine or blood screening.

Obesity.

Treatment: In children, the first step is to discover the underlying cause. If mild hypertension exists, treatment initially should be a nonpharmacologic regimen including weight reduction, moderate sodium reduction (80–100 mEq/day) increased calcium and potassium intake, aerobic exercise, and behavior modification.

If intervention is ineffective after a minimum of 3 months or a maximum of 6 months, drug treatment should be initiated. Single-agent therapy is preferred.

For young children, the drugs of choice are hydralazine (1–2 mg/kg per day bid) or propranolol (0.5–3.0 mg/kg per day tid). Other drugs used, in the order given, are clonidine (0.002–0.06 mg/kg per day bid), prazosin (0.05–0.1 mg/kg per day bid), catopril (0.3–2.0 mg/kg per day tid), nifedipine (0.25–1.0 mg/kg per day bid or qid).

Follow-up: Initially, weekly monitoring for 4–6 weeks, then every 2 months for 2–6 months, and finally every 6 months or when symptoms warrant a visit.

Sequelae: Headaches and epistaxis are common if the blood pressure is elevated. These should be reported immediately to the health-care provider. Stroke, although rare in children, is a possibility.

Prevention/Prophylaxis: Risk assessment, including hereditary factors, should be done on each child. Children should be taught to avoid cigarettes and drugs. The importance of aerobic exercise, decreasing salt, and decreasing fat should be stressed.

Early identification is essential; therefore, at each visit children aged 3 years and older should have their blood pressure taken.

Referral: Refer to a physician if secondary hypertension is suspected. Consult with a pediatrician and refer to a cardiologist if primary hypertension is suspected.

Education: Children and parents should be taught the dangers of obesity, drug use, smoking, and lack of exercise. Parents should be reassured that with adequate control, morbidity is significantly decreased. Adequate control also improves the growth and overall well-being of the child. Although heredity cannot be controlled, certain environmental and teratogenic agents can be avoided. The importance of maintaining the assigned regimen should be stressed.

Kawasaki Syndrome

Also called mucocutaneous lymph node syndrome, Kawasaki syndrome is an acute illness affecting multiple systems in infants and young children.

Etiology: Unknown. Possible causes include Epstein-Barr virus, retrovirus, Rickettsia, Group A streptococci, *Staphylococcus aureus*, *Propionibacterium* and *Candida*.

Occurrence: Most likely to occur in December through May.

Age: Most common in children under 2, with a total of 85% of all cases occurring by age 5.

Ethnicity: The incidence is highest in Asians and lowest in African-Americans.

Gender: More males than females contract the disease (1.5 : 1).

Contributing Factors: Ancestry and predisposing factors. Avoid contact with others known to have the disease.

Signs and Symptoms: There will be a history of a rash and fever greater than 103°F lasting for 5 or more days. Inspection reveals at least four or more of these features: polymorphic rash, bilateral conjunctivitis, changes in lips (cracked or dry), swollen lips, strawberry tongue, edema, erythema, desquamation or peringuinal desquamation of extremities.

Palpation reveals cervical lymphadenopathy and guarding in the right upper quadrant during assessment of the gallbladder. Auscultation may reveal a cardiac murmur.

Diagnostic Tests

Marked leukocytosis with a shift to the left
Elevated erythrocyte sedimentation rate (ESR)
Platelet count by week 3 greater than 800,000/mm^3
Moderately elevated serum IgE

An ECG should be done along with an echocardiogram to provide a baseline.

Differential Diagnosis

Measles, rubella, and *scarlet fever* are differentiated by characteristics of disease not present (e.g., platelet elevation, prolonged fever).
Rocky Mountain spotted fever is differentiated by laboratory tests.
Juvenile rheumatoid arthritis (JRA) usually have pain as the primary symptom.
Mercury poisoning is differentiated by laboratory test.

Treatment: The child diagnosed with or strongly suspected to have Kawasaki syndrome should be hospitalized. Consultation with pediatrician should also be initiated.

In the acute phase, aspirin is given in high doses (80–100 mg/kg per day) in 4 divided doses for 14 days. Intravenous gamma globulin 2000 mg/kg in one single dose is given IV over a 12-hour period.

After 14 days, if the patient is afebrile, aspirin (3–5 mg/kg per day) is given once per day for 6–8 weeks from the onset of disease. This should be done after an echocardiogram reveals *no* abnormalities.

Follow-up: An echocardiogram should be repeated 2–3 weeks after disease onset. Periodic physical examinations should be done until normal platelet, ESR, and liver function tests are obtained.

Sequelae: Cardiovascular findings, specifically myocarditis, pericardial effusion, mitral regurgitation, and—most important—coronary aneurysms, are the most serious complications.

Prevention/Prophylaxis: Prompt treatment and referral can prevent an aneurysm. Long-term cardiac follow-up should be offered to all children diagnosed with Kawasaki syndrome.

Referral: Immediate referral to a pediatrician when findings suggest the disease, with follow-up by a pediatric cardiologist.

Education: Parents should be taught the importance of maintaining the treatment regimens. They should be made aware that this disease lasts for 3–8 weeks, but that follow-up may be for life.

Rheumatic Fever

Rheumatic fever (RF), an inflammatory disease process, occurs after a Group A β-hemolytic streptococcal infection. There has recently been a resurgence of RF.

In the 1950s and 60s, RF and its major complications were significant worldwide health problems. The incidence declined until the late 1980s, when the increase was first noted; however, the reasons for this increase are not yet known. RF causes cardiac tissue damage and is thus a leading cause of acquired heart disease.

Etiology: The main agent is Group A β-hemolytic streptococcus.

Incidence: There is an increased number of RF cases in the fall, winter, and early spring. RF will develop in approximately 3–5% of patients with untreated or undertreated Group A β-hemolytic streptococcal infection.

Age: Occurs most often in children between ages 5 and 15.

Ethnicity: Not significant.

Gender: Occurs equally in males and females.

Contributing Factors: Groups who experience overcrowding, poverty, and social disadvantages are at increased risk for contracting the disease. Patients who have had a URI in which streptococcus was the causative agent and who have had inadequate or no treatment at all are predisposed to the development of RF.

Signs and Symptoms: The parent or child reports that the child has had a URI or sore throat for which there was either no treatment or ineffective treatment. They may report fever, joint pain, rash on the trunk and extremities, easily changeable moods, and a racing heart. They may also report that the child has a history of RF.

   The child appears ill, and the skin is warm or hot to the touch. A macular ecthymatous rash is present, mainly on the trunk and extremities. Palpation of the scalp, joints, and spine reveals (1) pea-sized nodules that are nontender and firm, called subcutaneous nodules; and (2) two or more joints with severe pain, tenderness, warmth, swelling, and redness.

   When percussing the chest, the NP may note (1) cardiomegaly or a heart size greater than expected; (2) a heart murmur that is new and fairly significant; and (3) an increased heart rate.

Diagnostic Tests: The gold standard remains a throat culture positive for Group A β-hemolytic streptococcus. ESR will also be increased. There are no specific tests that address RF, and therefore the diagnosis is determined based on the Jones criteria (Table 8–4). An ECG should also be performed in cases where there is a positive culture to see whether there is a prolonged P–R interval.

Differential Diagnosis

JRA, differentiated from RF by the following: (1) antistreptococcal agents produce no significant improvement in JRA; and (2) antinuclear antibody (ANA) test is positive in JRA.

Infective endocarditis, differentiated by blood cultures and endocarditis (in RF, there is pancarditis).

Connective tissue disease, particularly systemic lupus erythematosus, differentiated by a speckled ANA test result.

TABLE 8–4 JONES CRITERIA FOR
RHEUMATIC FEVER*

Major Criteria	Minor Criteria
Carditis	Fever
Migratory polyarthritis	Arthralgia
Erythema marginatum	Previous RF
Chorea	Elevated ESR
Subcutaneous nodules	Prolonged P–R interval on the ECG

*Diagnosis of RF may be made if the patient meets two major crite-
    ria or one major and two minor criteria and has had preceding
    Group A β-hemolytic streptococcal infection.
ECG = electrocardiogram; ESR = erythrocyte sedimentation rate;
    RF = rheumatic fever.

Lyme disease, differentiated by a positive Lyme titer.

Treatment: Treatment of the disease involves three major components. First, the Group A β-hemolytic streptococcal infection should be treated. Benzathine penicillin G, 1,200,000 units (600,000 if patient is less than 27 kg) should be given intramuscularly. Oral medicines may also be used, including penicillin V (250 mg/kg per day twice per day for 10 days) or erythromycin (40 mg/kg per day bid or tid; not to exceed 1 g in 24 hours). Second, anti-inflammatory agents should be used to reduce the arthralgia associated with the disease. These include steroids, given in a dosage of 2.5 mg/kg per day divided into two doses over a 2- to 3-week period. After treatment, the patient should be gradually weaned from the steroids. Salicylates should be given so that blood levels of 20–25 mg/dL are achieved. This requires giving about 90–120 mg/kg per day in four divided doses. Lastly, the patient should be given supportive therapy to treat other problems associated with RF, particularly CHF and carditis. Often the use of salicylates alone is effective for carditis, but a physician should be consulted to institute treatment for CHF.

Follow-up: Children who have been diagnosed with RF should have regular follow-ups at 1- to 2-week intervals for the first month and then about once per month; during these visits, antibiotic prophylaxis is given to ensure that the disease does not recur. Injections with benzathine penicillin G should be given once per month for up to 5 years after the diagnosis, although this is still controversial.

Sequelae: The most frequent sequela is the development of rheumatic valvular heart disease. Untreated, however, RF may result in death.

Referral: When cardiac involvement is suspected, the pediatric cardiologist should be consulted for treatment and follow-up. The NP should consult with a pediatrician for all children who have a presumptive diagnosis of RF.

Prevention/Prophylaxis: The best way to prevent this disease is to initiate prompt treatment of all cases of streptococcal infection.

Education: Parents and children should be taught the importance of compliance with drug regimens, especially antibiotic prophylaxis to prevent a recurrence of the disease.

Families should be taught that the child will need prophylaxis prior to dental work for the rest of his or her life.

Prompt identification and treatment of β-hemolytic streptococcal infections should be stressed to families.

Syncope

Commonly known as fainting, syncope is generally a benign event that may occur when a person experiences severe pain, anxiety, or high levels of emotion, or stands erect for a long period of time. If syncope occurs more than once, however, more serious etiologies must be ruled out.

Etiology: Syncope due to vasovagal stimulation results in a loss of consciousness, either partial or total, for a short period of time.

Occurrence: Common; about 50% of children have experienced at least one syncopal episode.

Age: Any age.

Ethnicity: Not significant.

Gender: Occurs equally in males and females.

Contributing Factors: Severe anxiety, stress, or standing for a long period of time.

Signs and Symptoms: The child or parent reports a period of partial or total unconsciousness that may be idiopathic in origin or can be related to stress, pain, or standing for a long period of time. Further evaluation is important if other family members have had the same problem (Fig. 8–5).

The syncopal event may be sudden or may have a prodromal period. The child may be diaphoretic and pale. The time the child is unconscious should be recorded; the time may vary from a few seconds to several minutes. There is a transient loss of muscle tone.

Skin will be cool and diaphoretic. Pulse rate can vary from absent to rapid and should be evaluated and recorded. Child may experience palpitations or bradycardia.

Diagnostic Tests: For the first episode, tests may be deferred. When syncope occurs in the absence of pain, anxiety, and standing for a long time, some tests should be performed. These tests include an ECG, which may be normal or may reveal a prolonged QT segment; Wolff-Parkinson-White syndrome (abnormal AV conduction problem); or tachycardia or bradycardia, which may suggest heart block.

A chest x-ray may reveal an enlarged heart, suggesting congenital heart disease or another underlying cardiomyopathy.

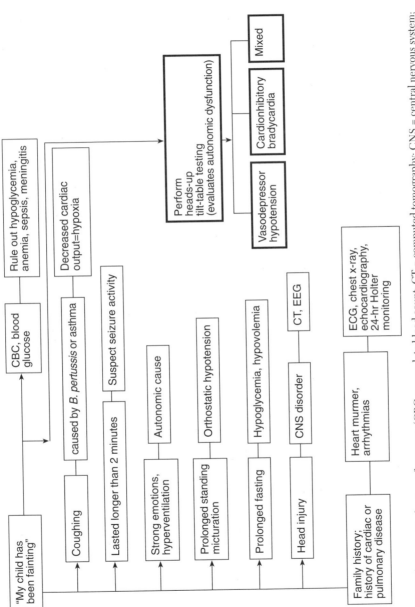

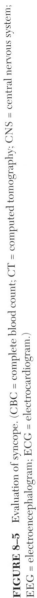

FIGURE 8–5 Evaluation of syncope. (CBC = complete blood count; CT = computed tomography; CNS = central nervous system; EEG = electroencephalogram; ECG = electrocardiogram.)

An echocardiogram should be ordered if a cardiomyopathy is suspected.

Differential Diagnosis

Prolonged QT syndrome, differentiated by an ECG, demonstrates this phenomenon.

Congenital cardiomyopathies, differentiated by history, abnormal ECG, echocardiogram demonstrating defect, or chest x-ray.

Severe autonomic disease, characterized by repeated episodes of syncope.

Wolff-Parkinson-White syndrome, differentiated by an ECG that demonstrates abnormalities in AV conduction.

Heart block, differentiated by an ECG.

Treatment: Protect the child from injury. Obtain a detailed history that includes questions related to the nature of the fainting spell, events that preceded the loss of consciousness, proximity to exercise, and any seizure activity during the event. If syncope is due to heart block, a pacemaker will be recommended. If the problem is related to a prolonged QT syndrome, a cardiologist may start β-blockers, steroids, or a combination of the two.

Follow-up: After initial episode, child should be reevaluated immediately if there is a repeat syncopal episode. If all tests are normal, follow-up should be done in accordance with the routine, recommended schedule.

Sequelae: Occasionally injury may occur as a result of the fall that occurs during syncope. Also, untreated or unrecognized cardiac abnormalities can result in death.

Prevention/Prophylaxis: Stress modification should be taught. If standing event was the problem, the child should be taught to alter pressure slightly in the legs and to move slightly during the period of time required to stand.

Referral: Unexplained or recurrent episodes of syncope should be referred to a pediatric cardiologist.

Education: Parents should be taught the importance of reporting the occurrence of syncopal events and of giving a detailed history of each episode.

Acute Life-threatening Event

An acute life-threatening event (ALTE) is a respiratory pause that lasts a minimum of 20 seconds or is associated with bradycardia (heart rate less than 100 beats/min). Formerly called near-miss sudden infant death syndrome (SIDS), ALTE now refers to pathological apnea that occurs in infants greater than 37 weeks' gestation.

Etiology: The etiology of ALTE is unclear. The condition appears to be related primarily to an unstable or depressed respiratory control system. Also implicated are depressed respiratory chemoreceptors, altered rapid eye movement (REM) sleep, and spontaneous airway obstruction.

Occurrence: The incidence of ALTE is not documented, but the incidence of SIDS-related deaths is 1.5–2 in 1000 live births per year. Approximately 80% of infants who die of SIDS have no identifiable risk and no history of ALTE. Siblings of infants who had SIDS are at increased risk for SIDS. Also at risk are infants born addicted to cocaine. Premature infants are especially prone to apnea.

Age: Most cases occur before age 9 months.

Ethnicity: Not significant.

Gender: Occurs equally in males and females.

Contributing Factors: Prematurity, congenital heart disease, hypoglycemia, hypocalcemia, electrolyte disorders, anemia, hypovolemia, intracranial hemorrhage, or seizures may be associated with apneic spells. No clear indicators for SIDS have been documented.

Signs and Symptoms: The parent reports that the baby was fine when it was put to bed, but was found either not to be breathing at all, or "breathing funny," having cool, bluish skin and not reacting to any stimulus. The following are the signs and symptoms seen in the infant with apnea: cessation of breathing, marked pallor or cyanosis, hypotonia, and bradycardia.

Diagnostic Tests: There is no test to diagnose ALTE. Tests done to rule out an underlying cause include the following:

A pneumogram is commonly done for premature infants or those with a sibling known to have had SIDS or ALTE. The results document apneic spells; a child is then given an apnea monitor for 9 months to wear whenever not being directly observed.
Electroencephalography (EEG) is done to rule out seizures.
CBC with differential is obtained to rule out underlying infection.
Electrolyte studies are ordered to determine alterations in electrolytes.
Glucose studies may indicate hypoglycemia.
Calcium may be low, indicating a depressed respiratory center.
Neck radiography is done to rule out obstruction.
Chest radiography may indicate pneumonia.
ABGs are ordered if the apnea is severe.

Differential Diagnosis

Sepsis, differentiated by fever, elevated white blood cells (WBCs), and progressive illness.
Seizures, differentiated by EEG.
Gastrointestinal (GI) reflux resulting in gagging or choking, differentiated by upper GI studies.
Metabolic disorders such as hypoglycemia and hypocalcemia, differentiated by serum and/or urine-specific tests.
Munchausen syndrome by proxy, differentiated by the presence of pinch marks on the nares.

Treatment: If a cause is found, treat the underlying cause. Infants with repeated episodes or siblings of infants who died of apnea may wear an electronic monitor in order to reassure the parents. The monitor is left in place usually until the infant has been alarm-free for 2 months, but the period may be as long as 9 months. Vigorous stimulation that consists of rubbing the trunk and thumping the feet is indicated during an episode; the infant should NEVER be shaken.

Follow-up: The infant should be seen at regular (e.g., monthly) intervals, depending on the needs of the family. If no ALTE occurs for 9 months, the monitor can be discontinued.

Sequelae: Infants who have experienced an ALTE requiring vigorous stimulation are at risk of dying. It is estimated that 25–30% will die of SIDS.

Prevention/Prophylaxis: For sleeping, place the child on the side or supine, rather than on the stomach.

Referral: Refer to the primary-care physician for consultation and perhaps admission to the hospital for observation and complete diagnostic evaluation.

Education: Parents should be instructed in cardiopulmonary resuscitation, and they should know the signs and symptoms of apnea.

Asthma

Asthma, a reversible obstructive airway disease, is characterized by hyper-responsiveness of the trachea and bronchi. Asthma has multiple triggers, but specific causes are often difficult to pinpoint. Although few children actually outgrow the disease during puberty, they usually experience a remission of symptoms.

Etiology: Specific etiology is unknown; however, there is a strong genetic predisposition.

Occurrence: Up to 12% in the United States.

Age: Thirty percent of affected children are symptomatic by age 1 year. The majority (70%) have symptoms by 4–5 years of age.

Ethnicity: Slightly higher incidence of asthma in African-American children.

Gender: Occurs in 10–15% of boys and 7–10% of girls. Before puberty, twice as many boys are affected; after puberty, the incidence equalizes.

Contributing Factors: Factors that may precipitate asthma include viral infection; allergens, either environmental or ingested; gastroesophageal reflux; emotional stress; and certain medications, specifically aspirin and β-adrenergic blockers.

Signs and Symptoms: Obtain a history including when the symptoms began, any factors that preceded the attacks, and the first signs noted. Also, determine whether there is a familial history of asthma or allergies. There will be complaints of wheezing, coughing, and dyspnea.

Signs and symptoms depend on whether the attack is acute or insidious. Signs that are generally progressive are cough, dyspnea, shortness of breath, wheezing, restlessness, and irritability. The child will have noisy respirations and may also have retractions, nasal flaring, and cyanosis. Other more general signs include atopic signs, chronic or serous otitis media; pale, blue-gray, and boggy nasal turbinates; and clear drainage from the nose. Additional signs include atopic dermatitis, tachycardia, and in chronic and recurrent asthma, barrel chest. High-pitched rhonchi and wheezing are noted on auscultation. Hyperinflation of the lungs is also noted.

Diagnostic Tests

Pulmonary function tests may be done for children over 6.

Inspiratory spirometry is useful.

Nasal cytology from a nasal smear with an eosinophil count greater than 10% is significant.

CBC is generally normal, but when associated with infection, WBC count may be elevated.

Chest x-ray, although not warranted with each attack, can be useful for diagnosing infiltrates.

Sinus x-rays or CT scans are helpful in diagnosing associated sinusitis.

Skin testing to detect specific irritants may be useful for severe or chronic asthma.

Peak flow meter values less than 70% of the expected baseline can indicate exacerbations of the disease.

Differential Diagnosis

Bronchiolitis is manifested by predisposition to wheeze; however, children having this problem will also have a positive RSV test.

Pneumonia is differentiated from asthma by the presence of fever, elevated WBCs, and a more acutely ill child.

Croup is associated with a barking cough and stridor.

Tuberculosis is differentiated by a positive tuberculosis (TB) test and lymphadenopathy.

Bronchitis is difficult to differentiate because many symptoms are similar.

Bronchopulmonary dysplasia is generally seen in premature infants and may progress to asthma.

Congenital heart disease may be accompanied by a heart murmur, feeding problems, poor weight gain, and progressive symptoms including digital clubbing.

Treatment: Inhaled β_2-agonists are commonly used for symptomatic asthma. Theophylline (3–8 mg/kg each night for nocturnal asthma) is also used for most asthma patients. For moderate asthma, cromolyn sodium (two puffs bid to qid) is recommended along with an inhaled β-agonist taken three to four times daily. Additionally, sustained-release theophylline is recommended to achieve a serum concentration of 5–15 μg/mL. Sometimes a short course of oral corticosteroids is also given (2 mg/kg qid for 1 week).

A metered-dose inhaler (MDI) or home nebulization machine may be used to deliver β-agonist and cromolyn sodium (Table 8–5). For children under 2, a nebulizer or an MDI with a spacer and mask is the most effective method of medication delivery. For children aged 2–4 years, an MDI with a spacer is the most useful; for children older than 5, MDIs and powdered inhaler preparations are the most effective.

The pediatric NP should treat asthmatics in close collaboration with a team of physicians, including a pulmonologist or allergist. For a complete therapy summary, see Table 8–5.

Follow-up: Parents should be instructed to return immediately to the clinic or emergency room if symptoms worsen. Routine follow-up should be scheduled in 1–2 weeks initially and then every month for 2 months. After that, a regular schedule should resume for health maintenance.

Sequelae: Possible complications include pulmonary atelectasis, pneumothorax, decreased growth, thoracic deformity, respiratory failure, psychological problems, and even death. Children often suffer from poor school performance, difficult relationships with peers, and a low self-esteem. In severe cases, depression and suicidal ideation are also seen.

Prevention/Prophylaxis: Avoidance of specific triggers, when known, is critical for all asthmatic patients. Adequate treatment of infections, which can trigger asthmatic attacks, is also important. Providing adequate rest, eating a balanced diet, avoiding stress, and promptly identifying symptoms can decrease the severity of the disease. A yearly TB test and influenza vaccine are recommended for all patients with asthma.

Referral: Children who have a relapse within 10 days of an asthmatic attack or those who do not respond to initial treatment should be referred to an allergist and/or pulmonologist.

Education: Educate parents in the use of peak flow meters and in the early signs of asthma, including breathing difficulty, coughing, wheezing, retractions, and dyspnea. Teach patients and families about potential complications and the signs and symptoms of problems such as severe hypoxia, dehydration, atelectasis, and pneumonia.

Teach parents the importance of giving extra fluids to maintain hydration and liquefy secretions (3000 mL/day unless contraindicated).

Educate parents regarding the purpose, dosage, side effects, and adverse and toxic effects of all medications. Teach families that they must continue medications and never abruptly stop any therapy. If steroid inhalers are used, the mouth should be rinsed to avoid candidiasis.

Teach patients relaxation techniques to improve breathing. Advise patients and families that regular exercise is needed, but that rest periods are also needed.

TABLE 8–5 ASTHMA MEDICATION THERAPY SUMMARY: DOSAGES FOR THERAPY IN CHILDHOOD ASTHMA

Medication	Dosage
β₂-Agonists	
Inhaled (*Examples*: albuterol, metaproterenol, bitolterol, terbutaline, pirbuterol)	
Mode of administration	
Metered-dose inhaler	2 puffs q 4–6 hr
Dry powder inhaler	1 capsule q 4–5 hr
Nebulizer solution*	Albuterol 5 mg/mL; 0.1–0.15 mg/kg in 2 mL saline q 4–6 hr; maximum 5.0 mg
	Metaproterenol, 50 mg/mL; 0.25–0.50 mg/kg in 2 mL saline q 4–6 hr; maximum 15.0 mg
Oral	
Liquids	
Albuterol	0.1–0.15 mg/kg q 4–6 hr
Metaproterenol	0.3–0.5 mg/kg q 4–6 hr
Tablets	
Albuterol	2- or 4-mg tablet q 4–6 hr
	4-mg sustained-release tablet q 12 hr
Metaproterenol	10- or 20-mg tablet q 4–6 hr
	2.5- or 5.0-mg tablet q 4–6 hr
Cromolyn Sodium	
Mode of administration	
Metered-dose inhaler	1 mg/puff; 2 puffs bid to qid
Dry powder inhaler	20 mg/capsule; 1 capsule bid to qid
Nebulizer solution	20 mg/2 mL ampule; 1 ampule bid to qid
Theophylline	
Liquid	
Tablets, capsules	
Sustained-release tablets, capsules	Dosage to achieve serum concentration of 5–15 µg/mL

Corticosteroids

Inhaled[†]

Beclomethasone	42 µg/puff, 2–4 puffs bid to qid
Triamcinolone	100 µg/puff, 2–4 puffs bid to qid
Flunisolide	250 µg/puff, 2–4 puffs bid

Oral[‡]

Liquids

Prednisone	5 mg/5 mL
Prednisolone	5 mg/5 mL
	15 mg/5 mL

Tablets

Prednisone	1, 2.5, 5, 10, 20, 25, 50 mg
Prednisolone	5 mg
Methylprednisolone	2, 4, 8, 16, 24, 32 mg

*Premixed solutions are available. It is suggested that the "per kilogram" dosage recommendations be followed until symptoms are controlled.

[†]Use spacer devices to minimize local adverse effects and systemic effects.

[‡]For acute exacerbations, doses of 1–2 mg/kg in single or divided doses are used initially and are then modified. Reassess in 3 days, as only a short burst may be needed. There is no need to taper a short (3- to 5-day) course of therapy. If therapy extends beyond this period, it may be appropriate to taper the dosage. For chronic dosage of oral steroids, the lowest possible alternate-day AM dosage should be established.

Bronchitis

Bronchitis is an inflammatory disease of the bronchi characterized by one or more of the following: hyperemia of the bronchial mucosa, increased production of mucus, and inflammatory exudate of mucus and WBCs.

Etiology: Viruses are the most common cause of acute bronchitis. Other common agents are the bacteria *Streptococcus pneumoniae, Haemophilus influenzae,* and *Mycoplasma pneumoniae.*

Occurrence: Seasonable occurrence has been noted, most frequently in the spring and winter.

Age: Not significant.

Ethnicity: Not significant.

Gender: Occurs equally in males and females.

Contributing Factors: Exposure to persons with URIs.

Signs and Symptoms: There will be a report of a dry, unproductive cough beginning a few days after rhinitis. There may also be complaints of low substernal discomfort or even a burning sensation in the chest. The parent may also state that the cough became productive after a few days. Substernal pain aggravated by coughing is also reported. Signs of nasopharyngeal infection, conjunctivitis, and rhinitis are common. There may be fever of less than 101°F. Some shortness of breath can be observed. Chest is clear on percussion. Coarse breath sounds and moist rales are heard in the upper part of chest. Rhonchi may be high-pitched and may be similar to the sounds of wheezing. Bacterial bronchitis is frequently characterized by copious sputum greater than 2 tbsp a day. Viral bronchitis rarely causes more than 2 tbsp of mucopurulent sputum.

Diagnostic Tests: Analysis and culture of sputum is initially negative in viral or mycoplasmal bronchitis, but purulent in other bacterial forms of bronchitis. Gram's stain and culture of sputum are not necessary unless sputum is purulent or pneumonia is suspected. A chest x-ray may be taken if the clinical assessment is equivocal, but generally is not necessary. In viral or mycoplasmal disease, the WBC count usually is normal; the count is rarely elevated even in bacterial bronchitis.

Differential Diagnosis

Bronchopneumonia, differentiated by x-ray.
Tuberculosis and other chronic pulmonary diseases, differentiated by skin tests (purified protein derivative, tine, histoplasmosis tests), and x-ray.
Bronchial asthma, differentiated by symptoms including marked inspiratory wheezing.

Treatment: Bronchitis with production of less than 2 tbsp mucoid or mucopurulent sputum per day requires rest, acetaminophen (Children's Tylenol), or ibuprophen (Children's Advil) for discomfort (Tables 8–6a and 8–6b), and a vaporizer or humidifier for increasing the humidity in the air, making it easier to breathe.

Cough suppressants such as dextromethorphan hydrobromide may be used sparingly (30 mg q 6–8 hours PO as needed; 240 mL is enough for 6 days). Expectorants may be used, although there is debate as to their efficacy. Guaifenesin (Tussi-Organidin NR) is available alone or in combination with cough suppressants; dosage is 200–400 mg (100 mg/tsp) PO q 4 hours PRN (comes in 4- and 8-ounce bottles).

Bronchitis with production of more than 2 tbsp purulent sputum per day (usually associated with systemic symptoms) requires rest. Children's Tylenol (325 mg PO, two tablets q 4–6 hours) *or* Children's Advil (200–400 mg PO q 6 hours for discomfort); an expectorant; a vaporizer or humidifier for moisture (this is of most value in winter); and antibiotic therapy. Some suggestions for antibiotics are as follows:

Cephalexin (Keflex) is indicated for treatment of *Escherichia coli*, Group A β-hemolytic streptococcus, *H. influenzae, S. pneumoniae*, and staphylococcus. Children's dosage is 6–12 mg/kg PO q 6 hours with a maximum dose of 25 mg/kg q 6 hours.

Amoxicillin is indicated for gram-negative and gram-positive organisms. Children's dosage is 20–40 mg/kg PO daily in divided doses q 8 hours.

Ampicillin is used for gram-negative and gram-positive organisms. Dosages are 50–100 mg/kg PO daily in divided doses q 6 hours.

Tetracycline is effective against gram-positive and gram-negative organisms. Children over 8 should be given 25–50 mg/kg PO q 6 hours.

Trimethoprim (TMP) and sulfamethoxazole (SMX) (Bactrim) is effective for children with penicillin allergy. Dosage is 8 mg/kg TMP and 50 mg/kg SMX PO q 24 hours.

TABLE 8–6a   IBUPROFEN SUSPENSION DOSAGES (100 mg/5 mL)

Age	Weight lb	Weight kg	Fever <102.5°F	Fever >102.5°F
6–11 mo	13–17	6–7.9	¼ tsp (25 mg)	½ tsp (50 mg)
12–23 mo	18–23	8–10.9	½ tsp (50 mg)	1 tsp (100 mg)
2–3 yr	24–35	11–15.9	¾ tsp (75 mg)	1½ tsp (150 mg)
4–5 yr	36–47	16–21.9	1 tsp (100 mg)	2 tsp (200 mg)
6–8 yr	48–59	22–26.9	1¼ tsp (125 mg)	2½ tsp (250 mg)
9–10 yr	60–71	27–31.9	1½ tsp (150 mg)	3 tsp (300 mg)
11–12 yr	72–95	32–43.9	2 tsp (200 mg)	4 tsp (400 mg)
Adult	96–154	44–70	2 tsp (200 mg)	4 tsp (400 mg)

TABLE 8–6b ACETAMINOPHEN DOSAGES

Age Caps/Gelcaps	Weight (lb)	Weight (kg)	Suspension Drops and Original Drops (80 mg/0.8 mL Dropperful [dppr])	Chewable Tabs (80-mg tabs)	Suspension Liquid and Original Elixir (160 mg/5 mL)	Junior Strength (160-mg caps/chewables)	Regular Strength (325-mg Caps/Tabs)	Extra Strength (500 mg)
0–3 mo	6–11	2.5–5.4	½ dppr (0.4 mL)					
4–11 mo	12–17	5.5–7.9	1 dppr (0.8 mL)		½ tsp			
12–23 mo	18–23	8.0–10.9	1½ dppr (1.2 mL)		¾ tsp			
2–3 yr	24–35	11.0–15.9	2 dppr (1.6 mL)	2 tab	1 tsp			
4–5 yr	36–47	16.0–21.9		3 tab	1½ tsp			
6–8 yr	48–59	22.0–26.9		4 tab	2 tsp	2 cap/tab		
9–10 yr	60–71	27.0–31.9		5 tab	2½ tsp	2½ cap/tab		
11 yr	72–95	32.0–43.9		6 tab	3 tsp	3 cap/tab		
Adults & Children ≥12 yr	96+	44.0+				4 cap/tab	1 or 2 caps/tabs	2 caps/gel

Clarithromycin (Biaxin) is effective against streptococcus and *S. pneumoniae*. Doses are 15 mg/kg per day in two divided doses.

Azithromycin (Zithromax) is effective against *H. influenzae, Moraxella, Staphylococcus* and *Streptococcus*.

If chest tightness and wheezing are present, metaproterenol or albuterol inhaler, two puffs q 4 hours, should be used.

To decrease respiratory problems, avoid bronchial irritants such as smoke.

Follow-up: Return visit if no improvement occurs in 72 hours, fever increases, or pleuritic pain develops.

Sequelae: Bronchitis can progress to more serious infections, such as pneumonia, but most cases resolve with no future problems.

Prevention/Prophylaxis: Avoid contact with persons with URIs.

Referral: Referral should be made if there is significant respiratory distress or failure to improve within 72 hours.

Education: To avoid progression of the disease, parents should be encouraged to report respiratory problems to health-care providers. Most of the time treatment is symptomatic; therefore, response needs to be monitored. Because bronchitis is usually caused by a viral infection, parents need to understand that antibiotics are not always needed.

Influenza

Influenza—an acute, contagious, viral illness—often occurs in epidemics. This disease is characterized by fever, malaise, myalgia, and respiratory symptoms.

Etiology: Caused by one of three myxoviruses having similar properties and categorized as influenza virus types A, B, and C. Influenza A viruses have shown an unusual ability to mutate, resulting in new antigenic strains that frequently produce worldwide epidemics.

Occurrence: Every 4–7 years.

Age: All ages.

Ethnicity: Not significant.

Gender: Occurs equally in males and females.

Contributing Factors: Epidemics occur usually in cooler weather and during the rainy season in the tropics.

Signs and Symptoms: Parents report that the child complains of a headache, malaise, lassitude, and occasional prostration. Some vomiting and diarrhea may be reported in young children. There will be a complaint of generalized myalgia. Clear nasal drainage is also noted. A nonproductive cough will be heard. Photophobia is often noted. Fever, often 102–103°F, will be present. Rhonchi and occasionally scattered rales will be auscultated. A rapid, weak pulse may be seen if myocarditis is present.

Diagnostic Tests: None.

Differential Diagnosis

Other viral respiratory infections, including *RSV,* are differentiated by a positive RSV test.

The symptoms of the common cold are much less severe, with fever less than 102°F.

Croup is differentiated by the classic barking cough, normal or only slightly elevated temperatures, and absence of generalized aching in joints.

Bacterial URIs cause elevated WBCs, with an increased band count and granulocytes; this does not occur in influenza.

Treatment

Symmetrel (given to children aged 1–9 in a dose of 5 mg/kg per day; maximum dose 150 mg/day) may decrease the severity of symptoms.

Acetaminophen (given to children over 10 years; children less than 40 kg receive 5 mg/kg day; children more than 40 kg receive 200 mg/day) may be given for fever.

Flumadine (100 mg bid for 5 days) is indicated for prophylaxis against influenza A in children over 12.

Fluid intake should be increased to help liquefy secretions.

A mild cough suppressant, such as guaifenesin plus dextromethorphan hydrobromide (Robitussin-DM) may be given to help the child rest and decrease the frequency of coughing spells.

Follow-up: As indicated. Generally the child should be seen within 2 weeks for follow-up to check for resolution of symptoms; the child should be seen sooner if condition worsens.

Sequelae: Influenza pneumonia and/or secondary bacterial pneumonia may be seen if disease progresses. Encephalitis and myocarditis rarely occur unless there is an underlying pathology or influenza is unresponsive to treatment.

Prevention/Prophylaxis: Children should avoid close contact with other children exhibiting flulike symptoms. Parents should consider keeping children home from day-care centers during epidemics. When appropriate, give influenza virus vaccine.

Referral: Refer to a pediatrician if patient is severely ill, experiences respiratory distress, or has widespread rales or rhonchi on physical examination. Pregnant patients should be referred to their Ob/Gyn physician.

Education: Parents should be taught that the disease is generally self-limiting. Symptoms should be treated as needed; worsening of symptoms may indicate progression of disease, requiring referral to a physician.

Pneumonia

Pneumonia, an infectious disease of the lower respiratory tract, can be classified in two ways—by the area it affects or by its cause. Classified by area, it can be subclassified as lobar, interstitial, and bronchopulmonary. Classified by cause, it can be subclassified as viral, bacterial, or aspiration. Pneumonia affects the lungs by altering normal lung secretions, inhibiting phagocytosis, changing the normal bacterial flora of the lungs, and disrupting the epithelial layer of the lungs. Children who have immunocompromised systems or chronic lung problems are often more susceptible to these infections.

Etiology: *S. pneumoniae* is estimated to cause approximately 90% of all bacterial pneumonia. Other bacterial agents that cause pneumonia include *Pneumococcus, Staphylococcus, H. influenzae, Klebsiella, Pseudomonas aeruginosa,* and *Mycobacterium tuberculosis.* Viral agents include cytomegalovirus and influenza virus. *Pneumocystis carinii, Coxiella burnetii, Mycoplasma pneumoniae, Treponema pallidum, Chlamydia,* and *Chlamydia psittaci* are still other causes. Finally, mycotic agents include *Aspergillus, Histoplasma, Candida,* and *Blastomyces.* Aspiration (e.g., amniotic fluids, food, foreign bodies, lipids or hydrocarbons) is still another cause of pneumonia.

Occurrence

		Incidence
Bacterial	Commonly acquired	1200/100,000
	Nosocomial	800/100,000
Mycoplasma	Commonly acquired	130/100,000
Viral	Nosocomial	60/100,000

Age: Can occur at any time, but children under 4 are more likely to acquire bacterial pneumonia. Mycoplasmal pneumonia is more likely to occur in children over 5.

Ethnicity: Not significant.

Gender: Occurs equally in males and females.

Contributing Factors: Chronic lung diseases, human immunodeficiency virus (HIV) infection (in infants), any other problem related to defects in swallowing or airway clearance, or altered secretions of the lung may increase the risk of pneumonia. Neonates born to mothers infected with *Chlamydia trachomatis* are at increased risk for this type of pneumonia. Bacterial pneumonia is more prevalent among persons living in overcrowded conditions.

Signs and Symptoms: In infants and young children with pneumonia, there will usually be a report of rhinitis or a stuffy nose, fever (up to 104°F), decreased appetite, cough, and restlessness accompanied by chills or shaking. For the older child and adolescent, there is a brief period of symptoms including a mild URI followed by the sudden onset of chills and a high fever. There will be a report of alternating periods of restlessness and sleepiness; a dry, hacking cough; and decreased appetite.

In chlamydial pneumonia in infants, there will be no fever but there may be a report of previous conjunctivitis. In viral pneumonia, there will be a slower, less dramatic progression of symptoms. Other facts may be given, such as a history of chronic lung or respiratory tract illnesses, exposure to another person with similar symptoms, HIV-positive history, or aspiration of a foreign body.

The infant with bacterial pneumonia appears ill, having nasal flaring, retractions, and grunting. Tachypnea and cyanosis may also be observed. There may be abdominal distention. Some nuchal rigidity is noted, indicating right upper lobe involvement but not meningitis. For the older child, retractions may also be noted with a splinting effect on the affected side. There may be circumoral cyanosis if the disease is severe. In bacterial pneumonia, there are fine crackling rales and diminished breath sounds over the area of the pneumonia.

In viral pneumonia, there is marked tachypnea, cough, and retractions. There are also rales, wheezing, and diminished breath sounds. If the causative agent is mycoplasmal pneumonia, the patient will have general symptoms of a URI—dry, hacking cough; sometimes a sore throat; and a fever. Infants with chlamydial pneumonia will have a repetitive cough, tachypnea, and air hunger, and, in some cases, conjunctivitis. In chlamydial pneumonia, rales are heard, but wheezing is a rare finding.

In mycoplasmal pneumonia, there are harsh breath sounds and rhonchi.

Diagnostic Tests: In bacterial pneumonia there is leukocytosis with a shift to the left. ABGs reveal hypoxemia. Blood cultures are positive for the specific agent. Chest x-ray will be diagnostically significant, showing lobar consolidation. In staphylococcal pneumonia, the right lobes are affected about 65% of the time. Nasopharyngeal swabs should also be taken. In mycoplasmal pneumonia, x-ray reveals increased bronchovascular markings and possible areas of atelectasis. In chlamydial pneumonia, x-ray findings may be consistent with hyperinflation of the lungs with diffuse infiltrates. The eosinophil count is 300–400/mm^3, with elevated IgM and IgG. In viral pneumonia, chest x-ray reveals patchy bronchopneumonia.

Differential Diagnosis

RSV in infants is differentiated by an RSV-positive nasopharyngeal swab.

Tuberculosis is differentiated by positive sputum cultures or chest x-ray.

Acute bronchiectasis due to aspiration of a foreign body may be detected on x-ray, but in small children this often necessitates consultation so that a bronchoscopy can be performed.

Because of the pain in the right lower quadrant of the abdomen, right lobar pneumonia may be confused with appendicitis; x-rays help differentiate this diagnosis.

Viral, fungal, and bacterial pneumonia can be differentiated with the appropriate cultures of nasopharyngeal secretions, sputum, or blood.

Treatment: Treatment depends on determination of the causative agent. For bacterial pneumonia, penicillin, methicillin, cefuroxime, and gentamycin are the drugs of choice. For viral pneumonia, supportive treatment of symptoms is all that is required. Erythromycin and TMP-SMX can be used for children who are allergic to penicillin. Erythromycin is used for mycoplasma and chlamydial pneumonia. Often humidified oxygen is used for infants; when necessary, supplemental oxygen is used for the child with severe hypoxemia. Intravenous fluids are used for any child who requires hospitalization and is not receiving the required amount of fluids by mouth. Specific doses of medications are found in Table 8–7.

Follow-up: A follow-up x-ray will probably not show significant improvement for about 6 weeks; therefore the x-ray should be done at that time. Repeat cultures are not necessary unless the child's symptoms worsen; then the cultures are done to see whether a new, previously unidentified bacterial infection is present. If the patient is treated on an outpatient basis, there should be close contact (every day or every other day) with the health-care provider.

Sequelae: Overall mortality rate is about 5%. In the otherwise healthy child or adult, improvement is noted within 1–3 days. Those with the poorest outcomes are the very young or the immunocompromised.

Possible complications include empyema, pulmonary abscess, pericarditis, pleurisy, and superinfections. A protracted course can occur when positive cultures are obtained or if the sensitivity and effectiveness of the medications are not adequate.

Prevention/Prophylaxis: Children considered at high risk for pneumonia (e.g., those with chronic lung disease, immunocompromise) should be given a yearly influenza immunization. A pneumococcal vaccine (Pneumovax) should also be given to all children who are over 2 and included in a high-risk group.

Referral: Refer when aspiration of a foreign object is suspected so that the child can undergo bronchoscopy to rule this out. Also, all children in a high-risk group should be referred to a pediatrician. Children requiring hospitalization should be treated collaboratively with a pediatrician.

Education: All parents of children who are at increased risk for serious complications should be taught the importance of immunizations to decrease or eliminate the possibility of pneumonia. Also, if a child is seen with a mild URI, parents should be taught when to bring the child back and what specific signs and symptoms may indicate that the disease is progressing. The importance of giving all medications on schedule and completing the course of therapy also should be stressed.

TABLE 8–7 COMMON ANTIBIOTIC THERAPY FOR PNEUMONIA

Medication	Dose	Causative Agent
Penicillin G	100,000 units/kg/day	*Streptococcus pneumoniae* or β-hemolytic streptococcus
	600,000 units IM followed by oral penicillin	
Erythromycin	30–50 mg/kg/day PO in divided doses qid	Penicillin-resistant patients
	15–20 mg/kg/day IV in divided doses q 4 or 6 hours	
Methicillin	200 mg/kg/day IV	*Staphylococcus aureus*
Cefuroxime	100 mg/kg/day	*Haemophilus influenzae*
Gentamycin	2.0–2.5 mg/kg IM or IV q 8 hr (if <1 week, q 12 hr)	*Pseudomonas, Escherichia coli*
		Klebsiella, Enterobacter, Staphylococcus
Trimethoprim-sulfamethoxazole	15 mg/kg/day in 3 divided doses	*Pneumocystis carinii*
Erythromycin	500 mg q 6 hr × 10–14 days if >9 years; 30–50 mg/kg/day for 10–14 days, if <9 years of age	*Mycoplasma Chlamydia*

Respiratory Syncytial Virus

RSV infection, an acute respiratory illness, is the most serious cause of bronchiolitis and pneumonia in infants and young children. Adults with RSV have minor symptoms of an upper respiratory tract illness. In infants and children, the symptoms may initially be minimal, but can progress to major signs requiring hospitalization and highly specialized treatment.

Etiology: This disease is caused by RSV, a large ribonucleic acid (RNA) virus seen in two major strains, A and B, usually occurring together. It is spread by human contact, namely exposure to infected droplets that are aerosolized. Incubation ranges from 2 to 8 days.

Occurrence: Annual epidemics are seen generally in the winter and early spring.

Age: Initial infection generally occurs in the first year of life.

Ethnicity: Not significant.

Gender: More prevalent in boys, by a ratio of 1.5 : 1.

Contributing Factors: Exposure to symptomatic or nonsymptomatic infected persons causes the disease. Nosocomial infection in hospitals often occurs during epidemics.

Signs and Symptoms: Mild to severe respiratory symptoms are reported. Other symptoms seen are lethargy, irritability, poor feeding, and apneic spells. Auscultation reveals diffuse rhonchi, fine rales, and wheezing. Chest x-rays are usually normal. Signs that the disease is severe include compromised cardiac, pulmonary, or immune function. Children with RSV exhibiting significant or severe symptoms should be hospitalized.

Diagnostic Tests: Nasopharyngeal cultures reveal the presence of RSV. If the disease is becoming exacerbated, a chest x-ray should also be obtained to detect pneumonia. WBC count is sometimes elevated, with a possible shift to the right or left. Blood cultures usually grow normal flora.

Differential Diagnosis

Bronchitis has a more insidious onset, with no wheezing or fever, and occurs in slightly older children.
Asthma is differentiated by increased wheezing and past history.
Pneumonia is a febrile illness with little or no wheezing.
Croup is characterized by a barking cough.

Treatment: Treatment should be given for symptoms; patients who exhibit respiratory distress should be hospitalized. Humidified oxygen with nebulization treatments should also be considered. Respiratory isolation should be instituted. Ribavirin, which is used only in severe cases for hospitalized patients, is administered by small-particle aerosol for 12–20 hours each day for 3–5 days.

Follow-up: For the hospitalized child, follow-up should occur 10–14 days after discharge.

Sequelae: Bronchitis, pneumonia, or even death have been reported.

Prevention/Prophylaxis: Control of nosocomial RSV is complicated because there is a continued chance of introduction of the virus by others not exhibiting any symptoms. Avoidance of contact with persons who may have the virus is perhaps the only control.

Referral: A child who continues to worsen after 24 hours of treatment should be referred to a pediatrician or pediatric pulmonologist.

Education: Parents should be taught the early signs of respiratory problems so they can seek early treatment and the appropriate diagnoses. Also, avoidance of contact with children who are known to be RSV-positive should be stressed.

Tuberculosis

TB is an infectious, inflammatory disease primarily affecting the lungs and is chronic in nature. Because of the danger TB poses to the community, it is a reportable disease, and when it is diagnosed, the health-care provider is mandated to report the case and all contacts to the local health department. Although the lung is the primary site, other sites are affected; in fact, the bacilli can lodge in any organ of the body. In the United States, the most common mode of transmission is inhalation of infected droplet nuclei. In other parts of the world, bovine spread is more common.

Etiology: The most common causative agent is *Mycobacterium tuberculosis.* Other more atypical causes are *M. bovis, M. avium, M. intracellulare, M. kansasii, M. simiae,* and *M. szulgai.*

Occurrence: Approximately 7.5 million cases of TB were reported in 1990; the incidence is growing. The World Health Organization has predicted that 4.5 million children will die of TB in this decade.

Age: Any age, but recent reports indicate that children under 15 years are at greater risk.

Ethnicity: Incidence is greater in nonwhite racial and ethnic minorities.

Gender: Occurs equally in males and females.

Contributing Factors: HIV, increasing world poverty, living in urban areas, and living in areas in Asia and Africa increase the likelihood of contracting TB. Other factors include chronic illness, diabetes, renal failure, advanced age, occupation (health-care workers), and race.

Signs and Symptoms: The primary caregiver may relate that the child has been in contact with someone who was diagnosed with TB. There may be reports of coughing, weight loss, and night sweats. Most children are asymptomatic, and therefore the diagnosis is accomplished by skin testing and chest x-ray. Infants, however, will have failure to thrive, coughing, fever, and rales. Children who have hypertension also exhibit significant pulmonary signs.

No obvious signs are seen except in infants, who look frail and exhibit signs of failure to thrive. Lymphadenopathy is the most common finding in children. Auscultation may reveal rhonchi, rales, or silence—indicating atelectasis. Because few overall symptoms or signs are seen, heard, or felt, a chest x-ray should be done to confirm the diagnosis.

Diagnostic Tests: The Mantoux purified protein derivative test (PPD) is the preferred test. It should be read in 48–72 hours and is considered positive when the area of induration is at least 15 mm. If the child is immunocompromised or HIV-positive, a reading of 10 mm or less is positive. An x-ray including a posterior, anterior, and lateral view should be taken if the child is positive or if a known exposure has been recognized. Sputum cultures are often negative for acid-fast bacilli in children.

Differential Diagnosis

Fatigue is related to disrupted sleep patterns.
Pneumonia is determined by x-ray and serum blood cultures that are negative for TB indicators.
Failure to thrive has a negative chest x-ray or PPD.

HIV is differentiated by Western blot and enzyme-linked immunosorbent assay (ELISA) tests, as well as viral load counts.

Treatment

Table 8–8 lists common dosages for TB drugs.

The routine regimen is isoniazid and rifampin for 4 months, and pyrazinamide for 2 months. If isoniazid resistance is known, Ethambutol or streptomycin may be used. When isoniazid or rifampin cannot be used because of demonstrated resistance, therapy is extended from 6 months to 12 months.

Directly observed therapy, which means that the health-care provider directly observes the patient taking the medicine, is the most effective therapy.

Follow-up: Children diagnosed with TB should have yearly chest x-rays taken.

Sequelae: In children under 6, tuberculous meningitis can occur 2–6 months after a diagnosis of TB. Tuberculomas (space-occupying lesions), bone and joint infections, and superficial lymphadenitis may also occur. Ultimately, TB can cause death.

TABLE 8–8 TUBERCULOSIS MEDICATIONS FOR CHILDREN

Drug	Dose	Adverse Reactions
Isoniazid	10–15 mg/kg/day *or* 20–40 mg/kg twice weekly	SGOT, SGPT Hepatitis Peripheral neuritis Hypersensitivity
Rifampin	10–20 mg/kg/day *or* 10–20 mg/kg twice weekly	Orange urine and bodily secretions Vomiting Hepatitis Thrombocytopenia Staining of contact lenses May inactivate birth-control pills
Pyrazinamide	20–40 mg/kg/day *or* 50–70 mg/kg twice weekly	Hepatotoxicity Hyperuricemia
Streptomycin (IM ONLY)	20–40 mg/kg/day *or* 20–40 mg/kg twice weekly	Ototoxicity Nephrotoxicity Skin rash
Ethambutol	15–25 mg/kg/day *or* 50 mg/kg twice weekly	Visual acuity Gastrointestinal disturbances Reversible optic neuritis

SGOT = serum glutamic oxaloacetic acid; SGPT = serum glutamic pyruvic transaminase.

Prevention/Prophylaxis: TB skin testing should be performed yearly on all children beginning at age 12 months. In a person who has signs and symptoms of TB, has had recent contact with a person with TB, has HIV or other chronic debilitating illness, or has recently immigrated to this country from Asia, Africa, Latin America, or Oceania, testing should be done at least every 6 months.

Referral: A physician should be consulted if there are signs of drug resistance or worsening of the condition.

Education: Communities and parents should be educated regarding the prevalence of TB. There has been a loss of vigilance regarding TB, but as poverty and HIV increase in children, there needs to be active participation of family and community in seeking out routine screening for all children and adults.

The importance of taking medicines according to the prescribed schedule should be stressed, as should the need for patients and families to reveal all contacts.

REFERENCES

General

Berhman, R, and Kleigman, R: Nelson's Essentials of Pediatrics. WB Saunders, Philadelphia, 1990.
Berman S: Pediatric Decision Making. BC Decker, Philadelphia, 1991.
Doenges, M, and Moorhouse, M: Nurses' Pocket Guide: Nursing Diagnoses with Interventions, ed 5. FA Davis, Philadelphia, 1995.
Fishman, A: Pulmonary Diseases and Disorders, ed 2. McGraw-Hill, New York, 1988.
Gessner, I, and Victoria, B: Pediatric Cardiology. WB Saunders, Philadelphia, 1993.
Green, M: Pediatric Diagnosis, ed 5. WB Saunders, Philadelphia, 1992.
Hoole, A: Patient Guidelines for Nurse Practitioners, ed 4. JB Lippincott, Philadelphia, 1995.
Jacobs, R: General problems in infectious diseases. In Tiernay LM, et al (eds): Current Medical Diagnosis and Treatment. Appleton-Lange, Norwalk, Conn, 1995, pp 1098–1099.
Krugman, S, et al: Infectious Diseases of Children. Mosby, St. Louis, 1992.
Nadas, A: Congenital heart disease. In Current Pediatric Therapy. WB Saunders, Philadelphia, 1990.
Peter, G, et al: The 1994 Red Book: Report of the Committee on Infectious Diseases. American Academy of Pediatrics, Elk Grove Village, Ill, 1994.

Chest Wall Trauma

Andrews, J: Difficult diagnoses in blunt thoraco-abdominal trauma. J Emerg Nurs 15(9):399, 1989.
Arajurvi, E, and Santavista, C: Chest injuries sustained in severe traffic accidents by seatbelt wearers. J Trauma 29(1):37, 1989.
Hammond, G: Chest injuries in the trauma patient. Nurs Clin North Am 3(25):35, 1990.
Lashowski-Jones, L: Meeting the challenge of chest trauma. Am J Nurs 95(9):22, 1995.
Pate, J: Chest wall injuries. Surg Clin North Am 69:59, 1989.

Congenital Cardiac Defects

Driscoll, D: Evaluation of the cyanotic newborn. Pediatr Clin North Am 37:1, 1990.
Hohn, A: Congenital heart disease—the first test. West J Med 156:435, 1992.
Lees, M, and King, J: Cyanosis in the newborn. Pediatr Rev 9:36, 1987.
Monett, Z, and Moynihan, P: Cardiovascular assessment of the neonatal heart. J Perinat Neonat Nurs 5(2):50, 1991.
Moss, A: Clues in diagnosing congenital heart disease. West J Med 156:392, 1992.

Norris, M, and Hill, C: Assessing congenital heart defects in the cocaine exposed neonate. Dimensions Crit Care Nurs 11(1):6, 1992.

Quinlan, W, et al: Congenital heart disease: Dr. Robert Anderson's systematic, sequential, analysis of morphologic features. Heart Lung 17(1):90, 1988.

Sapire, D: Understanding and diagnosing pediatric heart disease. Appleton-Lange, Norwalk, Conn, 1991.

Ventricular Septal Defect

Allen, H, et al: Heart murmur in children: When is a workup needed? Contemp Pediatr 11:31, 1994.

Carter, C, and Strauss, A: Cardiomyopathies: When to think of congenital causes. Contemp Pediatr 12:25, 1995.

Gessner, I, and Victoria, B: Pediatric Cardiology. WB Saunders, Philadelphia, 1993.

Hypertension

Adelman, RD: The hypertensive neonate. Clin Perinatol 15:567, 1988.

Barker, L, et al: Principles of ambulatory medicine, ed 4. Williams & Wilkins, Baltimore, 1993.

Coody, D, et al: Hypertension in children. J Pediatr Health Care 9:3, 1995.

Nadas, A: Congenital heart disease. In Current Pediatric Therapy. WB Saunders, Philadelphia, 1990.

Report of the Task Force on Blood Pressure Control in Children: Pediatrics 89:525, 1987.

Kawasaki Syndrome

Faubert, K, et al: A U.S. nationwide hospital survey of Kawasaki's disease and acute rheumatic fever. J Pediatr 119:279, 1991.

Fuit, L: Keeping up with Kawasaki syndrome. Contemp Pediatr 12:37, 1995.

Rheumatic Fever

Gooch, M: Alternatives to penicillin in the management of group A beta hemolytic streptococcus pharyngitis. Pediatr Ann 810, 1992.

Hollister, J: Rheumatic diseases. In Hay WW, et al (eds): Current Pediatric Diagnosis and Treatment, ed 12. Appleton & Lange, Norwalk, Conn, 1994.

Hosier, D, et al: Resurgence of rheumatic fever. Am J Disabled Child 141:730, 1989.

Markowitz, M, and Kaplan, E: Reappearance of rheumatic fever. Adv Pediatr 36:39, 1989.

Syncope

Almquist, A, et al: Provocation of bradycardia and hypotension by isoproterenol and upright posture in patients with unexplained syncope. New Engl J Med 320:346, 1989.

Hardy, C: Syncope and chest pain: To worry or not? Contemp Pediatr 11:19, 1994.

Rickman, R: Cardiac causes of syncope. Pediatr Rev 9:101, 1987.

Apparent Life-Threatening Event

American Academy of Pediatrics Task Force on Infant Positioning and SIDS: Positioning and SIDS. Pediatrics 89:1120, 1992.

Peter, G, et al: The 1994 Red Book: Report of the Committee on Infectious Diseases. American Academy of Pediatrics, Elk Grove Village, Ill, 1994.

Richard, R: Current Concepts: Sudden Death from Cardiac Causes in Children and Young Adults. Liberthson Source information from Harvard Medical School and Massachusetts General Hospital, Boston, Mass.

Asthma

Capen, C, et al: The team approach to pediatric asthma education. Pediatr Nurs 20:231, 1994.

Ferrante, S, and Painter, E: Continuous nebulization: A treatment modality for pediatric asthma patients. Pediatr Nurs 21(4):327, 1995.

Heermann, JA, and Wills, LM: Effect of problem solving instruction and health focus of control on the management of childhood asthma. Children's Health Care 21:76, 1992.

Kalinger, MA, et al: Asthma therapy: Into the 1990's. Patient Care 69:100, 1992.

Keenan, JM: Nedocromil: A new agent for the treatment of asthma in children. Am Fam 50:1059, 1994.

Moffitt, JE, et al: Management of asthma in children. Am Fam 50:1039, 1994.

Rachelefsky, G: Asthma update: New approaches and partnerships. J Pediatr Health Care 9:12, 1995.

Rachelefsky, G, et al: An update on the diagnosis and management of pediatric asthma. Nurse Pract 18:51, 1993.

Bronchitis

Crista, JR: Croup and related disorders. Pediatr Rev 14:19, 1993.

Urbach, A: What's behind that chronic cough: Contemp Pediatr 9:106,1993.

Welliver, J, and Welliver, R: Bronchiolitis. Pediatr Rev 14:134, 1993.

Pneumonia

Cassiere, H, et al: Delayed resolution of pneumonia: When healing is too slow. Postgrad Med 99:152, 1996.

Cunha, B: Community acquired pneumonia: Cost effective antimicrobial therapy. Postgrad Med 99:109, 1996.

File, T, et al: Community acquired pneumonia: What's needed for accurate diagnosis? Postgrad Med 9:95, 1996.

Levision, M: Pneumonia: Choosing empiric therapy. Patient Care 26:10, 1992.

Respiratory Syncytial Virus

Hall, C: Respiratory syncytial virus: What we know now. Contemp Pediatr 10:92, 1993.

Jondres, L: Respiratory syncytial virus infections. J Pediatr Health Care 8:277, 1994.

Tristnam, D, and Welliver, R: A vaccine for RSV: Is it possible? Contemp Pediatr 13:47, 1996.

Tuberculosis

Anon, P: Tuberculosis in children. Proceedings from the R.W. Johnson Workshop on Tuberculosis in Children. R.W. Johnson Foundation, Princeton, NJ, 1994, pp 2–32.

Peloquin, C, and Berning, S: Tuberculosis and multi-drug resistant tuberculosis in children. Pediatr Nurs 21:566, 1995.

Petue, G: The 1994 Red Book: Report of the Committee on Infectious Diseases. American Academy of Pediatrics, Elk Grove Village, Ill, 1994.

CHAPTER 9

ABDOMINAL

ASSESSMENT

Techniques of inspection, auscultation, percussion, and palpation specific for the abdomen may be used to evaluate abdominal disorders. In some cases, a rectal examination may be necessary

Young children may be examined in the mother's lap; in the very young, flexing the legs will help make the abdomen more relaxed. Using a pacifier to comfort a crying baby can make the examination easier. As the nurse practitioner (NP) begins the abdominal examination, older children, particularly if they are experiencing abdominal discomfort, benefit from the use of distraction and breathing techniques.

Assessment of the abdomen is done over the four abdominal quadrants because each quadrant contains specific structures. As the NP listens to the patient's history and palpates and auscultates the abdomen, he or she must be aware of which organs are located within each quadrant. It is easier to palpate the organs in children because the abdominal wall is less muscular. In children, the liver is larger and the urinary bladder is higher in the abdomen compared to adults.

In children, the most common symptoms of abdominal disease are nausea and vomiting, distention, change in bowel patterns, pruritus, and pain. Thus an appropriate history should explain the specific symptom in detail. The quality and location of pain is an important clue to the underlying cause (Fig. 9–1). Illness that induces vomiting may demonstrate specific characteristic patterns.

Remember to auscultate first and to examine the area of maximal pain last to prevent tightening of the abdominal muscles, which will make the examination more difficult. Because children do not always like to be touched, sometimes having them place a hand under the hand of the examiner facilitates the

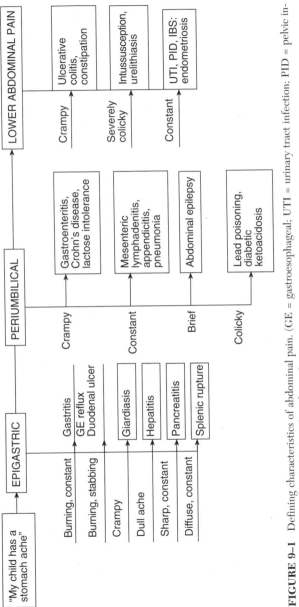

FIGURE 9–1 Defining characteristics of abdominal pain. (GE = gastroesophageal; UTI = urinary tract infection; PID = pelvic in-flammatory disease; IBS = irritable bowel syndrome.)

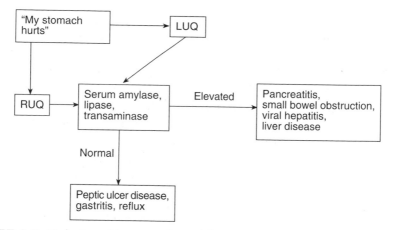

FIGURE 9-2 Evaluation of upper quadrant abdominal pain. (RUQ = right upper quadrant; LUQ = left upper quadrant.)

examination. Do not percuss over the area of the spleen. Watch and listen to the child for changes in crying, grimacing, or moving away from your hand, all of which are possible objective signs of abdominal tenderness (Fig. 9-2).

Intestinal parasites are not as common as they were a century ago. However, in disadvantaged areas in the United States and in developing countries, parasites are a common cause of gastrointestinal (GI) symptomatology. Telephone consultation is available from the Centers for Disease Control, Atlanta, Georgia (see Appendix).

Children have been taught, and rightly so, that it is not correct to allow "strangers" to examine their bottoms. Reassurance that the health-care provider is not a stranger in that sense helps make an examination of the rectal area more acceptable for the child. Preadolescent children are becoming aware of their bodies; therefore the proper use of drapes will do much to ease their embarrassment during the examination.

Ascariasis

Ascariasis is the infestation of the body by the parasite *Ascaris lumbricoides* due to accidental ingestion of the eggs.

Etiology: Ingestion of parasitic eggs through contaminated food, water, or dirt.

Occurrence: Common in endemic areas (Southern states).

Age: Usually seen in toddlers.

Ethnicity: Not significant.

Gender: Occurs equally in males and females.

Contributing Factors: Associated with day-care centers, infected pets, asymptomatic carriers, and travel to endemic areas.

Signs and Symptoms: Child presents with a cough, abdominal discomfort, or bloating depending on the stage of development of the parasite:

Pulmonary: Cough, blood-tinged sputum, and transient infiltrates on the lung (due to larvae migrating through the lung in the developmental processes.

Intestinal: abdominal discomfort and distention.

Sometimes the parent has observed the passage of the worms, either in the stool or in the sputum.

Diagnostic Tests

Stools for ova, cysts, and parasites (OCP). Stool samples will test positive for eggs.

Complete blood count (CBC). Eosinophil count may be elevated.

Differential Diagnosis

In *appendicitis,* white blood cell (WBC) count is elevated (greater than 15,000 cells/mm^3), neutrophils are elevated, and the patient presents with vomiting.

In *biliary colic,* pain is crampy and primarily in the right upper quadrant (RUQ); there is also occasional jaundice.

Treatment

Pharmacological

Pyrantel pamoate, 11 mg/kg single dose (maximum 1 g)

or

Mebendazole, 100 mg bid for 3 days.

Follow-up: Reevaluate in 2 weeks and perform a recheck stool examination.

Sequelae: Biliary obstruction due to migration of the worms to the biliary duct is rare, as is intestinal obstruction.

Prevention/Prophylaxis: Prevention may be enhanced by wearing shoes, not allowing children to play in possibly contaminated areas, and providing for adequate disposal of fecal material.

Referral: None.

Education: Instruct in proper handwashing techniques and disposal of fecal material.

Constipation

Constipation, the infrequent passage of dry, hard stools can be categorized into four types:

Organic (structural and disease-oriented).
Nonorganic (functional or retentive).
Dietary.
Related to drug or cathartic abuse.

Normal stool frequency for infants is as many as five stools per day to one stool every third day.

Etiology: There are varied causes for constipation (Fig. 9–3).

Organic causes include structural defects, such as spinal cord lesions and anorectal anatomical variances. Persons with hypothyroidism, hypercalcemia, or mental retardation are known to have constipation.

Nonorganic causes of retentive constipation include social factors such as lack of privacy at school, anxiety created by social events, and the development of the ability to ignore the sensation of rectal fullness.

Dietary causes are related primarily to excessive intake of milk and lack of bulk in the diet.

Drug and cathartic abuse is related to the intake of medications such as iron supplements, codeine, and theophylline.

Occurrence: Common.

Age: Occurs in all age groups.

Ethnicity: Ethnicity is not significant.

Gender: More common in males than females.

Contributing Factors: Psychological factors such as holding in anger, toilet training techniques, and diet all may contribute to constipation.

Signs and Symptoms: Child presents to clinic with the complaint of no stools for a variable number of days, straining at stool, and possibly blood-tinged stool. Investigate the child's usual bowel pattern and the changes noted that caused the office visit. Obtain a history of diet and medicines taken. Findings reveal a normal abdomen or one with mild distention. Abdominal palpation reveals a firm colonic mass. Rectal examination reveals firm to hard stool in the rectum. Rectal and perineal examinations reveal anal fissures, perianal abscesses, and diaper dermatitis, all of which may make it painful to pass stools.

Diagnostic Tests: None. Flat plate (x-ray) of the abdomen or kidney, ureter, and bladder (KUB) may reveal retained stool or signs of obstruction. For intractable constipation, refer patient for colonic manometry.

Differential Diagnosis

Aganglionic megacolon (Hirschsprung's disease) causes small, ribbonlike stools; rectal examination reveals no stool in the rectum.

Intestinal obstruction is suggested when a child is experiencing bile-colored vomitus and severe abdominal pain.

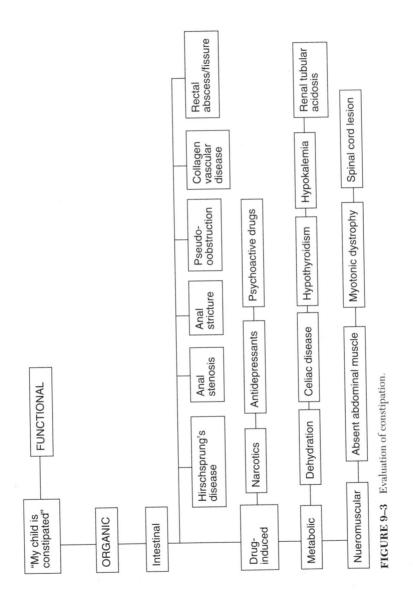

FIGURE 9–3 Evaluation of constipation.

Treatment: Treatment is focused on the suspected or identified underlying cause.

Nonpharmacological

Dietary causes may be treated by (1) increasing the intake of fluids, and (2) increasing bulk by adding fruits and vegetables (e.g., prune juice, tomatoes, olive oil, green vegetables). Manual removal of the impacted stool is another nonpharmacological alternative.

Pharmacological

Glycerin rectal suppositories to facilitate the passage of stool.
Bisacodyl (Dulcolax) suppository to aid in passage of stool (use one time).
Pediatric Fleet Enema to help pass a hard stool (use one time).
Mineral oil, 15 mL by mouth (PO), as a stool softener and to facilitate passage.

Follow-up: If no bowel movement in 2–3 days, return to clinic for further evaluation.

Sequelae: Chronic stool retention with increasing reliance on laxatives; anal fissures and fistulas.

Prevention/Prophylaxis: Changes in usual diet, fluid intake, and increased exercise are usually effective.

Referral: In cases of chronic constipation and/or fecal impaction, refer patient to the primary physician or psychiatrist.

Education: Instruct parents about normal bowel habits. Teach parents how to make dietary changes and when to become concerned about changes in their child's bowel habits.

Diarrhea

Diarrhea is an increase in the frequency, water content, and volume of feces that involves secretory, osmotic, and inflammatory processes. Causative agents may be viral, bacterial, or chemical, or the condition may be concomitant with other conditions; diarrhea may be accompanied by vomiting.

Etiology: Hand-to-mouth contact with viruses similar to rotavirus, adenovirus, echovirus, coxsackievirus, or parvovirus; or with enterotoxin-producing strains of *Escherichia coli*, cholera, *Clostridium perfringens*, *Staphylococcus* or *Yersinia*; or with nonentertoxin-producing bacteria, such as *Salmonella*, *Shigella*, and other strains of *E. coli*. Parasitic infections with *Entamoeba histolytica* and *Giardia lamblia* cause diarrhea. Common drugs that cause diarrhea are antibiotics and laxatives. Illnesses that may present with diarrhea are otitis media, urinary tract infection (UTI), and pneumonia. Neoplasms, aganglionic megacolon, and endocrinopathies are often accompanied by diarrhea.

Occurrence: Common; by the age of 3 years, a child will have had one to three episodes.

Age: All age groups.

Ethnicity: Not significant.

Gender: Occurs equally in males and females.

Contributing Factors: Environmental factors, such as exposure to others with the illness; and poor hygienic measures, such as inadequate handwashing by caregivers.

Signs and Symptoms: Child presents with a complaint of diarrhea. History includes a description of illness; onset, amount, number, color, and frequency of stools; presence of blood or mucus in the stool; and presence of fever or vomiting. Fluid intake and urinary output are explored. History of rash and other symptoms are investigated, as is history of exposure to similar illnesses (Fig. 9–4).

Findings may reveal generalized abdominal tenderness and hyperactive bowel sounds. Rebound tenderness indicates the possibility of appendicitis or peritonitis. If dehydrated, the child may be listless and lethargic, with dry mucous membranes, poor skin turgor, and weight loss.

Diagnostic Tests: None for diarrhea. Tests are ordered, if warranted, to determine the *cause* of diarrhea.

Stool cultures are indicated by the presence of blood or blood-tinged mucus in the stool, diarrhea lasting longer than 5 days, fever greater than 102°F, and the presence of a family or closed-population outbreak.

WBCs in the stool may be detected with a Wright's stain. Stool testing for occult blood.

A urinalysis with specific gravity to evaluate dehydration.

A stool for OCP if history warrants.

A WBC to assess for cause, whether viral or bacterial.

Differential Diagnosis

Intussusception: Characteristic acute onset, RUQ pain, and currant jelly–colored stools.

Appendicitis: In children, localized or point tenderness is diagnostically significant. Children with appendicitis often walk with a limp and lie with the right leg flexed; hyperextension of the right leg is painful (psoas sign).

Treatment: The goal is to restore and maintain fluid and electrolyte status.

Nonpharmacological

First 12 hours: If infant is breastfeeding, the mother should maintain infant at breast, but discontinue any supplemental feedings and give clear liquids. For older infants, parents should discontinue diet and formula, and give small amounts of clear liquids (e.g., water, Gatorade, Pedialyte, Kool Aid, ginger ale). Parents should offer liquids every 3–4 hours if child is not vomiting; otherwise, small amounts more frequently.

Second 12 hours: As diarrhea improves, parents should begin to offer formula at half strength; if well tolerated, it is safe to go to full strength. If unable to

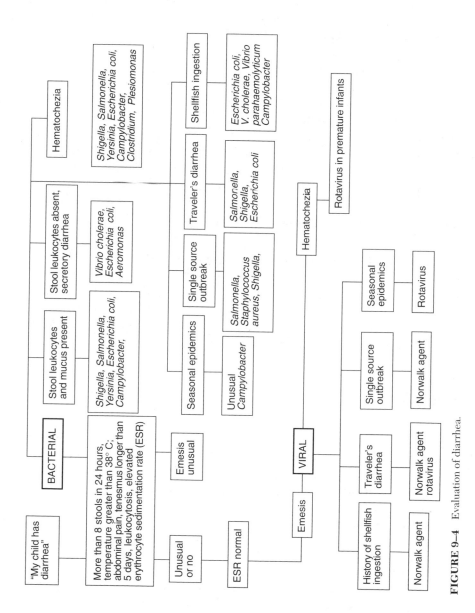

FIGURE 9–4 Evaluation of diarrhea.

tolerate, child should resume drinking clear liquids and then start lactose-free formula at half strength.

Next 24 hours: If diarrhea is subsiding, parents should add bananas, rice cereal, applesauce (not juice), and toast (the BRAT diet), and then increase the number of foods in diet as tolerated.

Pharmacological

Parents should increase child's fluid intake to rehydrate; if dehydration is sever, admit to the hospital for intravenous (IV) fluid replacement.

Antidiarrheal agents are usually unnecessary but can be dangerous in cases of inflammatory enteritis (shigellosis).

If diarrhea has a bacterial cause, antibiotics specific for the organism may be given. Do not treat salmonella with antibiotics, because they prolong the carrier state; however, treating shigellosis with antibiotics is usually indicated.

Follow-up: Child should return to clinic if not improved in 48 hours, particularly if under 3 years. Keep in contact with the caregiver by telephone.

Sequelae: Dehydration is to be considered. Milk intolerance may occur after recovery, probably as a result of secondary lactose intolerance.

Prevention/Prophylaxis: Avoid overfeeding of infants. Maintain good hygienic measures, such as handwashing. Prepare and store foods properly.

Education: Instruct parents in recording fluid intake, the number and characteristics of the stools, and the frequency of urination. Instruct parent and child in good handwashing techniques, and emphasize the importance of handwashing after diaper changing and defecation.

Encopresis

Encopresis is the daytime or nighttime incontinence of formed stools in children over ages 4–5 years. There are four types:

Retentive encopresis (psychogenic megacolon): Withholding of stool, development of constipation, fecal impaction, and seepage of stool. Examination reveals a large amount of feces in the rectal vault. Children are usually distressed by the soiling.

Continuous encopresis: Occurs in children who have never gained primary bowel control and have never received consistent bowel training; parents are usually disadvantaged.

Discontinuous encopresis: Usually occurs in response to a stressful situation after children have gained primary control, often as an expression of anger. Children are usually indifferent to the soiling.

Encopresis caused by toilet phobia: Infrequent cause. Toilet is viewed as a place to be avoided, and child fears being flushed away with the feces.

Etiology: Inefficient intestinal motility; overuse of laxatives, enemas, or suppositories, anal fissures or rashes that cause pain on defecation; and parental demands regarding bowel training.

Occurrence: Occurs in 1% of first and second graders.

Age: Occurs after ages 4–5 years; rare in adolescence.

Ethnicity: Not significant.

Gender: Primarily occurs in males (80% of cases).

Contributing Factors: Children often have no sense of the need to defecate; often associated with UTIs, psychosocial stresses or illness, and irrational fears of the toilet.

Signs and Symptoms: Child presents with a history of mild to severe soiling of underwear by feces. Obtain history of bowel patterns since birth, attempts to control or manage the incontinence, presence of stressors, and impact on the child and family.

A rectal examination reveals stool in the rectal vault. The child may or may not have abdominal pain.

Diagnostic Tests

Radiographic studies of the abdomen reveal feces in the colon and ampulla.
Urinalysis is normal.
Rectal examination will be positive for feces.

Differential Diagnosis

Patients with *Hirschsprung's disease* have a history of passing small, ribbonlike stools; disease is present from birth.
Chronic impaction may be related to dietary intake.
Anal fissures foster withholding of stool.
Childhood depression may be presenting symptom of encopresis.
Attention deficit hyperactivity disorder is often concomitant with encopresis.

Treatment

In Home (Immediate Catharsis)
For moderate to severe retention, three to four three-day cycles as follows:

Day 1: Hypophosphate enemas (Fleet Adult) bid
Day 2: Bisacodyl (Dulcolax) suppositories bid
Day 3: Bisacodyl (Dulcolax) suppositories given once

For mild retention:

Prescribe senna, one tablet daily for 7–14 days.
Take a follow-up abdominal x-ray to confirm adequate catharsis.
If child experiences discomfort, alter dosage and frequency. Give no lubricating agent at this time. Consider hospitalization if there is a small yield.

In Home (Maintenance)

Child sits on a toilet 10 minutes twice daily at the same time each day. A kitchen timer is helpful.

Light mineral oil, 2 tbsp bid, may be put into juice, cola, or any other food or beverage. Duration of mineral oil regimen may be as long as 4–6 months. Give multiple vitamins twice daily at times other than when mineral oil is administered. Give oral laxative (senna) for 2–3 weeks, then every other day for 1 month, and then discontinue.

Diet should be high in roughage (e.g., bran, cereal, fruits, vegetables).

Follow-up: Visits every 4–10 weeks to evaluate therapeutic response.

Sequelae: Relapses are common. Signs of relapse are excessive oil leaks, large stools, abdominal pain, decreased frequency of stools, and soiling.

Prevention/Prophylaxis: Teach parents developmental milestones related to bowel training.

Referral: In cases of relapse related to psychological stressors, referral to a mental health professional is advisable, as is a referral to a physician for further evaluation for organic disease syndromes. Consider referral for biofeedback training, as improvement has been noted with this technique.

Education: Teach parents normal growth and development. Bowel training is usually achieved between ages 2 and 3 years. Reassure parents by teaching about the disorder. Explain the treatment plan.

Enterobius (Pinworms)

Enterobius infestation is caused by accidental ingestion of the eggs of the intestinal nematode *Enterobius vermicularis.*

Etiology: Ingestion of the eggs of the causative parasite, *E. vermicularis.*

Age: Any age group, but usually seen in children under 10.

Ethnicity: Not significant.

Gender: Occurs equally in males and females.

Contributing Factors: Crowding and sleeping in an infested bed.

Signs and Symptoms: Child presents with a history of nocturnal anal pruritus and sleeplessness. Caregiver may have seen the parasites in the perianal area. May observe excoriations of the perianal area or vaginal discharge in females.

Diagnostic Tests: Collection of eggs from the perianal area by the use of adhesive tape.

Differential Diagnosis: None.

Treatment

Pyrantel pamoate, 11 mg/kg, single dose (maximum 1 g); repeat in 2 weeks
or
Mebendazole, 100 mg, single dose, repeat in 2 weeks
or
Albendazole, 400 mg, single dose; repeat in 2 weeks.

May need to repeat therapy because of reinfection. Treatment of all family members is recommended.

Follow-up: Reevaluate in 2 weeks and at 4 weeks for efficacy of treatment.

Sequelae: If appropriately treated, none; if untreated, vaginitis or salpingitis may develop as a result of worm migration.

Prevention/Prophylaxis: Handwashing; keeping the house dusted and cleaned, because eggs are laid in house dust and on bed clothes.

Referral: None.

Education: Teach parents that they must thoroughly clean the house on a regular basis.

Gastritis

Gastritis is an irritation of the lining of the stomach; may lead to ulcer formation.

Etiology: Illness may follow viral infections, ingestion of medications (aspirin, nonsteroidal anti-inflammatory drugs [NSAIDs]), chemotherapeutic agents, or corrosive agents.

Occurrence: Common.

Age: All age groups.

Ethnicity: Not significant.

Gender: Occurs equally in males and females.

Contributing Factors: Trauma, hypersensitivity drug reactions, and "acting out" behaviors are factors to be considered in younger children; in adolescents, chronic alcohol usage may be the cause.

Signs and Symptoms: Child presents with history of abdominal pain, nausea, vomiting, and possibly hematemesis. Palpation reveals epigastric or generalized abdominal tenderness. Hyperactive bowel sounds may be heard on auscultation.

Diagnostic Tests: Endoscopy and barium studies are not helpful. A CBC may indicate a viral or bacterial infection.

Differential Diagnosis: Peptic ulcer disease (PUD), which is more common in males and whites, can cause pain after eating; in PUD, however, the CBC is normal.

Treatment

Nonpharmacological

- Avoidance of irritating substances, such as aspirin.
- Liquid to soft diet for 24–48 hours.
- Avoidance of irritating foods.

Pharmacological

- Antacids:
  - In infants under 2 years, give 0.5–2.5 mL/kg q 1–2 hours; or 1–3 hours after meals and before bedtime. Alternate magnesium- and aluminum-based antacids to control diarrhea.
  - Antacids alone are used in children under 2 years. May be used in older children in conjunction with other therapies.
- H_2-*receptor antagonists* (not recommended for infants because they increase gastrin secretion):
  - Ranitidine, 2.5 mg/kg per day in divided doses.
  - Cimetidine, 5 mg/kg/dose at mealtime and bedtime.
- *Proton-pump inhibitors* (not recommended for infants because they increase gastrin levels):
  - Omeprazole, 20 mg daily.
  - Sucralfate, 1 g/dose qid.

Follow-up: Initially, patient should return in 1 week, and then every 2 weeks as therapy is continued for 6–8 weeks.

Sequelae: Untreated may result in PUD, perforation, obstruction, or uncontrolled bleeding.

Prevention/Prophylaxis: Observation for effects of drugs, proper storage of toxic agents, and avoidance of irritating substances.

Referral: Immediate referral for increased bleeding, or for medical intervention for ingestion of toxic agents.

Education: Instruct parents in proper storage of medicines and toxic agents.

Gastroenteritis (Acute Infectious Diarrhea)

This acute inflammatory process of the GI tract, which has a usual incubation period of 2–4 days, is manifested by severe diarrhea and occasional vomiting. Several organisms are causative agents. *Salmonella*, *Shigella*, *E. coli*, rotavirus, and Norwalk virus, *G. lamblia*, and *Staphylococcus aureus* are among the most common.

Etiology: Causative agents are spread by fecal contamination via hand-to-mouth contact.

Occurrence: Common. Occurs in outbreaks in day-care centers, schools, and hospitals and during the winter.

Age: All age groups.

Ethnicity: Not significant.

Gender: Equally in males and females.

Contributing Factors: Factors such as crowding, close contact, and improper handwashing have all been implicated.

Signs and Symptoms: Child usually presents with nonbilious, nonbloody vomiting (first 24–48 hours); degree of temperature elevation varies, and rash may be present in enteroviral infections. Stools are watery, frequent, and usually foul-smelling. A thorough history related to onset, activities prior to onset, number and frequency of stools, consistency, color, smell, and presence of blood or mucus is essential. History of vomiting, fluid intake, and urinary output is important. There is usually a history of a similar illness among friends or family (Figs. 9–5 and 9–6).

Skin turgor may be poor, based on the degree of dehydration; oral mucosa is dry if patient is dehydrated. Patient may have a fine, red, macular rash that is viral in origin. Abdomen may be distended, with increased bowel sounds. Child may appear listless.

Diagnostic Tests

Urinalysis and specific gravity to check for dehydration.
CBC to establish etiological agent, whether bacterial or viral.
Erythrocyte sedimentation rate, elevated in bacterial enteritis.
Stool sample for parasites, WBC, and culture and sensitivity.
Serum electrolytes to assess degree of dehydration.

Differential Diagnosis

Shigellosis is associated with high fever, febrile seizure, and change in mental status.

Severe abdominal pain indicates a more serious problem: *appendicitis, intussusception,* or *volvulus.*

Suspect *obstruction, poisoning,* or *hepatitis* when vomiting continues for 48 hours without diarrhea.

Treatment: The goal is to reestablish, correct, and maintain fluid and electrolyte status.

Nonpharmacological

First 12 hours: If infant is breastfeeding, mother should maintain infant at breast, but discontinue any supplemental feedings and give clear liquids instead.

For older infants, parents should discontinue diet and formula, and give small amounts of clear liquids (e.g., water, Gatorade, Pedialyte, Kool Aid, ginger ale). Parents should offer liquids every 3–4 hours if child is not vomiting; otherwise, small amounts more frequently.

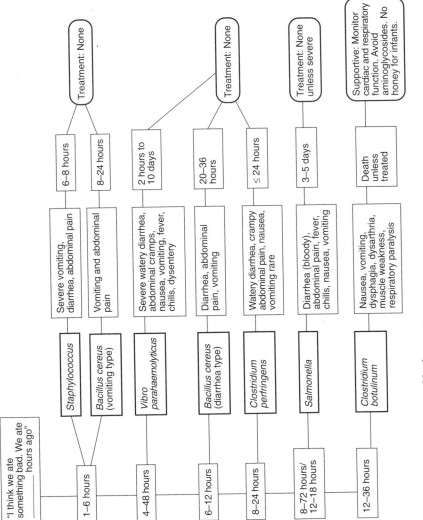

FIGURE 9–5 Evaluation of food poisoning.

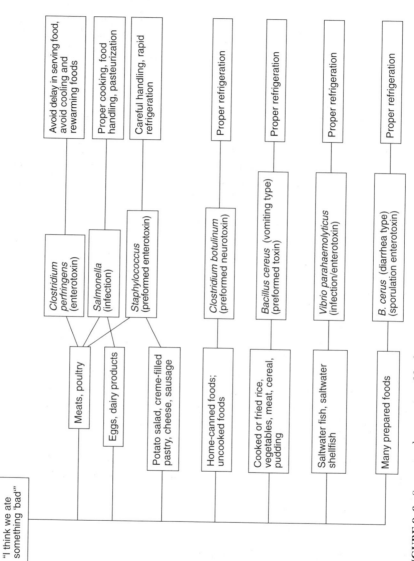

FIGURE 9–6   Sources and prevention of food poisoning.

Second 12 hours: As diarrhea improves, parents should begin to offer formula at half strength; if well tolerated, it is safe to go to full strength. If unable to tolerate, child should resume drinking clear liquids and then start lactose-free formula at half strength.

Next 24 hours: If no further vomiting occurs and diarrhea subsides, parents should give the BRAT diet, and then increase the number of foods in the diet as tolerated.

Pharmacological

Parents should increase fluid intake to rehydrate. If dehydration is severe, admit to the hospital for IV fluid replacement.

Antidiarrheal agents, which are usually unnecessary, can be dangerous in cases of inflammatory enteritis (shigellosis).

If diarrhea has a bacterial cause, antibiotics specific for the organism may be given. Do not treat a salmonella infection with antibiotics because they prolong the carrier state; however, treating shigellosis with antibiotics is usually indicated.

Follow-up: Patient should return in 24 and 48 hours for evaluation of progress, particularly hydration status.

Sequelae: Dehydration is the most important acute complication. Keeping the child on clear liquids may result in persistent loose stools and loss of weight. Occasionally, a milk protein allergy will follow a bout of gastroenteritis; an elemental formula should be given in such cases.

Prevention/Prophylaxis: Parents and children should use good handwashing techniques after diaper changing and defecating, respectively. A rotavirus vaccine is being evaluated.

Referral: Refer patient to primary-care physician for consultation regarding dehydration, severe abdominal pain, moderate amount of blood in the stool, failure to improve after 48 hours, and the need for hospital admission.

Education: Instruct parents and children in good handwashing techniques and the importance of good hygienic practices. Instruct parents in the normal bowel patterns of children and in the effects of diet or medication on bowel functioning. Instruct parents on how to monitor and record fluid intake, vomiting, and bowel movements.

Gastroesophageal Reflux

Gastroesophageal reflux (GER) is the flow back or return of acidic gastric contents into the esophagus; 85% of cases are self-limiting by age 12 months (because of child's erect posture and the addition of solids to the diet).

Etiology: May be caused by delayed gastric emptying, a large hiatal hernia, or inappropriate relaxation of the lower esophageal sphincter.

Occurrence: Common during the first year of life.

Age: Occurs in 3% of newborns.

Ethnicity: Not significant.

Gender: Occurs three times more often in males than females.

Contributing Factors: GER, which is common in neurologically impaired infants, may be associated with hiatal hernia.

Signs and Symptoms: Child presents with a history of effortless "spitting up," "projectile vomiting," difficulty feeding, and recurrent respiratory problems. Older child may complain of retrosternal burning and/or dysphagia, and may awaken with abdominal pain or discomfort. May observe Sandifer's syndrome (lateral head tilt with arching of back); otherwise, the physical examination is normal.

Diagnostic Tests: A barium swallow that reveals free regurgitation of barium from the stomach to the esophagus excludes anatomic causes, such as pyloric stenosis. A 24-hour monitoring of esophageal pH reveals prolonged periods where pH is less than 4 in the esophagus.

Differential Diagnosis: Pyloric stenosis, differentiated by the characteristic projectile vomiting and findings on the radiographic studies.

Treatment

Nonpharmacological

Positioning: To avoid aspiration, parents should elevate infant's head by 30° at all times. They should not involve infant in vigorous play after feeding.

Feeding: Parents should feed infant frequently with small amounts of thickened formula (e.g., ratio of 1 tbsp rice cereal to 6 ounces of formula). Parents should burp infant frequently and avoid giving carbonated beverages. Older children should avoid foods that reduce esophageal sphincter pressure, such as chocolate, fatty foods, and onions. Drugs such as calcium channel blockers, diazepam, theophylline, and progesterone-containing contraceptives also reduce esophageal sphincter pressure. Parents should not allow child to lie down until 4 hours after eating (i.e., bedtime snacks should be prohibited), and should elevate the head of the child's bed 4–6 inches.

Patients should avoid smoking and drinking coffee or alcoholic beverages. Tomato and citrus juices have also been implicated in GER.

Pharmacological

Antacids, 0.5 mL/kg with meals. Antacids alone are used in children under 2 years.

H_2-receptor antagonists (not recommended for infants because they increase excessive gastrin secretion).

Ranitidine, 2.5 mg/kg per day in divided doses.

Cimetidine, 5 mg/kg per dose at mealtime and bedtime.

Proton-pump inhibitors (not recommended for infants because they increase gastrin levels).

Omeprazole, 20 mg per day.

Prokinetic agents (may be helpful).

Metoclopramide, 0.1 mg/kg before meals

or

Bethanechol, 0.1 mg/kg before meals

or

Cisapride, 0.3 mg/kg three to four times per day.

Other

Acetaminophen, 0.1 mg/kg for pain q 4–6 hours as needed (PRN).

Surgical

Surgical intervention consists of a Nissen fundoplication, whereby the fundus of the stomach is wrapped around the distal esophagus. Thus, gastric distention after eating increases the pressure around the wrap and prevents reflux.

Follow-up: Follow patient weekly to assess weight gain.

Sequelae: Aspiration pneumonia, chronic cough, apneic spells, failure to thrive, esophagitis with bleeding, and anemia are all possible complications.

Prevention/Prophylaxis: None, except lifestyle changes and avoidance of foods known to cause discomfort.

Referral: Refer patient to surgeon in the following cases: medical intervention fails after 2–3 months, there is persistent vomiting with failure to thrive, patient has apneic spells or chronic pulmonary disease, or patient is over 18 months and has a hiatal hernia.

Education: Reassure parents that the condition is self-limiting. Instruct parents in appropriate feeding techniques.

Giardiasis

Giardiasis is the infestation of the GI tract by *G. lamblia,* caused by accidental ingestion of the cysts.

Etiology: Ingestion of cysts from a person with giardiasis or from contaminated food or water.

Occurrence: Common.

Age: All age groups.

Ethnicity: Not significant.

Gender: Occurs equally in males and females.

Contributing Factors: Contaminated water or food and crowded conditions are associated factors.

Signs and Symptoms: Child presents with a history of periumbilical pain, anorexia, nausea, abdominal distention, and diarrhea. On palpitation, there may be periumbilical tenderness. Auscultation may reveal distention.

Diagnostic Tests: Microscopic examination of stools, duodenal washings, or biopsy of the small bowel will reveal the causative organism.

Differential Diagnosis

Gastroenteritis is an acute, self-limiting illness usually lasting 3 days.

Patients with *school phobia* often present with abdominal pain. Discuss feelings related to the school situation with the child and parent.

Treatment

Quinacrine, 6 mg/kg per day tid after meals for 5 days (maximum 300 mg/day)
or
Furazolidone, 6–8 mg/kg per day in four doses for 7–10 days
or
Tinidazole, 50 mg/kg single dose (maximum 2 g)
or
Metronidazole, 15 mg/kg per day in three doses for 5 days
or
Paromomycin, 25–30 mg/kg per day in three doses for 7 days.

Follow-up: Reevaluate patient in 2 weeks to determine efficacy of treatment.

Sequelae: Usually none.

Prevention/Prophylaxis: Proper handwashing, proper preparation of food, and clean drinking water are all means of prevention.

Referral: None.

Education: Instruct parents in techniques of proper handwashing, proper food preparation, and water sterilization.

Inguinal Hernia

Inguinal hernia is the protrusion of abdominal structures into the scrotum or inguinal canal; patients present with a painless inguinal swelling. Unilateral, right-sided hernias account for 85–90% of the total number of hernia cases.

Etiology: The persistence of the peritoneal sac, which normally becomes fibrotic late in gestation, or a weakness of the musculature. Congenitally acquired cases are due to the incomplete closure of the processes vaginalis.

Occurrence: Inguinal hernias occur in about 2% of males with a small percentage (<0.5%) occurring in females.

Age: Any pediatric age group; 50% of cases are diagnosed during the first year of life, but most cases are diagnosed by age 3 months.

Ethnicity: Not significant.

Gender: Males or females, but mostly males (5–6 : 1 to as high as 9 : 1).

Contributing Factors: Coughing, vomiting, or standing for long periods of time may be factors. Prematurity may also be a factor; 5–30% of premature infants are born with inguinal hernias.

Signs and Symptoms: Child presents to clinic because the caregiver finds a mass in the inguinal canal, scrotum, or labia. This mass is particularly noticeable when the child cries. Usually the mass is reducible and there is no pain. Complaints of vomiting, small stools, melena, irritability, and abdominal distention are suggestive of incarceration.

Findings include the palpation of a mass in the scrotum or labia; the size of the mass is enhanced by the increase in intra-abdominal pressure when the child cries or strains. Attempts at transillumination are negative unless the bowel is filled with fluid. Most hernias are reducible; however if the neck of the sack closes over the herniated abdominal contents, the hernia may become incarcerated. If the area is tender and swollen, there is strangulation. Bilateral inguinal hernias with palpable contents in females should be investigated for an endocrine or genetic problem. Silk glove sign—a feeling of two surfaces sliding across each other during palpation along the inguinal canal—is evident.

Diagnostic Tests: An ultrasound helps to differentiate between a hydrocele and a hernia.

Differential Diagnosis

Patients with *inguinal lymph nodes* present with multiple, discrete masses. Transillumination is successful with a *hydrocele.*
Undescended testicle is movable along the canal and absent in the scrotum.
Lymphadenopathy may be accompanied by an increased WBC and lymphocyte count.
Neoplasms and other masses are differentiated by computed tomography (CT) or ultrasound.

Treatment: Surgical intervention to repair the intestinal obstruction.

Follow-up: Monitor patient at each well-child visit. Arrange a visit postoperatively.

Sequelae: Untreated, incarcerated hernia may develop into bowel gangrene. Incarceration or potential strangulation of hernia occurs in about two thirds of all hernias in children under 1 year.

Referral: In suspected cases of inguinal hernia, referral to a surgeon or urologist to be seen in 1–3 weeks. Suspected cases of incarcerated hernia should be referred to a surgeon immediately.

Prevention/Prophylaxis: None; this is a congenitally acquired condition.

Education: Teach the caregiver the technique for reducing the hernia. Teach the caregiver the signs and symptoms of incarceration and strangulation, including increased pain, erythema, vomiting, and abdominal distention. The parents should be instructed, if these symptoms arise, to call a surgeon or urologist or to go to the emergency room.

Irritable Bowel Syndrome

Irritable bowel syndrome (IBS) is a lifelong problem of continuous symptoms of abdominal pain and disordered defecation lasting at least 3 months. Diagnostic criteria as adapted by the International Congress of Gastroenterology are:

- Continuous or recurrent symptoms lasting at least 3 months, including:
  - Abdominal pain relieved with defecation or associated with a change in frequency or consistency of stool.
  - An irregular (varying) pattern of defecation at least 25% of the time (two or more of); altered stool frequency.
  - Altered stool from hard to loose or watery.
  - Altered stool passage (straining or urgency, feeling of incomplete evacuation).
  - Passage of mucus.
  - Bloating or feeling of abdominal distention.

Etiology: No universally accepted etiologic mechanism. The following have been suggested: altered colonic motility, abnormal colonic muscle tone, abnormal small-bowel motility, altered pain perception, and psychopathology.

Occurrence: Occurs in 5–15% of children.

Age: Occurs at any age, but typical onset is 5–15 years of age; has been seen between ages 6 and 20 months, clearing spontaneously at 36 months.

Ethnicity: Not significant.

Gender: Occurs more often in females than males.

Contributing Factors: Cultures that allow females to report somatic complaints but inhibit males from doing so; stress (e.g., entering high school, going to college, getting married, sibling rivalry); sexual abuse; menstruation; and familial history.

Signs and Symptoms: Child presents to clinic usually with a history of abdominal pain and bowel changes. Obtain a complete history, using the above-mentioned criteria for diagnosis of IBS as a guide. The history should include items related to diet, travel, laxative abuse, and psychological issues. Child may present with a history of nausea and vomiting, lethargy, and diarrhea. Nocturnal enuresis, fears, and sleep disturbances are noted in 30% of young children with IBS.

Physical findings are usually negative, except for abdominal tenderness, most often left lower quadrant.

Diagnostic Tests

CBC with erythrocyte sedimentation rate to rule out presence of infection.
Barium enema in older patients (diagnostic accuracy of 95% after 5 years).
Stools for OCP, fat, and blood (negative in IBS).
Flexible sigmoidoscopy (refer) to evaluate sigmoid musculature.

Differential Diagnosis

Lactose intolerance is differentiated by history and breath test.
Parasitic infection is differentiated by stool examinations isolating the parasite.
Diverticular disease is differentiated by muscular hypertrophy of the sigmoid
    colon.
Food intolerance is manifested by the presence of mucus and undigested food
    in the feces is differentiated in children under age 3 years, colic in the first 3
    months of life, history of food intolerance, loose feces with abdominal pain,
    pain relieved by evacuation, and presence of undigested vegetables in the
    feces is differentiated in children over 3 years.

Treatment: Dietary management, fiber supplementation to increase stool volume, psyllium agents, 1–2 tsp bid; loperamide (Imodium), 0.1–0.2 mg/kg per day in one to three doses to decrease urgency, stool frequency, loose stools, and pain.

Follow-up: Monthly initially to develop rapport with the patient and evaluate progress.

Sequelae: None.

Prevention/Prophylaxis: None.

Referral: Refer to primary-care physician or internist for flexible sigmoidoscopy and for diagnosis and treatment of depression, if indicated. Refer patient to a psychiatrist for short-term therapy to reduce stress and depression.

Education: Instruct patient in relaxation techniques to reduce pain. Instruct patient to increase intake of fruits, fiber, and fluids; to avoid caffeine, nicotine, and alcohol; and to avoid foods that seem to trigger episodes. Instruct patient to eliminate sources of stress and to increase exercise.

| Intussusception

Intussusception occurs when one segment of bowel telescopes into the distal segment. It usually starts proximal to the ileocecal valve; thus invagination is ileocecal, resulting in impairment of venous return causing swelling, hemorrhage, and incarceration with necrosis of the invaginated bowel. Prognosis depends on the duration of the condition.

Etiology: Unknown; lymphoid hyperplasia (Peyer patches) may form a lead point at the proximal segment.

Occurrence: The most frequent cause of intestinal obstruction in the first 2 years of life; after age 6, lymphomas are the most common lesion.

Age: Occurs primarily in infants aged 6–18 months; 10% of cases occur in children over 3 years.

Ethnicity: Not significant.

Gender: More prevalent in males (3 : 1).

Contributing Factors: Predisposing factors include cystic fibrosis, Schönlein-Henoch purpura, Meckel's diverticulum, lymphoma, and polyps.

Signs and Symptoms: Child presents with acute-onset, intermittent, colicky lower abdominal pain. During episodes of pain, child cries, draws up knees, and may vomit. Late findings may include lethargy, fever, and currant jelly–colored stools. A sausage-shaped mass may be palpated in the upper abdomen, which is tender and distended.

Diagnosis Tests: Barium enema to confirm diagnosis (in 75% of cases, barium enema will reduce the intussusception).

Differential Diagnosis

Incarcerated hernia is best differentiated by ultrasound and surgical consults, because diagnosis may be difficult.

Testicular torsion is best differentiated by ultrasound and surgical consults, because diagnosis may be difficult.

Acute gastroenteritis is differentiated by the presence of symptoms not present in intussusception, such as nausea, vomiting, and lymphocytosis.

Intestinal obstruction and *appendicitis* are differentiated by ultrasound; patient should be referred to the surgeon for a definitive diagnosis.

Treatment: Refer patient for hospitalization and medical intervention (hydrostatic reduction). Refer for surgical intervention in the following cases: clinical signs of peritonitis or shock, or likelihood of discovery of a pathological lead point.

Follow-up: After hospitalization, observe for signs of recurrence.

Sequelae: If intussusception is not treated promptly, shock or peritonitis may develop. Death may occur if untreated; mortality rate with treatment is 1–2%.

Recurrence rate is 3–4% after medical intervention—usually recurs within 24 hours.

Prevention/Prophylaxis: None.

Referral: Refer patient to pediatrician for medical intervention and/or to pediatric surgeon for surgical intervention.

Education: Reassure parents that they were not to blame.

Megacolon (Hirschsprung's Disease)

Megacolon is an aganglionic segment of variable length (5–20 mm) in the colon. In 75% of cases, the segment involved is the rectosigmoid colon, causing narrowing of the denervated segment with dilation of the proximal ganglionic colon.

Etiology: Failure of retrograde migration of neural crest–derived ganglion cells in the developing colon.

Occurrence: Accounts for 20% of neonatal intestinal obstruction.

Age: May be diagnosed at birth but obvious symptoms may not be noticed until the child is older.

Ethnicity: Not significant.

Gender: Occurs three times more often in males than females.

Contributing Factors: There may be a familial pattern; is associated with Down's syndrome (10–15%).

Signs and Symptoms: Child presents with no meconium stools in the first 24 hours of life, vomiting, and reluctance to feed. There is a repeated need for rectal stimulation to induce defecation. Stools are characteristically small and ribbon-like.

Findings may include failure to thrive (obtain height and weight), abdominal distention and prominent veins, and palpation of stool in the abdomen with an empty rectum.

Diagnostic Tests

Barium enema shows a transition zone between the narrow aganglionic segment of bowel and the dilated proximal segment. Obtain a lateral x-ray in 24 and 48 hours to assess passage of barium. In normal infants, the barium is passed in 24 hours; in infants with megacolon, the barium is retained and mixed with feces.

Anorectal manometry fails to show internal sphincter relaxation

Rectal biopsy demonstrates the absence of ganglion cells.

Obtain a CBC to determine the presence of anemia.

An erect lateral x-ray of the abdomen reveals dilated colonic loops and absence of gas below the pelvic colon.

Differential Diagnosis

Other causes of neonatal intestinal obstruction (e.g., *volvulus, intussusception*) should be investigated if radiographic studies are negative for megacolon.

Retentive constipation with colonic distention is differentiated by age of onset, presence of stool in the rectum, and size of the stool in the distended segment.

Celiac disease, a GI cause of failure to thrive, is differentiated by age of onset, chronic diarrhea, wasted skeletal muscle mass, and bowel biopsy.

Enterocolitis is differentiated by fever and diarrhea, which may be coexistent with megacolon and accounts for 30% of the mortality after surgery in infants.

Treatment: Surgical intervention is completed in two stages: First stage, a temporary colostomy or ileostomy to divert the feces; second stage, removal of the aganglionic segment and anastomosis at ages 12–14 months or, in an older child, 3–6 months after the initial procedure.

Follow-up: Immediate postoperative visits. Monitor growth and development to look for signs of failure to thrive.

Sequelae: Poor nourishment with associated anemia due to a defect in food assimilation. Anal stenosis is a postsurgical complication in 10–15% of cases.

Prevention/Prophylaxis: None.

Referral: Immediate referral for surgical intervention.

Education: For the older child, teach parents to implement a low-residue diet and to avoid serving the child milk, fried foods, and highly seasoned food. After surgery, the child will probably go home with instructions to eat a normal diet. Instruct parents in presurgery enema techniques. After surgery, instruct parents in colostomy care and skin care of the stoma.

Peptic Ulcer Disease

PUD is a circumscribed ulceration of the mucous membrane penetrating through a muscularis mucosa and occurring in areas exposed to acid and pepsin. There are two main kinds:

Duodenal: Located in the duodenum of the small intestine.
Gastric: Located in the stomach.

Close person-to-person contact has been implicated in the transmission of *Helicobacter pylori.*

Etiology: PUD is caused by an increased production of gastric acid. *H. pylori,* a multiflagellate, unipolar, spiral bacteria, is responsible for 50–60% of ulcer disease cases. PUD may be associated with the use of drugs such as aspirin, NSAIDs, tolazoline, and aminophylline. There is a breakdown of the normal gastric mucosal defense.

Occurrence: The incidence of PUD in children is unknown, but it is no longer a rare diagnosis in infants and neonates. The rise in prevalence is related to prolonged survival of critically ill neonates and infants at high risk of acute PUD, such as those with anoxia, hypotension, trauma, and sepsis.

Age: Occurs in any age group, but is more common in children aged 12–18 years.

Ethnicity: Increased incidence in whites.

Gender: After age 6 years, PUD is more common in males.

Contributing Factors: In 25–50% of patients, there is a family history of ulcers. Environmental factors such as crowding, climate, dietary habits, and emotional strain have been implicated. Associated conditions are pancreatitis, cystic fibrosis, uremia, hyperparathyroidism, multiple endocrine adenoma syndrome, and bleeding disorders. Consider chronic alcohol ingestion in adolescents.

Signs and Symptoms

Ages 0–3 years: Anorexia, vomiting, crying after meals, melena, or hematemesis. Hemorrhage or perforation may be the first sign.

Ages 3–6 years: Vomiting after eating, periumbilical or generalized abdominal pain, melena, hematemesis, and perforation.

Ages 6–18 years: Less than 50% have typical ulcer symptoms; 50% exhibit melena or hematemesis. Occult bleeding and anemia may be present. There may be some periumbilical or generalized tenderness. Child may be irritable.

Diagnostic Tests

Upper GI series to visualize lesion.

Gastroduodenoscopy to visualize the lesion; if lesions are multiple in the third or fourth portion of the duodenum or in the jejunum, suspect Zollinger-Ellison syndrome.

CBC to determine the presence of anemia.

Stool for occult blood to assess the presence of GI bleeding.

H. pylori titer (serum) to assess the presence of the organism, or the rapid ^{14}C urea breath test.

Differential Diagnosis

GER does not cause the patient to wake up with abdominal pain.

Patients with *Meckle's diverticulum* present with sharp pain from the periumbilical area to the lower abdomen, and painless rectal bleeding and obstruction.

Pancreatitis patients present with acute left upper quadrant pain, which is constant.

Patients with *inflammatory bowel disease* present with dull, crampy, intermittent pain, lasting 2 hours.

Appendicitis patients present with acute, sharp, steady pain located in the epigastric region, localizing to the right lower quadrant.

Treatment: The goal is suppression of gastric acid.

Nonpharmacological

Patient should avoid caffeine and foods that cause distress, avoid aspirin and NSAIDs, and eat three meals per day without between-meal snacks.

Pharmacological

- Antacids, 0.5–1.0 mL/kg 2–3 hours before feedings and at bedtime (antacids are used alone in children under age 2 years).
- H_2-receptor antagonists:
  - Ranitidine, 2.5 mg/kg q 12 hours
  or
  - Cimetidine, 5 mg/kg per dose, before meals and at bedtime.
- Proton-pump inhibitors:
  - Omeprazole (Prilosec; no dose provided for children); in adolescents, 20 mg daily.
- Prokinetic agents:
  - Metoclopramide, 0.1 mg/kg before meals.
  - Bethanechol, 0.1 mg/kg before meals.
  - Cisapride, 0.3 mg/kg three to four times per day.
- Others:
  - Sucralfate, 1 g/dose qid.
  - Acetaminophen, 0.1 mg/kg for pain.

H. pylori titer positive

H_2-antagonist for 6–8 weeks plus oral bismuth preparation, two tablets PO q 6 hours for 3 weeks (one tablet or liquid for smaller children); and amoxicillin, 40 mg/kg per day divided q 8 hours (maximum 1.5 g/day) for 3 weeks
or
Tetracycline 40 mg/kg per day divided q 6 hours (maximum 2 g/day) for 3 weeks. Metronidazole, 20 mg/kg per day divided q 8 hours (maximum 1.5 g/day) for 3 weeks
or
proton-pump inhibitors.
Omeprazole, 20 mg daily with clarithromycin (Biaxin), 250 mg bid to tid for 10–14 days (adolescents only).

Follow-up: Patient should return in 2 and 3 weeks and then monthly for 4–6 months.

Sequelae: Anemia, perforating peritonitis, or pancreatitis may be long-term sequelae.

Prevention/Prophylaxis: Patient should avoid caffeine and foods that cause distress, avoid aspirin and NSAIDs, and eat three meals per day without between-meal snacks.

Referral: If there is no improvement, or in cases of GI bleeding, weight loss, or signs and symptoms of appendicitis, refer patient to primary-care physician or surgeon.

Education: Inform child and parent that there is a possibility of recurrence; instruct regarding dietary and medication restrictions.

Pyloric Stenosis

Pyloric stenosis is an increase in the circular muscle of the pylorus resulting in abdominal distention and prominent gastric peristalsis.

Etiology: Unknown. The narrowing of the pyloric canal due to an increase in the circular muscle of the pylorus is the causative factor.

Occurrence: Occurs in 1 in 500 births; more common in twins or in a father and his sons.

Age: Occurs at birth.

Ethnicity: Ethnicity is not significant.

Gender: More common in males (1 in 150) than females (1 in 750).

Contributing Factors: Controversial suggested factors are birth order (increased prevalence in first born) and the season of birth (spring and fall).

Signs and Symptoms: Infant presents at age 2–4 weeks with a history of vomiting, usually projectile; poor weight gain or weight loss; and signs of being hungry, fretful, and constipated.
Poor weight gain or weight loss is verified. May palpate an olive-sized mass in RUQ, and may observe gastric peristaltic waves from left to right. There is abdominal distention after feeding.

Diagnostic Tests
Unconjugated bilirubin is elevated in 2–3% of cases.
Hemoglobin and hematocrit values are elevated because of hemoconcentration and potassium depletion.
Barium swallow reveals delayed gastric emptying and an elongated pyloric channel (string sign).

Differential Diagnosis
If there are no gastric contents, suspect *esophageal stenosis.*
If vomitus contains bile, suspect *volvulus* or *small bowel obstruction.*
UTIs may be checked by urine culture.

Treatment: If patient is dehydrated, restore fluid and electrolyte balance; surgical intervention for pyloromyotomy.

Follow-up: Monitor weight gain and relief of symptoms.

Sequelae: None, if treated promptly; if not, dehydration may develop.

Prevention/Prophylaxis: None.

Referral: Refer patient to a surgeon for appropriate intervention.

Education: Instruct parents in proper feeding technique: holding upright, not propping the bottle, feeding slowly, and burping infant after each ounce of formula. Reassure parents regarding the positive outcome of the surgery.

Umbilical Hernia

An umbilical hernia is a soft, bulging mass that is easily reducible and more prominent when a child is crying, rarely enlarges, and regresses spontaneously if no larger than 0.5 cm. Most larger ones disappear by school age; may be congenital or acquired.

Etiology: The incomplete closure of the fascia of the umbilical ring; acquired hernias are a result of an abnormal tumor or organomegaly.

Occurrence: Fairly common.

Age: Occurs in infancy.

Ethnicity: More common in African-American males; affects as many as 40% of black children under 1 year.

Gender: Occurs more often in males.

Contributing Factors: Occurs more frequently in premature infants and in children with Down's syndrome, hypothyroidism, or Hurler's syndrome.

Signs and Symptoms: During a well-child visit, parent comments on the status of the protruding umbilicus and may have even strapped the umbilicus. Findings reveal a soft, bulging, reducible mass at the umbilicus. The umbilical ring may be palpated.

Diagnostic Tests: None.

Differential Diagnosis: None.

Treatment: Surgical intervention to repair the defect if not closed by school age. Reducing and strapping do not hasten the healing process.

Follow-up: Observe patient at each visit to evaluate the progression of healing. Resume usual well-baby visits after the first posthospitalization visit *if* surgical intervention takes place.

Sequelae: Rarely becomes larger unless there is increased intra-abdominal pressure or ascites. In smaller hernias, incarceration is a possibility. If surgical intervention is done to repair the defect, there are no sequelae.

Prevention/Prophylaxis: None.

Referral: Refer patient to a surgeon if hernia persists up to school age or there is associated abdominal pain.

Education: Instruct parents in the signs and symptoms of incarceration: the hernia cannot be reduced, and abdominal pain is severe enough to cause the child to cry.

Volvulus

A volvulus is the twisting of the bowel that results in arterial obstruction, ischemia, and infarction. In 25% of cases the patients also have congenital cardiac anomalies.

Etiology: An anomaly of intestinal rotation occurs when the small intestine is not fixed in the abdomen and becomes suspended by a stalk containing the superior mesenteric artery.

Occurrence: Not noted.

Age: Occurs predominantly in infants: 80% within the first week of life and 75% within the first 3 weeks of life.

Ethnicity: Not significant.

Gender: Occurs equally in males and females.

Contributing Factors: Failure of the midgut to re-enter the fetal abdomen appropriately.

Signs and Symptoms: In the infant (first 3 weeks), a history of bile-stained vomitus and abdominal distention. In the older infant, a history of diarrhea and vomiting and intermittent abdominal obstruction, with vomiting and postprandial abdominal pain.

In the young infant, examination reveals visible gastric peristaltic waves and epigastric or generalized abdominal distention. In older children, there is also abdominal tenderness. In a sigmoid volvulus, a palpable mass is present.

Diagnostic Tests

Radiographic studies of the abdomen (upper GI series) show partial or complete small bowel obstruction.

A barium enema shows a mobile cecum located in the midline.

CBC with a peripheral smear; suspect a midgut volvulus when there are nucleated red blood cells in the peripheral blood.

Differential Diagnosis: The intestinal obstruction seen in Meckel's diverticulum is due in 10% of cases to volvulus or intussusception; thus the diagnoses overlap.

Characteristically the pain in Meckel's diverticulum is sharp in contrast to the pain of intestinal obstruction, which alternates between cramping (colicky) and painless periods. The pain in volvulus is intermittent and cramping.

Treatment: Refer patient to a surgeon. This condition constitutes a surgical emergency.

Sequelae: Intestinal obstruction, peritonitis, perforation, intestinal necrosis, and death.

Follow-up: As required postoperatively.

Prevention/Prophylaxis: None.

Referral: Pediatric surgeon for surgical intervention.

Education: Reassurance to the parents that they did not cause the problem.

REFERENCES

General

Berhman, R, and Kleigman, R: Nelson's Essentials of Pediatrics. WB Saunders, Philadelphia, 1990.
Doenges, M, and Moorhouse, M: Nurse's Pocket Guide: Nursing Diagnoses with Interventions, ed 5. FA Davis, Philadelphia, 1995.
Green, M: Pediatric Diagnosis: Interpretation of Symptoms & Signs in Infants, Children, and Adolescents. WB Saunders, Philadelphia, 1992.
Hay, W, et al: Current Pediatric Diagnosis & Treatment, ed 12. Appleton & Lange, Norwalk, Conn, 1995.
Steele, R: The Clinical Handbook of Pediatric Infectious Disease. Parthenon, New York, 1994.

Constipation

DiLorenzo, C, et al: Use of colonic manometry to differentiate causes of intractable constipation in children. J Pediatr 120:690, 695.

Encopresis

Cox, DJ, et al: Some electromyographic biofeedback treatment for chronic pediatric constipation/encopresis: Preliminary report. Biofeedback Self Regul 19:41, 1994.
Rockney, R: The plain abdominal roentgenogram in the management of encopresis. Arch Pediatr Adolesc Med 149:623, 1995.

Gastroesophageal Reflux

Berube, M, and Parrish, R: Home care of the infant with gastroesophageal reflux and respiratory disease. J Pediatr Health Care 8:173, 1994.
Stephen, TC, et al: Diagnosis of gastroesophageal reflux in pediatrics. J Ky Med Assoc 92:188, 1994.

Inguinal Hernia

Nahayomia, D, and Rowe, M: Inguinal hernia and acute scrotum in infants and children. Pediatr Rev 11:87, 1989.
Rosenstein, B, and Fosarelli, P: Pediatric Pearls, ed 2. Mosby-Year Book, St. Louis, 1993.
Ryan, D, and Doody, E: Genital pain. In Dershewitz, R (ed): Ambulatory Pediatric Care. JB Lippincott, Philadelphia, 1993.
Skoog, SJ, and Conlin, MJ: Pediatric hernias and hydroceles: The urologist's perspective. Urol Clin North Am 22:119, 1995.

Irritable Bowel Syndrome

Bonamico, M, et al: Irritable bowel syndrome in children: An Italian multicentre study: Collaborating centres. Ital J Gastroenterol 27:13, 1995.
Hyams, JS, et al: Characterization of symptoms in children with recurrent abdominal pain: Resemblance to irritable bowel syndrome. J Pediatr Gastroenterol Nutr 20:209, 1995.
Nostrant, T: Irritable bowel syndrome. Female Patient 20:48, 1995.

Peptic Ulcer Disease

Danish Omeprazole Study Group: Omeprazole and cimetidine in the treatment of ulcers of the body of the stomach: A double-blind comparative trial. Br Med J 298:645, 1989.
Chong, SK, et al: Helicobacter pylori infection in recurrent abdominal pain in childhood: Comparison of diagnostic tests and therapy. Pediatrics 96:211, 1995.

George, D, and Glassman, M: Peptic ulcer disease in children. Gastrointest Endosc Clin North Am 4:23, 1994.

Steele, R: The Clinical Handbook of Pediatric Infectious Disease. Parthenon, New York, 1994.

Webb, P, et al: Relation between infection with Helicobacter pylori and living conditions in childhood: Evidence for person to person transmission in early life. Br Med J 308:750, 1994.

Yamshiro, Y, et al: Helicobacter pylori colonization in children with peptic ulcer disease III. Diagnostic value of the 13C-urea breath test to detect gastric H. pylori colonization. Acta Paediatr Jpn 37:12, 1995.

CHAPTER **10**

RENAL AND

UROLOGIC

ASSESSMENT

Renal problems commonly occur in children, whether due to diseases primary to the kidney or to dysfunction secondary to systemic diseases, malfunctions of the urinary system, or injury.

Assessment of the kidney and urinary tract begins with a thorough history. Data should be gathered concerning prenatal care, birth experience, and family history—including a history of congenital disease or a past acute or chronic illness. Investigate any past history of rashes or joint pain that might signal a post-streptococcal glomerulonephritis. Note any problems in growth and development; history of urinary problems (e.g., frequency, dysuria, enuresis) or pain (e.g., abdominal, flank); and exposure to chemical or toxic substances.

The physical examination includes vital signs: height, weight, and blood pressure. Observe the patient for café au lait spots, skin color, and the presence of edema. The abdomen and flank should be palpated for masses, tenderness, and ascites.

The first clue to renal difficulties is usually a change in the urine: amount, color, and odor. Usually one of these changes causes the parent to bring the child to the clinic, rather than the symptoms of flank or suprapubic pain. The amount excreted, polyuria or oliguria, are indicative of systemic diseases such as diabetes mellitus, sickle cell anemia, dehydration, or nephritis. A change in color is suspicious of bleeding, excretion of pigment, or intake of certain medications or food (Fig. 10–1). For more definitive workups, a urinalysis including culture and sensitivity and renal function studies is often indicated. (*Note:* Small children have

235

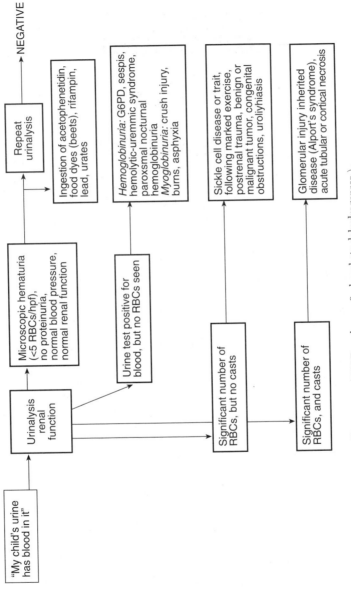

FIGURE 10–1   Evaluation of hematuria. (G6PD = glucose-6-phosphate dehydrogenase.)

different creatinine levels thus effecting the glomerular filtration rate.) Dark, strong-smelling urine may be indicative of infection or dehydration.

Girls are at greater risk than boys for the development of urinary tract infections (UTIs) because of their shorter urethra and the greater potential for perineal contamination. In boys, the presence of a foreskin is a risk factor for UTI. Changes in hygienic practices contribute greatly to the reduction of UTIs.

Enuresis

Involuntary urinary incontinence occurring in a child age 5 or older is categorized as follows:

> *Primary nocturnal enuresis:* Has never been dry at night; wet only at night and during sleep.
> *Secondary nocturnal enuresis:* Has had bladder control, but now wets at night (continent period of 6–12 months).
> *Diurnal enuresis:* Wets during the day, 60–80% also wet at night.

Etiology: Nonorganic causes include:

> Positive family history (usually fathers).
> Genetic causes (chromosome 13).
> Times of emotional stress.
> Anxiety or psychiatric disorder.

Organic causes include:

> Deficiency in antidiuretic hormone.
> Fecal impaction.
> UTIs.
> Seizures.
> Illness such as diabetes.
> Structural abnormalities.

Occurrence: Primary nocturnal enuresis occurs in 15–30% of 6-year-old children. Secondary enuresis occurs in 20% of bed wetters over age 4. Diurnal enuresis occurs in 1% of children aged 6–12.

Age: Children over 5; may extend throughout the pediatric age span.

Ethnicity: Occurs more often in African-American males.

Gender: Three times more often in males than females.

Contributing Factors: Maturational lag, emotional stress, anxiety, timidity or shyness, family history of bed wetting (usually fathers; if both parents were "wetters," 77% of children will have problems).

Signs and Symptoms: Parents may be reluctant to reveal this problem. Inquiries at routine visits as to toileting habits may lead to identification of the problem.

History may reveal past involuntary urinary incontinence. Additionally, there may be a history of UTIs, bladder spasms, dysuria, hematuria, and increased frequency. Talk to the child, and elicit his or her feelings and perceptions of the problem. Ask about recent emotional stressors: a recent move, divorce, or school problems. Ask about interventions that the family may have initiated.

Assess the genitalia for signs of sexual abuse. Observe the urinary stream for dribbling and small stream. On palpation of the abdomen, a pelvic mass could indicate a fecal impaction.

Diagnostic Tests

Urinalysis to determine specific gravity and glucose level. This assesses for predisposing medical conditions, such as diabetes insipidus and diabetes mellitus.

Culture and sensitivity of urine to assess for covert infection, particularly in females. A covert infection may indicate urinary tract malformations.

Voiding cystourethrography, renal ultrasonography, or intravenous pyelography to assess for urinary tract malformation.

Evaluation of bladder capacity; small bladder capacity is classified as 10 mL/kg or 1 ounce per year of age +2 (1 oz × age + 2 = bladder capacity).

Differential Diagnosis

Behavioral problems, such as depression and anger. These children, most often, have diurnal enuresis and void voluntarily.

Diabetes and *urinary tract abnormalities and infections* must be considered.

Emotional problems, such as those found in cases of sexual abuse.

Treatment: Specific treatment is not recommended for children under 6 because of spontaneous remission. For children over age 6 and if the parent and/or child is concerned:

Behavioral

The goal is for the child to take a responsible, active role in dealing with the enuresis. The following are recommendations for the child:

Keep a calendar of wet and dry nights.

Urinate immediately before bedtime.

Change wet bed linens and clothing and, if age-appropriate, launder them.

The following are recommendations for the parent:

Do not give more than 2 ounces of fluid after dinner.

Provide positive reinforcement for dry nights (gold stars or some prearranged reward, praise).

Avoid punishments and angry responses.

Nonpharmacological

For children with urgency incontinence, instruct on how to practice stream-interruption exercises. For children with small bladder capacity, recommend en-

uresis alarms and bladder stretching exercises. For children who can read, *Dry All Night* may be of assistance in teaching the child to awaken during the night.
The following are some sources of enuresis alarms:

Nite Train'r Alarm: 1-800-544-4240.
Nytone Medical Products: 1-801-973-4090.
Wet Stop Alarm: 1-800-346-4488.

Pharmacological

Imipramine HCl (Tofranil PM), 25–50 mg at bedtime for children aged 6–12; 50–75 mg for children over 12. After 1 month of dryness, decrease dosage by tapering off over a 2–4 week period.

DDAVP (desmopressin acetate), 20 μg, 1 hour before bedtime (10 μg in each nostril) for 1–2 weeks; increase 10 μg every 2 weeks. Maximum dose is 40 μg. Child is classified as nonresponder if unresponsive after several weeks at a dose of 40 μg.

Oxybutynin (Ditropan), for children aged 1–5; 0.2 mg/kg bid or qid for enuresis.

Follow-up: Every 2–6 weeks during interventions for progress reports; complete blood counts every 2–4 weeks while on imipramine.

Sequelae: Child will experience a decline in self-esteem. Social events, such as parties and sleepovers, become a problem.

Prevention/Prophylaxis: Reduction of stress; identification and treatment of organic cause.

Referral: Obtain a urology consult for children with suspected urinary tract abnormalities. Consider mental health referral in cases of children with daytime wetting and secondary enuresis.

Education: Instruct families that patience is a virtue (15% of children have spontaneous remission after age 6). Assist families in identifying appropriate strategies and interventions. To alleviate their self-blame and guilt, reassure parents as to the etiology and prognosis.

Glomerulonephritis

Glomerulonephritis is a clinical syndrome of glomerular hematuria associated with hypertension, edema, proteinuria, and decreased urinary output and renal function. Glomerular diseases encountered in childhood may be categorized as follows:

Postinfection glomerulonephritis: Onset 10–14 days after an acute illness, usually streptococcal.

Membranoproliferative glomerulonephritis: Etiology unknown.

IgA nephropathy: Asymptomatic gross hematuria.

Schönlein-Henoch purpura glomerulonephritis: Varied renal involvement.

Glomerulonephritis of systemic lupus erythematosus (SLE): On rare occasions, it is the first sign of SLE.

Hereditary glomerulonephritis (Alport's syndrome): Transmission is autosomal-dominant/X-linked and there is a family history of end-stage renal disease, especially in young males. Sometimes associated with deafness and eye abnormalities.

Etiology: Most common cause is poststreptococcal infection.

Occurrence: Worldwide.

Age: Occurs in any pediatric age group, but usually in children aged 3–7.

Ethnicity: Not significant.

Gender: Occurs equally in males and females.

Contributing Factors: Additional factors to be considered are a past history of streptococcal infection (impetigo, streptococcal throat infection, and family history of urinary abnormalities, genetics).

Signs and Symptoms: Parents describe a history of hematuria and decreased urinary output. Many patients complain of headache or malaise. Obtain a past medical history, particularly including streptococcal infections and family history of renal problems.

Physical examination may reveal periorbital edema. Hypertension may be discovered. The patient usually has no fever. In severe cases, ascites will be noted.

Diagnostic Tests

Urinalysis for red blood cell casts, gross hematuria ("coffee- or tea-colored" urine)

Serum complement level (decreased).

24-hour urine for creatinine and protein (1 g proteinuria/24 hours).

Throat culture and sensitivity.

Complete blood count with differential to assess for continuing infection.

Glomerular filtration rate (decreased).

Differential Diagnosis

Nephrotic syndrome: persistent 4+ proteinuria, hyperlipidemia.

Acute renal failure.

Treatment: Mild to moderate disease state should be treated with supportive therapy and restrictions regarding salt and water intake. Treatment for severe disease may include dialysis and renal failure transplant.

Follow-up: Weekly follow-up for monitoring blood pressure, proteinuria, and edema.

Sequelae: Untreated, glomerulonephritis can result in infection, renal failure, growth failure, anemia, and hypertension.

Prevention/Prophylaxis: Adequate treatment of streptococcal infections as a preventive measure.

Referral: Refer child to a pediatric urologist/nephrologist.

Education: Instruct parents in the importance of completion of the antibiotic regimen, the signs and symptoms of renal infection, the methods for monitoring intake and output, and the nutritional requirements and restrictions.

Urethritis

Urethritis is an infection of the urethra resulting from contact with a pathogen during sexual contact.

Etiology: Most common bacterial pathogens are *Neisseria gonorrhoeae* and *Chlamydia trachomatis*. *Ureaplasma urealyticum* and *Mycoplasma genitalium* are implicated in possibly one-third of nongonococcal urethritis cases.

Occurrence: Common.

Age: Usually occurs in adolescents; 15–24 year age group has highest incidence of sexually transmitted diseases.

Ethnicity: Not significant.

Gender: Occurs equally in males and females.

Contributing Factors: Multiple sexual partners, failure to use contraceptives, and failure to seek early treatment.

Signs and Symptoms: Patients complain of dysuria and urethral discharge. History of sexual activity should be obtained. In females particularly, suspect sexual abuse. Obtain a history related to trauma, sexual abuse, and masturbation. Males may complain of urinary frequency, urgency, and priapism. There may be a clear, white, or purulent discharge from the urethra, as well as suprapubic tenderness. Some infections are asymptomatic.

Diagnostic Tests

First-void urine demonstrating at least 10 white blood cells (WBCs) per high-power field. Gram's stain of urethral secretions with at least five WBCs per oil-immersion field. First-void urine with a positive leukocyte esterase test.

Collect pelvic and penile cultures for identification of a specific organism.

Culture for *N. gonorrhoeae* using chocolate agar or Thayer-Martin medium.

Culture, enzyme-linked immunoassay (ELISA) or monoclonal antibody.

Immunofluorescence test for *Chlamydia*.

Differential Diagnosis

Topical irritants.

Pinworms, identified in the discharge.

Treatment:

N. gonorrhoeae

For children who weigh less than 45 kg:

      Ceftriaxone, 125 mg IM in a single dose.

Alternative: Spectinomycin 40 mg/kg (maximum 2 g) in a single dose (may not be reliable).

For adults and adolescents:

      Cefixime, 400 mg PO in a single dose

      or

      Ceftriaxone, 125 mg IM in a single dose

      or

      Ofloxacin, 400 mg PO in a single dose

      or

      Azithromycin, 1 g PO in a single dose

      or

      Doxycycline, 100 mg PO bid for 7 days.

Alternative: Spectinomycin 2 g IM in a single dose

      or

      Ceftizoxime, 500 mg IM in a single dose

      or

      Cefotaxime, 500 mg IM in a single dose

      or

      Cefoxitin, 2 g IM in a single dose

      or

      Cefotetan, 1 g IM in a single dose

      or

      Enoxacin, 400 mg PO in a single dose

      or

      Norfloxacin, 800 mg PO in a single dose.

Chlamydia   Azithromycin, 1 g PO in a single dose *plus*

      Doxycycline 100 mg PO bid for 7 days

Alternative: Erythromycin base 500 mg PO qid for 7 days

      or

      Erythromycin ethylsuccinate 800 mg PO qid for 7 days

      or

      Ofloxacin 300 mg bid for 7 days.

For those unable to tolerate high doses of erythromycin:

      Erythromycin base 250 mg PO qid for 14 days

      or

      Erythromycin ethylsuccinate 400 mg PO qid for 14 days.

For recurrent or persistent chlamydia:

      Metronidazole 2 mg PO in a single dose *plus*

      Erythromycin 500 mg PO qid for 7 days

      or

      Erythromycin ethylsuccinate 800 mg PO ID for 7 days.

Follow-up: Return in 1 week for evaluation of therapeutic response.

Sequelae: If untreated or inadequately treated, urethritis can result in cervicitis in females; in males, it can result in prostatitis, epididymitis, or orchitis.

Prevention/Prophylaxis: Preventive measures include practicing safe sex and using appropriate contraceptives. Treatment of both partners is important to prevent reinfection.

Referral: Report sexually transmitted diseases to the local health department.

Education: Emphasize abstinence until both partners have been treated adequately. Teach proper handwashing technique, and instruct patients to wash hands accordingly after voiding.

Urinary Tract Infections

UTIs are caused by the introduction of bacteria or irritants into the urinary tract (bladder and/or kidneys), resulting in an infection.

Etiology

Bacterial: Most common organisms are *Escherichia coli, Klebsiella, Proteus,* enterococci, and staphylococci.

Nonbacterial: Residual urine, foreign bodies, vesicoureteral reflux, and urinary stasis have been implicated.

Occurrence: Most common of the genitourinary problems of childhood: found in 1% of premature infants and newborns, 3–7.8% of school-age girls, and 1–1.7% of boys.

Age: All age groups.

Ethnicity: Not significant.

Gender: During the first months of life, more common in males; from age 2 months to adulthood, more common in females.

Contributing Factors: Short urethra in females, use of bubble baths, colored and/or perfumed toilet paper, perianal infection (pinworms), improper wiping after defecating, too-tight undergarments, congenital defects, sexual activity in females, and masturbation.

Signs and Symptoms: Presenting symptoms and physical findings depend on age (Fig. 10–2).

Neonates: Feeding problems, diarrhea, vomiting, fever, failure to thrive, hyperbilirubinemia.

Ages 1 month to 2 years: Feeding problems, diarrhea, fever of unknown origin, colic, irritability and screaming periods, failure to thrive.

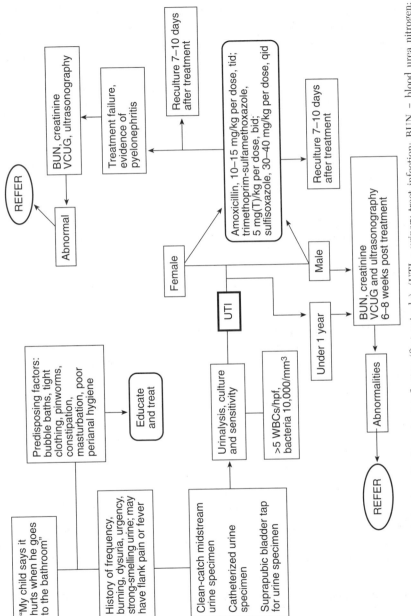

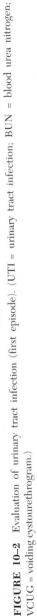

FIGURE 10–2 Evaluation of urinary tract infection (first episode). (UTI = urinary tract infection; BUN = blood urea nitrogen; VCUG = voiding cystourethrogram.)

Ages 2–6 years: Urgency, dysuria, frequency, abdominal pain, strong-smelling urine.

Ages 6–18 years: Frequency, dysuria, urgency, abdominal or flank pain.

Diagnostic Tests

Urinalysis reveals more than five WBCs per high-power field.

Culture and sensitivity shows 10^2 colonies/mL.

Radiographic studies (intravenous pyelogram or voiding cystourethrogram). Criteria for conducting such studies are UTI in a male, UTI in the first year of life, and UTI in a female with treatment failure and/or evidence of pyelonephritis. Radiographic studies usually done 6–8 weeks post-treatment.

Differential Diagnosis

Upper UTIs, as opposed to lower UTIs, show glitter cells and WBC casts; patient has high fever and anatomical abnormalities.

Patients with *anatomical abnormalities* such as neurogenic bladder, vesicoureteral reflux, and urinary stasis may initially present as having a UTI.

Pyelonephritis shows elevated C-reactive protein and high fever.

Treatment

Trimethoprim (TMP) and sulfamethoxazole (SMX): 2 mg/kg TMP plus 10 mg/kg SMX per day at bedtime or 5 mg TMP plus 25 mg SMX twice per week

or

Nitrofurantoin: 1–2 mg/kg per day in divided doses q 12 hours

or

Sulfisoxazole: 10–20 mg/kg per day in divided doses q 12 hours

or

Nalidixic acid: 30 mg/kg per day in divided doses q 12 hours

or

Methenamine mandelate: 75 mg/kg per day in divided doses q 12 hours.

(*Note:* In children under 2 months, do not use sulfonamide antibiotics or nitrofurantoin because of the risk of displacing bilirubin from albumin.)

Follow-up: Follow-up urinalysis in 3 days and again in 10 days to evaluate clinical response. Follow-up urinalysis in 1–2 months until patient is infection-free for 1 year.

Sequelae: If not treated promptly, the infection can result in renal scarring and pyelonephritis.

Prevention/Prophylaxis: Instruct parent and/or patient as follows:

Increase water intake to 1–2 L/day.

Empty bladder every 3–4 hours during the day.

Use improved hygienic measures.

Use white, unscented toilet paper.

Avoid taking bubble baths.

Prescribe suppressive antibiotic therapy for children with recurrent infections or those at high risk for reinfection (e.g., children under 5, those with urinary tract abnormalities).

Referral: Refer female patients to a urologist after treatment failure. Treatment failures often suggest an anatomical abnormality. Refer any male with UTI to a urologist.

Education: Instruct parents in measures to promote a healthy environment, such as avoiding bubble baths, using unscented toilet paper, properly cleansing after voiding, and dressing child in white cotton panties with no aniline dyes. Instruct parents as to the importance of completing the therapeutic regimen.

REFERENCES

General

Berhman, R, and Kleigman, R: Nelson's Essentials of Pediatrics. WB Saunders, Philadelphia, 1990.
Doenges, M, and Moorhouse, M: Nurse's Pocket Guide: Nursing Diagnoses with Interventions, ed 5. FA Davis, Philadelphia, 1995.
Engle, J: Pocket Guide to Pediatric Assessment, ed 2. Mosby, St. Louis, 1992.
Hay, W, et al: Current Pediatric Diagnosis & Treatment, ed 12. Appleton & Lange, Norwalk, Conn, 1995.

Assessment

DeGowin, R: DeGowin & DeGowin's Diagnostic Examination. McGraw-Hill, New York, 1994.
Steele, R: Clinical Handbook of Pediatric Infectious Diseases. Parthenon, New York, 1994.
Swartz, M: Textbook of Physical Diagnosis: History and Examination, ed 2. WB Saunders, Philadelphia, 1992.

Enuresis

Garber, K: Enuresis: An update on diagnosis and management. J Pediatr Health Care 10:202, 1996.
Mack, R: Dry All Night. Little, Brown & Co, Boston, 1989.
Moser, R: Those wee hours of the night: Nocturnal enuresis in children. Adv Nurse Pract 2(7):14, 1994.

Urethritis

U.S. Department of Health and Human Services, Centers for Disease Control and Prevention. 1998 Guidelines for treatment of sexually transmitted diseases. MMWR 47(RR-1), 1998.

CHAPTER 11

ASSESSMENT OF

THE REPRODUCTIVE

SYSTEM

Generally, when discussing reproductive health issues, the nurse practitioner (NP) thinks of females and the problems related to the gynecological system. However, the NP also should consider males and their reproductive health issues, because approximately the same number of males and females are seen in the primary-care clinic.

Assessment should always include a thorough history. The NP should ask questions related to familial patterns or problems; for the female patient, the NP should also ascertain maternal age of menarche or any history of dysmenorrhea or endometriosis. The NP should ask the female patient whether she has any history of bleeding disorders, malignancy, diethylstilbestrol (DES) exposure, or other genetic disorders that might affect the reproductive system. If menses has begun, the NP should obtain a thorough menstrual history including questions regarding age of onset, duration of menses, time between cycles, and any dysmenorrhea. For the male patient, the NP must ascertain any history of sexual dysfunction or testicular cancer.

A sexual history from both male and female adolescent patients should be obtained in an atmosphere of privacy and confidentiality. NPs should ask their patients whether they use any form of contraception, whether safe sex is practiced, whether they have or have had multiple partners, how many, and their frequency of sexual intercourse. Questions should include whether they have had sexual relations with persons of the opposite or same sex, or both, and whether those encounters involved oral, anal, and/or vaginal sex. For females, the NP should take an obstetrical history, including any abortions or pregnancies that they may have had. The NP should also conduct a complete review of systems, including vaginal (in females), urinary, abdominal, pelvic (in females), testicular (in males), and any general concerns.

For the prepubertal child, either the knee-chest or the frog-leg position is the most comfortable and most commonly used. In females, applying gentle traction on the labia and pulling it forward and lateral allow the best visualization. An otoscope provides adequate light and magnification to conduct a complete examination. In both males and females, the NP should examine the breasts, abdomen, and inguinal areas. Hernias, the presence and distribution of hair, and the state of hygiene can be assessed at this time. In females, the NP should measure the size of the clitoris; the average size is about 3×3 mm. Prepubertal mucosa is generally thin and red; one sign of estrogenization is a moist or dull mucosa. In males, the NP should evaluate the size and appearance of the penis and testes. Position of the urethra is important; a previously undetected hypospadias or epispadias can be detected at this time. If one or both testes are enlarged, transillumination should assist in determining whether a hydrocele is present or whether there is some other pathology that needs further evaluation. In females, the NP should examine and describe the hymen. Hymenal opening is correlated with age, and a 1-mm increase for each year of age is considered normal. A hymen that is 10–15 mm open is abnormal, and the cause should be investigated further.

Examination of both male and female adolescents should include a breast examination (Fig. 11–1); this is also an excellent time ot teach self-examination of the breast. The NP should inspect the external genitalia and perform Tanner staging (Table 11–1).

In sexually active female adolescents, the NP should use a speculum in conducting the examination. Bilateral palpation of the uterus and adnexa is also necessary. The NP should question males regarding any penile discharge, sores, or growths and should perform the appropriate cultures and examinations if any of these symptoms are present.

Reproductive health issues, such as family planning, risk-taking sexual behaviors, and strategies to reduce the spread of sexually transmitted diseases (STDs), should be addressed with the sexually active patient in a nonjudgmental manner. Issues related to sexual preference should also be discussed.

For parents as well as male and female adolescents, discussions regarding reproductive health issues are often uncomfortable. Education aimed at making the transition into puberty an easier one for all involved can help promote healthy reproductive practices and hence a healthy reproductive system.

Amenorrhea

Amenorrhea, the absence of menses, can occur in either a primary or a secondary form. Primary amenorrhea is diagnosed when the onset of menses has

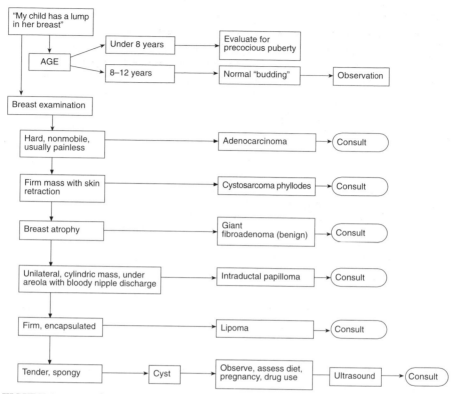

FIGURE 11–1 Evaluation of breast lumps in female patients.

not occurred by age 17. Secondary amenorrhea is diagnosed when menses has not occurred for at least 3 months.

Etiology: There is no genetic predisposition for either primary or secondary amenorrhea. Primary amenorrhea may be caused by an imperforate hymen, agenesis of the uterus, Turner's syndrome, or constitutional delay. Secondary amenorrhea may be due to pregnancy, a corpus luteum cyst, menopause, or breastfeeding. Other causes of secondary amenorrhea include diabetes, hypothyroidism or hyperthyroidism, chemotherapy, stress, weight loss, or polycystic ovaries.

Occurrence: Amenorrhea occurs in 3.3% of the female population.

Age: Amenorrhea can occur from menarche to menopause.

Ethnicity: Not significant.

Gender: Occurs only in females.

Contributing Factors: Strenuous athletic exercise or training, eating disorders including bulimia and anorexia, psychological problems, and emotional crisis may contribute to the incidence of amenorrhea.

TABLE 11–1   STAGES OF PUBERTY—TANNER STAGES

Stage	Female Breasts	Female and Male Pubic Hair	Male Penis	Male Testes
1	Diameter of areolae increases	None	Prepubertal	Prepubertal
2	Breast buds develop	Light, straight, sparse	Enlarges	Testes enlarge, scrotum becomes red and coarse
3	Areolae and breasts enlarge	Darker, curling, slight increase in amount	Lengthens	Continuation of stage 2
4	Contour differentiates between areola and breast	Coarse, curly, moderate amount	Increases in diameter	Scrotum darkens
5	Breasts fully developed	Adult distribution and amount, spread to medial thighs; thickening will continue	Fully developed	Testes and scrotum fully developed

Source: Adapted from Tanner, JM: Growth at Adolescence, ed 2. Blackwell Scientific, Oxford, 1962.

Signs and Symptoms: In primary amenorrhea, the patient, who is at least 17, reports that she has never had a menstrual period. She may state that this has occurred in other members of her family.

In secondary amenorrhea, the patient may state that it has been a minimum of 3 months since her last menstrual cycle. She may relate signs and symptoms suggestive of pregnancy, including bloating, enlarged and tender breasts, nausea and vomiting at different periods of the day (usually in the morning on awakening), and increased lethargy. She may state that she has had unprotected sexual intercourse. Other complaints may include weight gain, polyuria, polydypsia, an emotional crisis, or a recent increase in an athletic training schedule.

Inspection reveals few findings unless the patient is pregnant. In hypothyroidism, the skin may be extremely dry, periorbital edema may be noted, and there may be some apparent voice changes (hoarseness). When a Pap smear and vaginal examination are performed, an imperforate hymen (rare) may be noted. The cervix may be blue or purple, suggestive of changes seen in pregnancy; other changes include breast enlargement and darkened areolae. When constitutional delay is suspected, the NP should carefully evaluate breast development and pubic hair distribution to determine the Tanner stage (see Table 11–1).

Palpation and percussion may reveal breast tenderness, increased uterine size, and increased height of the fundus. Thyroid size should be evaluated for enlargement when thyroid disease is suspected (Fig. 11–2).

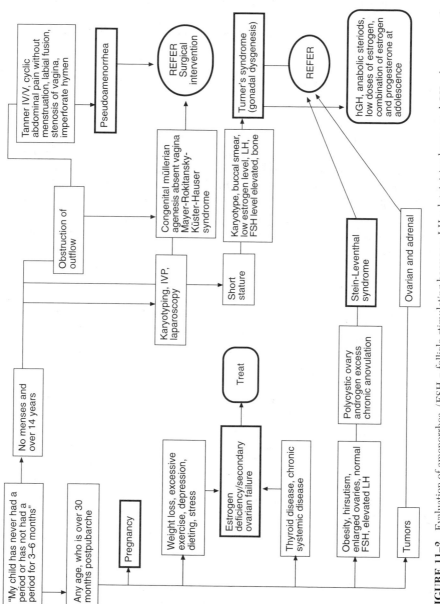
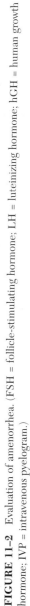

FIGURE 11–2 Evaluation of amenorrhea. (FSH = follicle-stimulating hormone; LH = luteinizing hormone; hGH = human growth hormone; IVP = intravenous pyelogram.)

Diagnostic Tests

A serum pregnancy test is done to differentiate amenorrhea from pregnancy.

Follicle-stimulating hormone (FSH) and luteal hormone (LH) levels are normal in amenorrhea.

Thyroxine (T_4) and thyroid-stimulating hormone (TSH) levels may indicate a thyroid dysfunction, if abnormal.

Laparoscopy may be done to evaluate the presence and state of the ovaries.

Ultrasound of the pelvis and ovaries is done to detect cysts, masses, and other abnormalities.

Differential Diagnosis

Pregnancy is differentiated by a serum pregnancy test.

Overtraining is determined from the history. Menses returns when the training schedule is moderated and there is less physical stress on the body.

Eating disorders are determined from the history but may often be missed by the health-care provider, especially during an initial visit; also, subtle changes in weight cannot be known unless the patient shares these facts.

Turner's syndrome is differentiated by physical examination (webbed neck, pectus excavatus, short stature, heart murmur) and/or genetic screening.

Pituitary diseases and uncontrolled endocrinopathies, which can suppress menses, can be detected by hormonal studies.

Because some *medications and medical treatments* can suppress menses (e.g., GH-RH analog, donazol, medroxyprogesterone acetate [Depo-Provera], chemotherapy), the patient's medication history should be obtained.

Treatment: If the cause is imperforate hymen, surgery is indicated. If overweight or underweight, proper nutritional counseling is needed. In all cases, hormone replacement therapy is indicated for 6 months to reduce the risk of osteoporosis. Medroxyprogesterone acetate, 10 mg daily for 10 days of each month, is a good mode of treatment. Conjugated estrogens, 1.25 mg daily for 21 days, with medroxyprogesterone acetate, 10 mg daily during the last 7 days of the month, is another treatment modality.

Follow-up: Ninety-nine percent of all cases of secondary amenorrhea spontaneously resolve; therefore, routine health-care visits are all that is needed. If the patient is not pregnant and hormone replacement therapy is used, further assessment is suggested in 6 months; the therapy should be stopped and the patient referred if the menses does not return spontaneously.

Sequelae: Estrogen-deficiency symptoms, such as hot flashes and vaginal dryness along with signs of osteoporosis, can occur if amenorrhea is prolonged.

Prevention/Prophylaxis: Maintenance of proper body weight, moderation in athletic training, and the use of prophylaxis for sexual intercourse can prevent secondary amenorrhea.

Referral: If amenorrhea persists for 6 months after treatment has been instituted, refer to a gynecologist. If pregnancy is suspected or proved by tests and examination, refer immediately to a midwife or gynecologist. If an endocrine disorder is suspected, refer to an endocrinologist.

Education: The patient must be fully informed of all the findings, including pregnancy. If needed, refer to a gynecologist. The need for regular prenatal care should be stressed. The effects of long-term amenorrhea should be fully explained to the patient. Explain treatment options (e.g., hormonal replacement therapy, lubricants for vaginal dryness, other medication regimens) to the patient, and allow the patient an opportunity to ask questions. As menses returns, offer contraceptive counseling.

Cryptorchidism

Cryptorchidism is the failure of one or both testes to descend into the scrotum.

Etiology: This disorder may be related to some interference with descent of the testes between the seventh and ninth prenatal month. Because it is a congenital defect, the exact cause is unknown.

Occurrence: Found in 3% of all newborns and up to 17% of premature males. Thirty percent of premature males exhibit this condition. Ten percent of patients with cryptorchidism have an associated upper urinary tract abnormality.

Age: Present at birth.

Ethnicity: Not significant.

Gender: Males.

Contributing Factors: Unknown: congenital anomaly.

Signs and Symptoms: The parent reports that the scrotal area looks "different" from that of other children, or that the sac feels or looks empty. The cremasteric reflex is absent or weak at birth. The testis(es) cannot be palpated in the scrotum. The scrotal sacs appear smaller (bilateral) or asymmetrical (unilateral).

Diagnostic Tests: A sonogram is indicated if the defect is bilateral to see whether the testes are absent or undescended.

Differential Diagnosis

Anorchia is differentiated by sonogram, which will demonstrate the absence of one or both testicles.

Retractile testis occurs when one testis remains retracted the majority of the time, but is palpable on examination. It may respond to cold.

Ambiguous genitalia may be confused with bilateral cryptorchidism, but the testes are usually absent while the scrotum is present. Additionally, both female and male genitalia are present.

Treatment: Hormone therapy, which may be instituted by a urologist to facilitate surgery, is followed by an orchiopexy between 1 and 3 years of age.

Follow-up: By age 1 year, a child with unilateral cryptorchidism should be seen by a urologist. If surgery is performed, the child should be seen at 6-month intervals for 1–2 years.

Sequelae: Infertility, atrophy of the testicle, and an increased risk of developing a malignant testicular tumor.

Prevention/Prophylaxis: None: congenital abnormality.

Referral: Patients with bilateral and/or nonpalpable cryptorchidism should be referred to a urologist. Unilateral cryptorchidism should be referred to a urologist by age 1 year.

Education: Parents should be taught to palpate the child's testes so they can detect any abnormality. Also, they should be shown the difference between a retractile testicle and one that is absent. An open discussion with the child and parent should be done so that all involved are aware of the possible sequelae.

Dysmenorrhea

Dysmenorrhea is painful menstruation characterized by lower abdominal cramping usually occurring during the first few days of bleeding. Dysmenorrhea is divided into two types: primary, which occurs in the absence of any pelvic pathology; and secondary, which is associated with a specific pelvic pathology.

Etiology: Primary dysmenorrhea has no known causative agent, but it is suspected that painful menses occurs when there is an increase of prostaglandin $F_{2\alpha}$ ($PGF_{2\alpha}$) and $PGE_{2\alpha}$. Secondary dysmenorrhea is usually caused by pelvic inflammatory disease (PID), endometriosis, uterine myomas, polyps or adhesions, adenomyosis, ovarian cysts or tumors, the presence of an intrauterine device (IUD), cervical stenosis or strictures, or congenital malformations.

Occurrence: Seventy-five percent of adolescent females experience some pain with menses, 10–15% of whom have pain so severe that it limits normal activities.

Age: Dysmenorrhea occurs from about 6–12 months after menarche begins to the mid 20s, with a very few women experiencing cramping until a more advanced age.

Ethnicity: Not significant.

Gender: Females.

Contributing Factors: Underlying pathologies, along with emotional stress and certain hormonal abnormalities; familial tendency.

Signs and Symptoms: When obtaining a history, ask the following questions:

What is the pain like (sharp, dull, pressure)?
When did you first start having the pain?
Are there associated symptoms, such as nausea and vomiting?

Does the pain cause you to miss school or work?
What remedies have you used, and were they successful?
Is there a maternal or sibling history of painful menses?

The adolescent will report that her first few menstrual cycles were without pain, but that recently she experienced lower abdominal and back pain during the first 1–3 days of her cycle.

Inspection reveals the patient to be guarding, in pain, and rubbing the abdomen. The skin should be observed for hirsutism, bruising, or petechia. Palpation and percussion of the abdomen and kidneys should be done to detect masses and tender areas. In primary dysmenorrhea, few findings will be noted.

In secondary dysmenorrhea, the history may reveal other symptoms, such as fever (PID); pain that lasts beyond the menstrual cycle (endometriosis); heaviness in the lower abdomen, swelling, or heavy bleeding (cysts or tumors); and a vaginal discharge and odor (STD).

Inspection reveals a white to brown vaginal discharge along with an odor. There may be a string visible if the pain is the result of an IUD. Palpation and percussion may reveal tenderness or a mass in the abdomen or suprapubic area. In the adolescent who is not sexually active, a speculum may not be needed and therefore should not be insisted upon for the examination.

Diagnostic Tests: No tests are needed if underlying pathology is not suggested by the examination. Otherwise, appropriate tests for the detection of masses and cysts (e.g., sonogram of the abdomen and pelvis) should be performed. Cultures and smears should be done for a suspected infection. If there is heavy bleeding, a hemoglobin and hematocrit should be ordered.

Differential Diagnosis

Abdominal, uterine, or bladder *mass* is differentiated by sonogram or computed tomographic (CT) scan.
STD is differentiated by vaginal cultures and/or a blood test.
Endometriosis is differentiated by endometrial biopsy.

Treatment: Treatment for mild dysmenorrhea includes ibuprofen, aspirin, or acetaminophen. The most commonly prescribed drug is ibuprofen, 400 mg q 4–6 hours for 24–72 hours. For moderate to severe dysmenorrhea, nonsteroidal anti-inflammatory drugs (NSAIDs), given for 3–4 months, are the treatment of choice:

Naproxen (Aleve, Naprosyn), 500 mg for the first dose and then 250 mg q 4–6 hours
or
Mefenamic acid (Ponstel), 500 mg for the first dose and then 250 mg q 6–8 hours
or
Naproxen sodium (Anaprox), 500 mg at the first dose and then 275 mg q 6–8 hours for the duration of the symptoms.

If NSAIDs are not effective or if the adolescent is sexually active, low-dose combination oral contraceptives (OCs) should be used. They may be used alone or in combination with the NSAIDs. OCs are about 90% effective in severe dysmenorrhea. Heating pads, mild exercise, and maintenance of a good diet also may help to alleviate or decrease the symptoms.

Follow-up: At 3 months, if the symptoms have not worsened, the patient should be seen to evaluate the effectiveness of the treatment. If the patient is sexually active, a yearly Pap smear and examination should be scheduled.

Sequelae: Usually there is no serious physical sequela; however, adolescents may miss school or work because of severe pain, which in turn results in poor school performance or the loss of a job.

Prevention/Prophylaxis: A mild exercise program, good diet, and proper use of medications (NSAIDs and OCs) can prevent serious pain. A menstrual diary may help patients anticipate their menstrual cycle.

Education: Most patients will be symptom-free after 3–4 months of therapy, so their education should include reassurance. The importance of a good diet, mild to moderate exercise, and regular use of medications should be stressed.

Epididymitis

Epididymitis is a painful, acute inflammation of the epididymis. The epididymis is a small, elongated body that rests on the surface of each testis, serving as the excretory duct.

Etiology: Commonly, epididymitis is caused by *Neisseria gonorrhoeae* and *Chlamydia*, but it can also occur along with an infection in the urethra or bladder.

Occurrence: Fairly common; not influenced by seasonality.

Age: Epididymitis is a very rare occurrence prior to puberty, but it can occur any time after a child becomes sexually active. In extremely rare cases, it can occur in children under 2 who have congenital anomalies associated with the urologic system.

Ethnicity: Not significant.

Gender: Occurs only in males.

Contributing Factors: Congenital anomalies of the kidney, bladder, or urethra and engaging in unprotected sex can increase the risk.

Signs and Symptoms: The child reports painful swelling of the scrotum that can be either acute or insidious. The scrotum is painful to touch and manipulate. The child reports having a fever, dysuria, and increased frequency of urination. The child admits having had unprotected sex within 45 days of the onset of the problem.

On inspection, the NP notes scrotal swelling and redness; the scrotum feels warm to touch. During palpation of the scrotum, the child reports pain. The epididymis feels hard and enlarged, and tenderness to touch can be elicited. Prehn's sign, relief of pain when the testes are elevated, is positive. There may also be a urethral discharge. A rectal examination, which elicits tenderness of the prostate, can produce urethral discharge.

Diagnostic Tests

A urinalysis to determine the presence of leukocytes and bacteria (positive in epididymitis).

A urethral culture and Gram's stain to reveal the causative agent.

If available, a Doppler ultrasound to differentiate between epididymitis and torsion of the testicle.

If sexual activity is denied, a follow-up voiding cystourethrogram to rule out congenital anomalies.

Differential Diagnosis: *Testicular torsion,* differentiated by the Prehn's sign: in torsion, elevation of the scrotum produces pain.

Treatment: Measures to relieve pain should be instituted, including elevation of the scrotum, bed rest, and application of ice packs to the area. NSAIDs can be used.

Antibiotic therapy is essential; the first-line treatment is one dose of ceftri-axone 250 mg intramuscular (IM) followed by doxycycline 100 mg bid for 10 days. If the patient cannot tolerate ceftriaxone, then ofloxacin 300 mg bid for 10 days or ciprofloxin 500 mg in one dose plus doxycycline 100 mg bid for 10 days should be used. One dose of ofloxacin 400 mg plus doxycycline 100 mg bid for 10 days can also be used.

Follow-up: If sexual activity is denied, a voiding cystourethrogram should be performed. Otherwise, no follow-up is necessary if symptoms resolve.

Sequelae: If untreated or incompletely treated, infertility, abscess, or even atrophy of the testis can occur.

Referral: If the patient does not have a prompt response to treatment, a referral should be made.

Education: Patient should be taught that unprotected sexual activity is the mode of transmission and that, to prevent epididymitis, a condom should be worn. It should also be stressed that reinfection can occur when sexual partners have not been treated.

Gynecomastia in Males

Gynecomastia in males is a benign, self-limiting breast enlargement during Tanner stages II and III. Twenty percent of cases have bilateral involvement; resolution may take up to 2 years.

Etiology: Testosterone-estrogen imbalance, increased prolactin level, and abnormal serum-binding protein levels are suggested causes.

Occurrence: Occurs in 50–60% of males during early adolescence.

Age: Boys aged 12–14.

Ethnicity: Not significant.

Gender: Only in males.

Contributing Factors: Klinefelter's syndrome, use of certain prescription and illegal drugs.

Signs and Symptoms: Child is brought to clinic with the complaint, "He is growing breasts." Obtain a history as to other sexual developmental signs: growth of body hair, family history for familial pattern, past and present medical history, and medication history.

Physical findings include a 1–3 cm, round, freely mobile, firm mass immediately beneath the areola.

Diagnostic Tests: None. If mass gets larger or does not resolve in 2 years, obtain a thyroid panel, liver function studies, and urinary gonadotrophins if indicated.

Differential Diagnosis

Pseudogynecomastia, differentiated by excessive fat tissue and prominent pectoralis muscles.

Drug-induced gynecomastia, caused by ingestion of amphetamines, marijuana, meprobamate, opiates (e.g., codeine, heroin, morphine), prescription drugs (e.g., amitriptyline, cimetidine, diazepam, haloperidol, imipramine, isoniazid, tricyclic antidepressants), hormones, and chemotherapy.

Tumors (e.g., testicular, adrenal, pituitary), differentiated by elevated prolactin, or a CT or MRI scan.

Hypothyroidism or hyperthyroidism, differentiated by a thyroid panel.

Hepatic dysfunction, differentiated by abnormal liver function tests.

Klinefelter's syndrome, differentiated by the clinical picture: tall eunuchoid build, diminished facial hair, normal to borderline low IQ, micro-orchidism, and high levels of urinary gonadotropins.

Treatment: None. If condition worsens and associated psychological problems develop, the NP may give bromocriptine, a drug that suppresses lactation. Surgical intervention is rarely indicated.

Follow-up: Patient should return to clinic in 3 months for reevaluation.

Sequelae: If unresolved, investigate further as to the cause.

Prevention/Prophylaxis: None.

Referral: Refer patient to primary-care physician if there are any large, hard, or fixed enlargements or masses with any discharge.

Education: Reassure parent and child that idiopathic gynecomastia is a benign condition that usually resolves within 2 years.

Herpes Simplex Virus Type 2

Herpes simplex virus type 2 causes a vesicular eruption of the skin and mucous membranes that can be a primary or recurrent problem in the sexually active. In the very young child presenting with these symptoms, sexual abuse should be ruled out.

Etiology: Herpes, which is caused by human herpesvirus, usually affects the skin below the umbilicus. After a primary infection, the virus can remain latent in the cells that are in the area of the original eruption, but can become reactivated at various intervals.

Occurrence: Occurs when the patient is sexually active or in contact with another person who has active lesions.

Age: Any age when the patient is sexually active.

Ethnicity: Not significant.

Gender: Occurs equally in males and females.

Contributing Factors: Primary infection is due to exposure to a known carrier. Stress (either emotional or physical), fever, or exposure to sun may cause a later eruption.

Signs and Symptoms: Mild to severe discomfort may be present. If old enough, the patient describes a prodrome phase in which there was some mild paresthesia (e.g., burning, tingling). Dysuria and urinary retention, tenderness of the affected area, dyspareunia, and increasing pain is also described. There may be low-grade fever, headache, and malaise. Inguinal lymphadenopathy, maceration in moist areas, and a cluster of blisterlike eruptions can be found at the site of infection. In recurrent episodes, the signs tend to be less severe, although eruptions tend to ulcerate.

Inspection of a primary or recurrent episode reveals vesicular eruptions that are fluid-filled, reddened, and tender to palpation. Patients may have frequent or very infrequent eruptions.

Diagnostic Tests: Diagnosis is made on the basis of clinical symptoms; tests are not indicated. Cultures are available, but rarely done.

Differential Diagnosis

Chickenpox is differentiated by vesicular eruptions above and below the umbilicus. Eruptions are widespread over the entire body.
Coxsackievirus and echovirus are differentiated by the appearance of the rash, which is flat, pink, and sometimes lacy in appearance.
Herpangina is not sexually transmitted; usually occurs in or on the mouth.

Treatment: Pain medication may need to be prescribed. The use of acetaminophen or ibuprofen for children is appropriate. Viscous lidocaine may also be directly applied for relief of symptomatic pain. Both oral and topical acyclovir are primary medications in the management of herpes type 2. Topical acyclovir can be used every 2 hours for the first 2–3 days and then every 6 hours. Oral dosing should be based on weight (20 mg/kg per day in four divided doses).

Follow-up: Each exacerbation should be treated. The patient should be seen by the health-care provider; otherwise, routine health maintenance should be continued.

Sequelae: Spread of the infection to other parts of the body is a frequent problem, which can then lead to a generalized eruption of the disease. Secondary bacterial infection (staphylococcal or β-hemolytic streptococcal), which requires appropriate medication, is also a complication of herpes type 2. Immunosuppressed persons are at high risk for contracting the disease, so they should be extremely careful to avoid contact with herpes type 2 patients during the active phase of the disease. If an affected patient becomes pregnant, a cesarean section may be considered for delivery of the baby.

Prevention/Prophylaxis: Avoidance of contact with persons who have the disease and certainly of open lesions. If any of the lesions are present above the umbilicus (e.g., face, mouth), no direct contact with the person or items used by the person (e.g., drinking cups) should occur. Use of condoms among sexually active persons is of utmost importance in preventing the spread of this disease. If the disease occurs during pregnancy, either as a primary infection or as a recurrent eruption, the obstetrician should be made aware of this factor so that a decision can be made regarding the mode of delivery (vaginal versus cesarean section).

Referral: Infected immunocompromised patients or those who do not respond to topical or oral treatment should be referred to an infectious disease specialist. All pregnant females should be referred to an obstetrician or midwife so that care can be monitored; the fetus must also be carefully monitored.

Education: All patients should be educated that barrier methods of protection, specifically condoms, can reduce the spread of the disease. Herpes patients should begin treatment at the first sign of recurrent eruption of a herpetic lesion.

Hydrocele

A hydrocele is a collection of fluid in the scrotum causing asymptomatic swelling. When the amount of fluid varies, there is communication between the scrotum and the peritoneal cavity. This condition may or may not be accompanied by a hernia; it usually resolves by age 1 year.

Etiology: A congenital hydrocele results from a failure of the processus vaginalis peritonei to close at birth. Acquired hydrocele may result from a trauma or tumor of the scrotum.

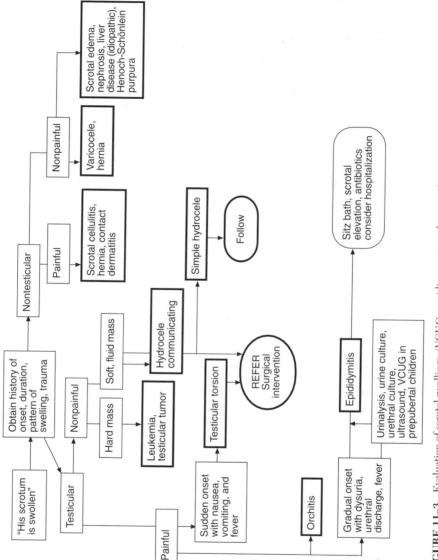

FIGURE 11–3 Evaluation of scrotal swellings. (VCUG = voiding cystourethrogram.)

Occurrence: Unknown.

Age: May occur at birth if congenital or at any age if related to trauma or tumor.

Ethnicity: Not significant.

Gender: Occurs in males.

Contributing Factors: Trauma, tumor, or congenital defect.

Signs and Symptoms: The parent will state, or the NP will note, that the scrotal sac is enlarged but does not appear discolored or painful. The testes can be palpated in the scrotal sac. There is no discomfort or discoloration associated with the hydrocele. The scrotal sac can be transilluminated.

Inspection reveals a swollen testis (or testes), which can be transilluminated. Palpation reveals no hardness or tenderness.

Diagnostic Tests: None.

Differential Diagnosis: Inguinal hernia, neoplasm, infectious process of the testes, trauma, hematoma, hematocele orchitis, and a cystic lesion should all be considered in the differential diagnosis of hydrocele (Fig. 11–3).

Infectious process, differentiated by laboratory data.
Trauma and hematoma, differentiated by the appearance of bruising or discolorations.
Lesions or mass, differentiated by ultrasound or CT scan.

Treatment: Monitor patient for 1 year for changes. Expect the hydrocele to resolve within that year. If resolution does not occur or if pain, scrotal redness, warmth, or hardness occurs, refer patient to a urologist.

Follow-up: Routine health-care visits.

Sequelae: Rare.

Prevention/Prophylaxis: None in cases of congenital malformation. Testicular self-examination can be performed each month to detect a mass. Males involved in contact sports should be mandated to wear protective gear to protect the scrotum from injury.

Referral: Refer patient to a urologist after 1 year of age.

Education: By adolescence, males should be taught how to perform testicular self-examination.

Hypospadias and Epispadias

Hypospadias occurs when the opening for the urethral meatus is on the ventral surface of the penis instead of at the top of the glans penis. The opening most often occurs near the glans, but may appear farther along the shaft. This condition is often accompanied by a ventral curvature of the penis (chordae) and/or a

hooded appearance of the penis. Epispadias occurs when the opening of the urethral meatus is placed somewhere along the dorsal side of the penis.

Etiology: There is a familial tendency for these conditions (7%); however, some
cases can be related to maternal exposure to progesterone at 8–14 weeks' gestation.

Occurrence: Hypospadias occurs in 1 in 250 live male births. Epispadias is a
rare occurrence (less than 1% of live births).

Age: Present at birth.

Ethnicity: Not significant.

Gender: Occurs in males.

Contributing Factors: Familial tendency (up to 14% recurrence); maternal exposure to progesterone at 8–14 weeks' gestation.

Signs and Symptoms: Inspection of the penis reveals misplacement of the urethral meatus opening, possibly accompanied by a hooded or curved appearance of the penis. Urethral opening can be seen on either the dorsal or ventral
surface of the penis. Note where along the shaft the opening appears.

Diagnostic Tests: None specifically for hypospadias or epispadias, but if other
abnormalities are suspected, an ultrasound of the renal organs should be ordered.

Differential Diagnosis: Ambiguous genitalia by virtue of inspection.

Treatment: Withhold circumcision. Between 12 and 18 months, refer infant to
a urologist for possible surgical repair.

Follow-up: Routine health-care visits should be made. If surgery is performed,
follow-up is generally at 2 weeks and again at 6 months by the surgeon.

Sequelae: Ten percent of boys who have hypospadias have undescended testes as
well. Unrepaired hypospadias may interfere with urination and sexual function,
and may induce psychological problems related to malformed external genitalia.

Prevention/Prophylaxis: None: congenital defect.

Referral: By age 1 year, or no older than 2, patient should be referred to a urologist.

Education: Parents should be told that this is not a life-threatening condition.
At about age 2 surgical repair can be done to correct the defect, and there will
be no long-term problems.

Labial Adhesions

Labial adhesions occur when there is partial or complete closure of the external
vaginal opening as a result of adhesions of the medial edges of the labia minora.
It is an asymptomatic, benign condition seen from age 2 months to menarche.

Etiology: This condition can be the result of hypoestrogenization, trauma (including rape), inflammation, or an infectious process. In adolescence, as the pH becomes more acidic, this is rarely seen.

Occurrence: Labial adhesions can occur in females from infancy to menarche.

Age: Labial adhesions can occur in females from infancy to menarche.

Ethnicity: Not significant.

Gender: Females.

Contributing Factors: It is believed that when children have low levels of estrogen, there is an increased frequency of labial adhesions. Another factor may be local irritation or scratching, which denudes the thin skin covering the labia, resulting in an adhesion as healing occurs. Sexual abuse must also be considered.

Signs and Symptoms: History of trauma, difficulty urinating, or discomfort with urination may be related by the child or parent.

Inspection reveals that the labia minora is medially connected by a thin layer of tissue, thereby closing or partially closing the external vaginal opening. Recurrent urinary tract infections (UTIs) may also be a sign of an adhesion.

Diagnostic Tests: None.

Differential Diagnosis: Imperforate vagina (rare), differentiated by physical examination.

Treatment: Often no treatment is indicated, because this is a self-limiting problem. When symptomatic, estrogen cream is topically applied for 2–4 weeks. A topical antibiotic ointment is also helpful and applied each evening. Petroleum jelly should be applied for 1–2 months after adhesion is separated. Mechanical separation should *not* be done because of the risk of trauma to the area.

Follow-up: Follow up 2–4 weeks after the use of estrogen cream. A routine health-care visit schedule should be maintained.

Sequelae: Frequent UTIs and urinary discomfort may result from a labial adhesion.

Prevention/Prophylaxis: Improved perineal hygiene and removal of irritants may decrease the incidence of labial adhesions. Discourage scratching the pubic area. Treatment of external genitalia with estrogen creams is recommended.

Referral: When topical application with estrogen is not successful, or if severe urinary symptoms exist, surgery is then indicated and the patient should be referred to a urologist.

Education: Parents should be taught to examine child's external genitalia or to be alert for signs and symptoms of urinary difficulty. Also, because this is a fairly benign and self-limiting condition, parents need to know that there are no long-term sequelae.

Pelvic Inflammatory Disease

PID includes an inflammatory disorder of the female upper genital tract that can include salpingitis, endometritis, and pelvic peritonitis. Patients may present either as symptomatic or asymptomatic. PID, the result of undetected or inadequately treated STD of the endocervix, is often seen as a complication of common STDs.

Etiology: Generally, the etiology is considered polymicrobial. Sexually transmitted organisms, however, are implicated in most cases. Currently *Neisseria gonorrhoeae, Chlamydia trachomatis, Gardnerella vaginalis, Streptococcus* Groups A and B, coliform bacteria, and genital tract mycoplasmas should all be suspected as causative agents.

Occurrence: Any age at which a female is sexually active.

Age: PID rate is highest among sexually active adolescents.

Ethnicity: Highest in African-American females.

Gender: Occurs in females.

Contributing Factors: Multiple sexual partners, use of douches, or a previous episode of PID.

Signs and Symptoms: Patients may present with fever and complaints of lower abdominal pain, vaginal discharge, and irregular bleeding. They are sexually active, and they may have more than one partner. They may also have specific complaints related to the genitourinary system, including dysuria and vaginal discharge.

Inspection reveals an affect of discomfort, guarding of the lower abdomen, fever, chills, or sweating. Palpation and percussion reveal tenderness of the lower abdomen, pain on movement of cervix or adnexa. Guarding on palpation. Vital signs should also be assessed. When performing the vaginal examination, look for friability or erosion of the cervix, pain on movement of the cervix, or adnexal tenderness.

Diagnostic Tests: C-reactive protein is positive. Erythrocyte sedimentation rate is elevated. Complete blood count (CBC) reveals a white blood cell count (WBC) greater than 10,500. Cultures to demonstrate the presence of *N. gonorrhoeae* or *Chlamydia* in cervical secretions, a pregnancy test, and HIV testing should be done. Ultrasound may be performed to rule out ectopic pregnancy.

Differential Diagnosis

STDs, differentiated by cultures.

Ectopic pregnancy, confirmed by ultrasound.

Appendicitis, confirmed by examination, pain only in the lower quarter of the abdomen, (worse on right side), and ultrasound or CT of abdomen (Fig. 11–4; Table 11–2).

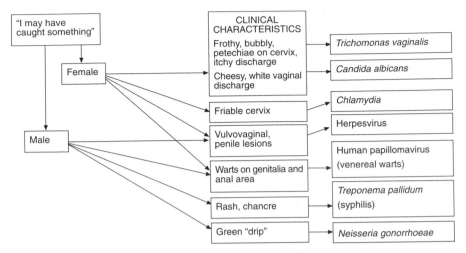

FIGURE 11–4   Differential diagnosis of sexually transmitted diseases.

Treatment: Treatment is given according to symptoms; because the specific organisms are generally not identified, treatment should be broad enough to cover all common etiologic agents. Prompt initiation of treatment with broad-spectrum antibiotic therapy is indicated to reduce the risk of exacerbation of the disease. If the patient fails to respond in 48 hours of outpatient treatment, she should be hospitalized. Advise the patient to abstain from sexual intercourse until treatment is complete. Medications currently suggested include: (Table 11–3)

Outpatient
Cefoxitin 2 g IM once and probenecid 1 g by mouth (PO) once, or ceftriaxone 250 mg IM once, both followed by docycycline 100 mg bid for 10 days

TABLE 11–2   DIFFERENTIAL DIAGNOSIS OF SEXUALLY TRANSMITTED DISEASES

Organism	Laboratory Test	Rule Out
Trichomonas	Wet prep	*Candida*
Candida	KOH prep	Cervical cancer
Herpesvirus	Viral cultures	
Chlamydia	Viral culture	
Papillomavirus		Melanoma
Neisseria gonorrhoeae	Gram's stain, culture	Nonspecific urethritis
Treponema pallidum	Blood test	

or metronidazole (Flagyl) 500 mg PO bid for 14 days with oxfloxacin 400 mg PO bid for 14 days.

Inpatient

Intravenous (IV) antibiotics, including clindamycin IV 900 mg q 8 hours plus gentamicin 1.5 mg/kg q 8 hours following a loading dose of 2 mg/kg.

Follow-up: All contacts should be treated, and follow-up cultures should be done in 4–6 weeks.

Sequelae: Sterility may result from incomplete or unsuccessful treatment. Chronic pelvic pain and/or ectopic pregnancy may also result from PID.

Prevention/Prophylaxis: Patient should avoid engaging in unprotected sex and having multiple sexual partners. She should not douche after sexual intercourse.

Referral: Patient should be referred to gynecologist if no improvement is seen in 48 hours.

Education: Patient should be educated not to have sexual intercourse until therapy is complete. Partners must be notified and treated. Furthermore, instructions regarding the consequences of PID and modes of transmission should be reviewed. The need to use condoms and the dangers of having multiple sexual partners and/or unprotected sex should be stressed.

Phimosis/Paraphimosis

Phimosis is the inability to retract the prepuce (foreskin) by the age of 3 years. Paraphimosis occurs when the foreskin has been retracted behind the sulcus and cannot be reduced. This condition may warrant immediate surgical intervention (circumcision).

Etiology: Phimosis is either congenital or acquired (i.e., when followed by an inflammation of the foreskin).

Occurrence: Paraphimosis occurs in 0.9% of the male population; phimosis occurs in approximately 10% of the population of uncircumcised males.

Age: Phimosis generally is noted before age 3, when the foreskin cannot easily be retracted.

Ethnicity: Not significant.

Gender: Occurs in males.

Contributing Factors: None.

Signs and Symptoms: The parent may report that the child's urinary stream is thin, and that he often states that he cannot go to the bathroom.

Phimosis is diagnosed by age 3, when the foreskin still cannot be retracted. It is confirmed when the foreskin cannot be retracted and returned to its original position.

TABLE 11-3 SUMMARY OF STD TREATMENT GUIDELINES CDC (JANUARY 23, 1998)

Disease	Recommended Regimens	Alternative Regimens
CHANCROID	<ul><li>Azithromycin 1 g PO in a single dose, or</li><li>Ceftriaxone 250 mg IM in a single dose, or</li><li>Ciprofloxacin 500 mg PO bid for 3 days, or[1]</li><li>Erythromycin base 500 mg PO qid for 7 days</li></ul>	
GENITAL HERPES SIMPLEX VIRUS (HSV) First Clinical Episode	<ul><li>Acyclovir 400 mg PO tid for 7–10 days, or</li><li>Acyclovir 200 mg PO 5× per day for 7–10 days, or</li><li>Famciclovir 250 mg PO tid for 7–10 days, or</li><li>Valacyclovir 1 g PO bid for 7–10 days</li></ul> Treatment may be extended if healing is incomplete after 10 days	
Recurrent Episodes	<ul><li>Acyclovir 400 mg PO tid for 5 days, or</li><li>Acyclovir 200 mg PO 5× per day for 5 days, or</li><li>Acyclovir 800 mg PO bid for 5 days, or</li><li>Famciclovir 125 mg PO bid for 5 days, or</li><li>Valacyclovir 500 mg PO bid for 5 days</li></ul>	
Severe Disease	<ul><li>Acyclovir 5–10 mg/kg body weight IV q8h for 5–7 days or until clinical resolution</li></ul>	
GRANULOMA INGUINALE (DONOVANOSIS)	<ul><li>Trimethoprim-sulfamethoxazole 1 double-strength tablet PO bid for a minimum of 3 weeks, or</li><li>Doxycycline 100 mg PO bid for a minimum of 3 weeks</li></ul> Add an aminoglycoside (gentamicin 1 mg/kg IV q8h) if lesions do not respond with the first few days of therapy.	<ul><li>Ciprofloxacin 750 mg PO bid for a minimum of 3 weeks, or</li><li>Erythromycin base 500 mg PO qid for a minimum of 3 weeks</li></ul> Add an aminoglycoside (gentamicin 1 mg/kg IV q8h) if lesions do not respond with the first few days of therapy.

LYMPHOGRANULOMA VENERUM

SYPHILIS

Primary and secondary syphilis
- Doxycycline 100 mg PO bid for 21 days
- Benzathine penicillin G 2.4 million units IM in a single dose

In patients with penicillin allergy
- Erythromycin base 500 mg PO qid for 21 days
- Doxycycline 100 mg PO bid for 2 weeks
- Tetracycline 500 mg PO qid for 2 weeks

Latent syphilis

Early latent syphilis
- Benzathine penicillin G 2.4 million units IM in a single dose

In patients with penicillin allergy
- Doxycycline 100 mg PO bid, or
- Tetracycline 500 mg PO qid

Late latent syphilis
- Benzathine penicillin G 7.2 million units total, administered as three doses of 2.4 million units IM each at 1 week intervals

Administer drugs for 2 weeks if the duration of infection is known to have been <1 year; otherwise, administer for 4 weeks

Tertiary syphilis
- Benzathine penicillin G 7.2 million units total, administered as three doses of 2.4 million units IM each at 1 week intervals

Neurosyphilis
- Aqueous crystalline penicillin G 18–24 million units a day. Administered as 3–4 units IV q4h for 10–14 days
- Procaine penicillin 2.4 million units IM OD plus probenecid 500 mg PO qid both for 10–14 days

Primary and secondary syphilis in HIV-infected persons
- Benzathine penicillin G 2.4 million units IM in a single dose. Some experts recommend additional doses of three weekly doses.

Latent syphilis in HIV-infected persons
- Benzathine penicillin G 7.2 million units total, administered as three doses of 2.4 million units IM each at 1 week intervals

Congenital syphilis during first month of life
- Aqueous crystalline penicillin G 100,000–150,000 units/kg per day, administered as 50,000 units/kg per dose IV q12h during the first 7 days of life, and q8h thereafter for a total of 8 days, or
- Procaine penicillin G 50,000 units/kg per dose IM OD in a single dose for 10 days

Continued on following page

269

TABLE 11-3 *Continued*

Disease	Recommended Regimens	Alternative Regimens
URETHRITIS AND CERVICITIS Nongonococcal urethritis	• Azithromycin 1 g PO in a single dose, or • Doxycycline 100 mg PO bid for 7 days	• Erythromycin base 500 mg PO qid for 7 days, or • Erythromycin ethlysuccinate 800 mg PO qid for 7 days, or • Ofloxacin 300 mg bid for 7 days For those patients who cannot tolerate high doses of erythromycin • Erythromycin base 250 mg PO qid for 14 days, or • Erythromycin ethlysuccinate 400 mg PO qid for 14 days
Recurrent and persistent urethritis	• Metronidazole 2 mg PO in a single dose, *plus* • Erythromycin base 500 mg PO qid for 7 days, or • Erythromycin ethlysuccinate 800 mg PO qid for 7 days	
CHLAMYDIAL INFECTION In adults and adolescents	• Azithromycin 1 g PO in a single dose, or • Doxycycline 100 mg PO bid for 7 days	• Erythromycin base 500 mg PO qid for 7 days, or • Erythromycin ethlysuccinate 800 mg PO qid for 7 days, or • Ofloxacin 300 mg bid for 7 days
In pregnancy	• Erythromycin base 500 mg PO qid for 7 days, or • Amoxicillin 500 mg PO tid for 7 days	• Erythromycin base 250 mg PO qid for 14 days, or • Erythromycin ethlysuccinate 800 mg PO qid for 7 days, or • Erythromycin ethlysuccinate 400 mg PO qid for 14 days, or • Azithromycin 1 g PO in a single dose

In infants

Infant pneumonia caused by *C. trachomatis*

- Erythromycin 50 mg/kg per day PO divided in four equal doses daily for 10–14 days
- Erythromycin base 50 mg/kg per day PO divided in four equal doses daily for 10–14 days

Infants born to mothers who have a chlamydial infection

Children who weigh <45 kg:
- Erythromycin base 50 mg/kg per day PO divided in four equal doses daily for 10–14 days[2]

Children who weigh ≥45 kg but are <8 years of age:
- Azithromycin 1 g PO in a single dose

Children ≥8 years of age:
- Azithromycin 1 g PO in a single dose, or
- Doxycycline 100 mg PO bid for 7 days

GONOCOCCAL INFECTION

Uncomplicated gonococcal infections of the cervix, urethra, and rectum

- Cefixime 400 mg PO in a single dose, or
- Ceftriaxone 125 mg IM in a single dose, or
- Ofloxacin 400 mg PO in a single dose, or
- Azithromycin 1 g PO in a single dose, or
- Doxycycline 100 mg PO bid for 7 days

- Spectinomycin 2 g IM in a single dose, or
- Ceftizoxime 500 mg IM in a single dose, or
- Cefotaxime 500 mg IM in a single dose, or
- Cefotetan 1 g IM in a single dose, or
- Cefoxitin 2 g IM with probenecid 1 g PO in a single dose
- Enoxacin 400 mg PO in a single dose, or
- Lomefloxacin 400 mg PO in a single dose, or
- Norfloxacin 800 mg PO in a single dose

Uncomplicated gonococcal infection of the pharynx

- Ceftriaxone 125 mg IM in a single dose, or
- Ciprofloxacin 500 mg PO in a single dose, or
- Ofloxacin 400 mg PO in a single dose, *plus*
- Azithromycin 1 g PO in a single dose, or
- Doxycycline 100 mg PO bid for 7 days

Gonococcal conjunctivitis

- Ceftriaxone 1 g IM in a single dose, and lavage the infected eye with saline solution once.

Continued on following page

TABLE 11-3 *Continued*

Disease	Recommended Regimens	Alternative Regimens
Disseminated gonococcal infection	• Ceftriaxone 1 g IM or IV every 24 hours for 24–48 hours after improvement	• Cefotaxime 1 g IV q 8 hours, or • Ceftizoxime 1 g IV q 8 hours, or For persons allergic to β-lactam drugs: • Ciprofloxacin 500 mg IV q 12 hours, or • Ofloxacin 400 mg IV q 12 hours, or • Spectinomycin 2 g IV q 12 hours. All for 24–48 hours after improvement, at which time may be switched to one of the following regimens to complete a full week of antimicrobial treatment: • Cefixime 400 mg PO bid, or • Ciprofloxacin 500 mg PO bid, or • Ofloxacin 400 mg PO bid
Gonococcal meningitis or endocarditis	• Ceftriaxone 1–2 g IV every 12 hours for 10–14 days for meningitis and for at least 4 weeks for endocarditis	
Ophthalmia neonatorum caused by *N. gonorrhoeae*	• Ceftriaxone 25–50 mg/kg IV or IM in a single dose, not to exceed 125 mg	
Disseminated gonococcal infection and gonococcal scalp abscess in newborns	• Ceftriaxone 25–50 mg/kg IV or IM in a single daily dose for 7 days, with a duration of 10–14 days if meningitis is documented, or • Cefotaxime 25 mg/kg IV or IM every 12 hours for 7 days, with a duration of 10–14 days if meningitis is documented	
Prophylactic treatment for infants whose mothers have gonococcal infection	• Ceftriaxone 25–50 mg/kg IV or IM in a single dose, not to exceed 125 mg	

Gonococcal infection in children

For children who weigh ≥45 kg:
- Use one of the regimens recommended for adults except for quinolones since they are not approved for use in children

For children who weigh <45 kg and who have uncomplicated gonococcal vulvovaginitis, cervicitis, urethritis, pharyngitis, or proctitis:
- Ceftriaxone 125 mg IM in a single dose

For children who weigh <45 kg and who have bacteremia or arthritis:
- Ceftriaxone 50 mg/kg (maximum dose: 1 g) IM or IV in a single daily dose for 7 days

For children who weigh ≥45 kg and who have bacteremia or arthritis:
- Ceftriaxone 50 mg/kg (maximum dose: 2 g) IM or IV in a single daily dose for 10–14 days

- Spectinomycin 40 mg/kg (maximum dose: 2 g) in a single dose but this treatment may be unreliable

Ophthalmia neonatorum prophylaxis
- Silver nitrate (1%) aqueous solution in a single application, or
- Erythromycin (0.5%) ophthalmic ointment in a single application, or
- Tetracycline ophthalmic ointment (1%) in a single application
Treatment should be instilled into both eyes as soon as possible after delivery

BACTERIAL VAGINOSIS
Nonpregnant women
- Metronidazole 500 mg PO bid for 7 days, or
- Clindamycin cream 2%, one full applicator (5 g) intravaginally at bedtime for 7 days, or
- Metronidazole gel 0.5%, one full applicator (5 g) intravaginally bid for 5 days
- Metronidazole 250 mg PO tid for 7 days

- Metronidazole 2 g PO in a single dose
- Clindamycin 300 mg PO bid for 7 days

High-risk pregnant women
- Metronidazole 2 g PO in a single dose
- Clindamycin 300 mg PO bid for 7 days

Continued on following page

TABLE 11–3 *Continued*

Disease	Recommended Regimens	Alternative Regimens
Low-risk pregnant women	• Metronidazole 250 mg PO tid for 7 days	• Metronidazole 2 g PO in a single dose • Clindamycin 300 mg PO bid for 7 days, or • Metronidazole gel 0.75% one full applicator (5 g) intravaginally bid for 5 days • Metronidazole 500 mg PO bid for 7 days
TRICHOMONIASIS VULVOVAGINITIS CANDIDIASIS	• Metronidazole 2 g PO in a single dose Intravaginal agents: • Butoconazole 2% 5 g intravaginally for 3 days,[3,4] or • Clotrimazole 1% cream 5 g intravaginally for 7–14 days,[3,4] or • Clotrimazole 100 mg vaginal tablet for 7 days,[3] or • Clotrimazole 100 mg vaginal tablet, two tablets for 3 days,[3] or • Clotrimazole 500 mg vaginal tablet, one tablet in a single application,[3] or • Miconazole 2% cream 5 g intravaginally for 7 days[3,4] • Miconazole 200 mg vaginal suppository, one suppository for 3 days,[3,4] or • Miconazole 100 mg vaginal suppository, one suppository for 7 days,[3,4] or • Nystatin 100,000-unit vaginal tablet, one tablet for 14 days, or • Tioconazole 6.5% ointment 5 g intravaginally in a single application,[3,4] or • Terconazole 0.4% cream 5 g intravaginally for 7 days,[3]	

- Terconazole 0.8% cream 5 g intravaginally for 3 days,[3] or
- Terconazole 80 mg vaginal suppository, one suppository for 3 days[3]

Oral agent:

- Fluconazole 150 mg oral tablet, one tablet in single dose

PELVIC INFLAMMATORY DISEASE

Parenteral regimen A

- Cefotetan 2 g IV q 12 hours, or
- Cefoxitin 2 g IV q 6 hours, or
- Doxycycline 100 mg IV or PO q 12 hours

Parenteral therapy may be discontinued 24 hours after clinical improvement and then

- Doxycycline 100 mg bid should continue for a total of 14 days

Parenteral regimen B

- Clindamycin 900 mg IV q 8 hours, plus
- Gentamicin loading dose IV or IM (2 mg/kg of body weight), followed by a maintenance dose (1.5 mg/kg) q 8 hours. Single daily dosing may be substituted

Parenteral therapy may be discontinued 24 hours after clinical improvement and then

- Doxycycline 100 mg bid should continue for a total of 14 days, or
- Clindamycin 450 mg PO qid to complete a total of 14 days of therapy

Oral regimen A

- Ofloxacin 400 mg PO bid for 14 days, plus
- Metronidazole 500 mg PO bid for 14 days

Regimen B

- Ceftriaxone 250 mg IM once, or
- Cefoxitine 2 g IM plus
- Probenecid 1 g PO in a single dose concurrently once, or

- Ofloxacin 400 mg IV q 12 hours, plus
- Metronidazole 500 mg IV q 8 hours, or
- Ampicillin/sulbactam 3 g IV q 6 hours, plus
- Doxycycline 100 mg IV or PO q 12 hours, or
- Ciprofloxacin 200 mg IV q 12 hours, plus
- Doxycycline 100 mg IV or PO q 12 hours, plus
- Metronidazole 500 mg IV q 8 hours

Continued on following page

TABLE 11-3 *Continued*

Disease	Recommended Regimens	Alternative Regimens
	• Other parenteral third-generation cephalosporin (eg ceftizoxime or cefotaxime), *plus* • Doxycycline 100 mg PO bid for 14 days (Include this regimen with one of the above regimens)	
EPIDIDYMITIS Most likely caused by gonococcal or chlamydial infection Most likely caused by enteric organisms or for patients allergic to cephalosporins and/or tetracyclines	• Ceftriaxone 250 mg IM in a single dose, *plus* • Doxycycline 100 mg PO bid for 10 days • Ofloxacin 300 mg PO bid for 10 days	
HUMAN PAPILLOMAVIRUS INFECTION External genital warts	• Podofilox 0.5% solution or gel. Apply bid to visible genital warts for 3 days, followed by 4 days of no therapy. Repeat as necessary for a total of 4 cycles. Total wart area treated not to exceed 10 cm² and a total volume of podofilox not to exceed 0.5 ml/day, or • Imiquimod 5% cream. Apply at bedtime, 3 times per week for as long as 16 weeks. Wash area with mild soap and water 1–10 hours after treatment. • Cryotherapy with liquid nitrogen or cryoprobe. Repeat applications every 1 to 2 weeks, or • Podophyllin resin 10%–25% in a compound tincture of benzoin. Repeat weekly if necessary, or	• Intralesional interferon, or • Laser surgery

Vaginal warts

- TCA or BCA 80%–90%. Apply a small amount to warts and allow to dry, at which time frosting develops; powder with talc or sodium bicarbonate to remove unreacted acid if an excess amount is applied. Repeat weekly if necessary, or
- Surgical removal either by tangential scissor excision, tangential shave excision, curettage, or electrosurgery
- Cryotherapy with liquid nitrogen, or
- TCA or BCA 80%–90%. Apply a small amount to warts and allow to dry, at which time frosting develops; powder with talc or sodium bicarbonate to remove unreacted acid if an excess amount is applied. Repeat weekly if necessary, or
- Podophyllin resin 10%–25% in a compound tincture of benzoin applied to a treated area that must be dried before the speculum is removed. Treat with ≤2 cm² per session. Repeat weekly.

Urethral warts

- Cryotherapy with liquid nitrogen, or
- Benzoin applied to a treated area that must be dried before contact with normal mucosa. Repeat weekly.

Anal warts

- TCA or BCA 80%–90%. Apply a small amount to warts and allow to dry, at which time frosting develops; powder with talc or sodium bicarbonate to remove unreacted acid if an excess amount is applied. Repeat weekly if necessary, or
- Surgical removal

Continued on following page

TABLE 11-3 *Continued*

Disease	Recommended Regimens	Alternative Regimens
Oral warts	• Cryotherapy with liquid nitrogen, or • Surgical removal	
PROCTITIS, PROCTOCOLITIS, AND ENTERITIS	• Ceftriaxone 125 mg IM (or another agent effective against anal and genital gonorrhea), *plus* • Doxycycline 100 mg PO bid for 7 days	
ECTOPARASITIC INFECTIONS Pediculosis pubic	• Permethrin 1% crème rinse applied to affected areas and washed off after 10 minutes, or • Lindane 1% shampoo applied for 4 minutes to the affected area, and then thoroughly washed off. This regimen is not recommended for pregnant or lactating women or for children ≤2 years • Pyrethrins with piperonyl butoxide applied to the affected area and washed off after 10 minutes	
Scabies	• Premethrin cream 5% applied to all areas of the body from the neck down and washed off after 8–14 hours	• Lindane 1% precipitated in ointment applied thinly to all areas nightly for 3 nights. Previous applications should be washed off before new applications are applied. Thoroughly wash off 24 hours after the last treatment.

1. Contraindicated for pregnant and lactating women and for persons aged <18 years.
2. Effectiveness of treatment is approximately 80%; a second course of therapy may be indicated.
3. Creams and suppositories are oil-based and might weaken latex condoms and diaphragms.
4. Over-the-counter preparations.

Source: U.S. Department of Health and Human Services, Centers for Disease Control and Prevention, Morbidity and Mortality Reports, *1998 Guidelines for Treatment of Sexually Transmitted Diseases.* Vol 41. No. RR-1, January 23, 1998.

Paraphimosis results in swelling and pain due to the inability to reduce the foreskin. There is also a possibility of a visibly poor urinary stream. Accumulation of smegma, although not pathological, is also present.

Diagnostic Tests: None.

Differential Diagnosis: Traumatic injury to penis, differentiated by the presence of bruising or swelling.

Treatment: Circumcision.

Follow-up: Regular health-care visits.

Sequelae: Phimosis: interference with sexual and urinary function. Paraphimosis: venous statis distal to the corona.

Prevention/Prophylaxis: If congenital, none. If acquired, early treatment of inflammatory infections.

Referral: Refer to a surgeon and/or urologist.

Education: Parents should be told that 90% of all uncircumcised males will be able to retract the foreskin by 2 years of age.

Pregnancy

Pregnancy is a normal physiological event that spans from conception to birth and lasts approximately 280 days or 40 weeks. The time period between conception and the onset of labor is referred to as the antepartal period, whereas the time period between conception and the birth of the baby is referred to as the prenatal period. The expected date of delivery is calculated by beginning with the first day of the last menstrual period, adding 7 days and then subtracting 3 months. Pregnancy is divided into three trimesters: 0–12 weeks, 13–28 weeks, and 29–40 weeks. Although pregnancy is a normal event, its occurrence in the very young creates a multitude of problems or potential problems. Pregnant children often have school and family problems.

Etiology: Pregnancy results from the fertilization of an ovum by a sperm and the successful implantation of this fertilized egg into the uterus.

Occurrence: Current statistics indicate that the incidence of teen-age pregnancy nationwide has decreased slightly in the last 5 years; however, in areas where there is increased poverty and in the African-American population, the teen-age pregnancy rate continues to increase.

Age: Eight years to 50+ years.

Ethnicity: There is a significantly higher incidence of pregnancy in children aged 8–16 in the African-American population.

Contributing Factors: Poverty, illiteracy, poor access to health care, rape, and incest all contribute to the occurrence of pregnancy in children.

Signs and Symptoms: The child presents with a report of a missed period (menstrual suppression), feeling tired, nauseated in the morning (morning sickness) or throughout the day, and other presumptive signs, such as urinary frequency, breast tenderness, dark blue discoloration of the vaginal mucosal membrane (Chadwick's sign), pigmentation of the skin, and abdominal striae.

Probable signs include enlargement of the abdomen, changes in the size and shape of the uterus (Hagar's sign), changes in the cervix, and a positive pregnancy test.

Positive signs include fetal heart sounds, fetal movements felt by the examiner, and ultrasound demonstrating the presence of a fetus.

Diagnostic Tests: Serum radioimmunoassay is positive 7 days after conception and urine human chorionic gonadotropin (hCG) is positive 38–42 days after the last menstrual period.

Differential Diagnosis

Amenorrhea, acute infection, pseudocyesis, hyperestrinism, and STDs can be differentiated by serum hCG.

Physical examination can also exclude pregnancy by the absence of an enlarged uterus or lack of any other presumptive or suggestive signs.

Treatment: All confirmed pregnancies should be referred to either a nurse midwife or an obstetrician. Pregnant adolescents are at high risk for complications and should be referred as soon as possible to ensure the healthiest outcome for both the mother and the infant.

Follow-up: Follow-up is conducted by an obstetrician or midwife.

Sequelae: Multiple problems may result from a teen-ager's pregnancy, including alienation from her family, poor fetal outcome, and increased risk to the mother. There is some evidence to support an increased occurrence of neglect and abuse of infants born to young mothers.

Prevention/Prophylaxis: One way to decrease the number of unplanned teenage pregnancies is to begin sex education in the very early years, preferably during grade school. Other solutions include parental involvement, open communication, development of life goals, and increasing teen-agers' knowledge regarding pregnancy and condoms. With the assistance of both parents and schools, children can be educated regarding the ways to protect themselves from unplanned pregnancies. The regular use of any contraceptive method is essential for success in reducing the teen-age pregnancy rate. In conjunction with the use of condoms (to reduce STDs) any of the following methods are acceptable for female teen-agers: OCs, medroxyprogesterone acetate injections, and barrier methods. As with any medical regimen, care must be taken to follow up with regularly scheduled visits with a health-care provider. The pediatric NP is an ideal provider of both education and health-care supervision for birth control.

Referral: Refer patient to an obstetrician or midwife.

Education: Methods of safe sex and family planning should be done early by both family and schools. The need for early health care to ensure healthy outcomes for both baby and mother should be stressed.

Primary Gonococcal Infections

Gonorrhea, an infection of the genitourinary tract, oropharynx, or anorectal tract that may or may not be characterized by pain, is classified as a reportable STD. When detected in very young children, sexual abuse should be suspected.

Etiology: The bacterium *N. gonorrhoeae.*

Occurrence: Recent reports show a marked increase in the incidence of gonorrhea; of even more concern, many infections are penicillin resistant, which makes treatment more difficult. The annual incidence in 10- to 14-year-old boys is about 35.7 in 100,000; in females, it is 1175 in 100,000.

Age: Occurs at any age, even in newborns.

Ethnicity: Not significant.

Gender: Occurs in both males and females, but more commonly in females.

Contributing Factors: Unprotected sexual intercourse and multiple partners.

Signs and Symptoms: In males, urethritis is the most frequent acute presentation. The patient complains of dysuria and frequent urination, and a purulent discharge is present. History may include multiple sexual partners and high-risk or unprotected rectal, oral, or vaginal sexual intercourse. If the contact is a result of orogenital contact, the chief complaint is pharyngitis. With anorectal infection, there is burning in the rectal area, a mucopurulent discharge, and painful defecation. In females, urethritis (with dysuria and frequent urination) is the chief complaint. When salpingitis is present, there is bilateral lower abdominal pain, adnexal tenderness, and tenderness when the cervix is manipulated. In some cases the patient has an elevated temperature and chills. Occasionally, the female patient reports right upper quadrant pain.

Diagnostic Tests: Gram's stain of urethral discharge in both males and females should be done to confirm the diagnosis of *N. gonorrhoeae.* A Venereal Disease Research Laboratory (VDRL) test for syphilis should also be done. Cultures should be obtained for the area under suspicion, but in the case of suspected child abuse, cultures should be obtained from oral, vaginal, or urethral and anal areas. For females, the endocervix is the best area for screening and obtaining the cultures. A saline wet mount, urinalysis, and *Chlamydia* test should also be performed to rule out other STDs.

Differential Diagnosis

Acute abdominal problems: salpingitis (acute pain) in females and nongonococcal prostatitis in males, differentiated by examination.

UTI, differentiated by urinalysis and culture.

Treatment: Drugs of choice include amoxicillin 3.0 g and probenecid 1 g by mouth, aqueous penicillin G 4.8 million units IM with probenecid 1 g PO, or tetracycline 500 mg PO for 5 days. For oral gonorrhea, ceftriaxone sodium 250 mg IM in a single dose is the suggested treatment. All sexual contacts should be located and treated. There should be no sexual intercourse for the period of treatment and until all cultures are negative.

Follow-up: Follow-up cultures should be performed in 7–14 days to validate the absence of the disease.

Sequelae: Urethral or rectal strictures may occur. Sterility, although rare, may also result. Other complications include monarticular septic arthritis, disseminated gonococcal infection manifesting primarily as skin lesions, and gonococcal endocarditis.

Prevention/Prophylaxis: Stress the use of condoms to all patients who are sexually active. Stress the importance of avoiding all persons suspected of having the disease and reporting all who may have been exposed to the disease so that adequate treatment may be instituted, helping to decrease the spread of the disease.

Referral: Gonorrhea is a reportable STD. Refer patient to a physician if treatment is not effective in 14 days.

Education: Teach patients that the use of condoms can reduce the spread of this disease.

Syphilis

Syphilis is a bacterial STD that begins at the primary site and then, when untreated, becomes systemic. There are two forms of syphilis. Congenital syphilis results from transplacental transmission, which can occur at any stage of pregnancy, but most likely in the third trimester. Acquired syphilis results almost exclusively from unprotected sexual transmission. In acquired syphilis, the signs and symptoms can be divided into three stages: primary, secondary, and tertiary. When seen in very young children, sexual abuse should be suspected.

Etiology: Syphilis is caused by *Treponema pallidum,* a bacterial spirochete.

Occurrence: Since 1986, the incidence of both acquired and congenital syphilis has decreased dramatically in the United States.

Age: In the pediatric age group, this disease is most common during adolescence as a result of unprotected sexual practices.

Ethnicity: Syphilis is more prevalent among inner-city and minority populations.

Gender: More prevalent in males (2 : 1).

Contributing Factors: In acquired syphilis, unprotected sexual intercourse.

Signs and Symptoms: Congenital syphilis can be an asymptomatic illness, especially during the first weeks of life. If the disease is symptomatic, the symptoms are usually osteitis, hepatitis, lymphadenopathy, pneumonitis, mucocutaneous lesions, anemia, and hemorrhage.

The symptoms of acquired syphilis vary according to stage. In the primary stage, the patient usually presents with one or more painless, indurated ulcers, also known as chancre of the skin and mucous membrane, at the site of inoculation. The most common site is the genitalia. The patient will relate having had unprotected intercourse or contact with a person who has recently been diagnosed with syphilis.

In the secondary stage, the patient presents with a polymorphic rash, classically on the hands and feet, that is generalized and maculopapular. There may also be lymphadenopathy, fever, malaise, sore throat, headaches, splenomegaly, and arthralgia.

In the tertiary stage of syphilis, various manifestations of neurosyphilis are seen. This stage takes about 15 years to manifest after the primary infection.

Diagnostic Tests

Dark-field examination, VDRL, and gonococcal culture for diagnosis of syphilis.

Additionally, a urinalysis, saline wet mount, herpesvirus culture, and *Chlamydia* culture should also be done to differentiate this problem from other diseases.

Diagnosis is based on a positive VDRL test and identifying the spirochete by microscopic dark-field examination.

HIV testing should be done on all patients with gonorrhea.

Differential Diagnosis: Herpes, venereal warts, and other STDs, differentiated by cultures and/or serologic testing.

Treatment: The preferred treatment is either penicillin G benzathine, 2.4 million units IM, repeated in 1 week; or aqueous procaine penicillin G, 600,000 units IM for 10 days. Syphilis is a reportable STD: It should be reported to the state public health department, and all contacts should be identified and treated.

Follow-up: In congenital syphilis, follow-up should continue until nontreponemal serologic tests are negative. In adults, follow-up continues until cultures are negative and quantitative serology is negative.

Sequelae: Untreated, syphilis can affect multiple organs including the liver, spleen, heart, and skin. In congenital syphilis, teeth are affected with notched or barrel-shaped incisors, abnormal enamel, and tooth destruction. Meningitis can result in both adults and infants. Neurosyphilis and cardiovascular disease resulting in death are also complications of this disease.

Prevention/Prophylaxis: Early identification of the positive pregnant female assists the health-care provider in preparing for treatment of the newborn. Identification of all contacts also assists in decreasing the spread of the disease.

Referral: Patients with the congenital form of the disease should be referred to a pediatrician or local health department. When multiple organs are involved in the adult, the patient should be referred.

Education: Education of adolescents regarding safe-sex practices and barrier methods, such as condoms and foam, is important for preventing the spread of syphilis. Education concerning multiple partners and decreasing the risks of contracting STDs should begin early in childhood.

Vulvovaginitis

Vulvovaginitis is an inflammation of the vulva and vagina caused by an infection or an irritating substance. It is often accompanied by vaginal discharge.

Etiology: Often, the etiology of vulvovaginitis depends on the age of the patient. Maturational factors figure in closely with the causes of this problem. In the prepubertal child, the lack of estrogen causes a thin, atrophic vaginal mucosa. Because of the lack of pubic hair and the thickness of the labia, there is no barrier to protect against irritants or invading organisms. Proximity of the vaginal opening to the anus provides yet another cause of vulvovaginitis. In adolescent girls, vulvovaginitis may be due to normal leukorrhea, bacterial vaginosis, *Trichomonas, Monilia,* β-hemolytic streptococcus, or pinworms. In both prepubertal and adolescent girls, foreign bodies should also be considered as a cause of this disease.

Occurrence: More prevalent among females who use douches or contraceptive foams and creams; take bubble baths; or have a recent history of antibiotic use, diabetes mellitus, or an immunosuppressive disease.

Age: All ages.

Ethnicity: Usually not significant, but current studies suggest a higher prevalence among African-American females.

Gender: Females.

Contributing Factors: Factors that contribute to the manifestation of the disease are emotional stress, poor personal hygiene, multiple sexual partners, and the use of tampons, irritating douches, condoms, contraceptive foams, and creams. Foreign bodies, (often tampons) are often responsible for vulvovaginitis in the adolescent girl; tissue, toilet paper, or other objects contribute to the occurrence in the young girl. Rape should be considered when this disease is diagnosed.

Signs and Symptoms: In both the prepubertal and adolescent girl, there may be a complaint of genital irritation, itching, pain or redness, and swelling of the labia. There may be a complaint of vaginal discharge. Ask the following questions:

When was this first noted?

How much discharge is present, what color is it, and is there an odor?

What is the consistency of the discharge, and how long has it been present?

Occasionally there is a further complaint of pain on urination. The parent and/or child may recall the child's recent use of antibiotics. Question the patient about the use of bubble baths and the type of soap used. Also, there may be a complaint of perianal itching, and it should be noted when this symptom is most problematic (e.g., day or night). For the adolescent, a menstrual and sexual history should be obtained, as well as whether there has been a possible exposure to an STD. The recent use of tampons or contraceptive creams or foams should also be noted.

For the prepubertal child, use the frog-leg or knee-chest position. Examine not only the external labia and genitalia, but also the anus. If further evaluation is needed, an otoscope may be used to provide a more thorough evaluation of the internal genitalia. Sexually active adolescents should have a complete bimanual pelvic examination, including inspection and palpation.

The type of discharge depends on the causative agent:

Normal leukorrhea: A white-gray, odorless, nonirritating discharge; occurs prior to puberty.

Chemical or mechanical vulvovaginitis: A scant amount of discharge that is clear to yellow, sometimes blood tinged; there is some external inflammation of the genitalia.

Foreign body, such as toilet paper or other object: A purulent, foul brown discharge.

Bacterial infection (usually streptococcal): Copious, foul-smelling discharge and bleeding accompanied by a fever and abdominal pain.

Bacterial vaginosis is accompanied by a thin, gray-clear discharge that has a fishy odor when exposed to a potassium hydroxide (KOH) test.

Candidiasis: A thick, white, curdlike, odorless discharge accompanied by pruritus, dysuria, and dyspareunia.

Trichomoniasis: A foul-smelling, yellow-gray, profuse discharge accompanied by persistent hemorrhagic lesions on the cervix.

There may also be irritation caused by itching, and redness and swelling of the external genitalia may be observed.

Diagnostic Tests

Urinalysis is done to detect increased WBCs, yeast cells, or trichomonads.

pH of vaginal secretions is checked: if greater than 4.5, the infection is most likely vaginosis or trichomoniasis; if less than 4.5, it is most likely candidiasis.

Wet preparation with saline and 10% KOH of vaginal secretions will elicit a positive amine (Whiff) test.

The presence of flagellated parasites on a saline wet mount or Pap smear is diagnostic of trichomoniasis.

Differential Diagnosis

Concomitant STDs, cervicitis, PID, and *foreign body* are determined by cultures and examination.

In the infant or prepubertal child, *sexual abuse* should be investigated.

Referral: If the symptoms do not resolve, or if they recur, after the prescribed therapy, refer the patient. If sexual abuse is suspected, refer the patient *immediately* to the child protection agency and the police. Often the most effective way to accomplish this is while the child is in the clinic. Call 911, and the police generally send an officer immediately to interview the NP, child, and accompanying adult. Erring on the side of protecting the child is much more important than waiting so that no one is embarrassed or angered by your suspicion.

Treatment: Bacterial infections are treated with penicillin, 125–250 mg tid for 10 days; in penicillin-allergic patients, erythromycin, 30–50 mg/kg per day tid for 10 days.

Bacterial vaginosis is treated with metronidazole, 2 g PO one time or 500 mg bid for 10 days. Another treatment may be clindamycin, 300 mg bid for 7 days. In lieu of oral medication, topical clindamycin 2% cream can be used for 7 days at night.

For candidiasis, use a local external medication such as clotrimazole, miconazole, or butoconazol, which can be applied once or twice daily for 7 days.

Trichomoniasis is treated with oral metronidazole, 2 g PO one time or 500 mg bid for 7 days. Partners should always be treated; abstinence from sexual intercourse is required until about 1–2 weeks after treatment is completed for both partners.

Follow-up: A follow-up examination is usually not necessary unless there is a return of symptoms or continued complaints.

Sequelae: In some cases, sterility may result from untreated or fulminating infections. Additionally, secondary infections of the skin may develop, which affect the skin's integrity and result in open wounds.

Prevention/Prophylaxis: Condoms may reduce the risk of contracting STDs. Maintaining monogamous relationships can also help decrease one's risk. Patients should be told to urinate after sexual intercourse and to undergo regular examinations if they are sexually active so that if an infection is present, it can be treated early.

Education: Patients should be told that they are at increased risk for contracting STDs when they engage in unprotected sex or sex with multiple partners. Teaching the patient to urinate after intercourse and to avoid douching may further decrease the incidence of STDs. The importance of treating sexual partners with some of these problems needs to be stressed; the patient should be informed of the risks for reinfection if their partner is not treated. Patients should be taught the importance of completing their prescribed treatment regimens.

REFERENCES

General

Berhman, R, and Kleigman, R: Nelson's Essentials of Pediatrics. WB Saunders, Philadelphia, 1990.
Carpenter, S, and Roch, J: Pediatric and Adolescent Gynecology. Raven, New York, 1992.
Doenges, M, and Moorhouse, M: Nurse's Pocket Guide: Nursing Diagnoses with Interventions, ed 5. FA Davis, Philadelphia, 1995.
Green, M: Pediatric Diagnosis: Interpretation of Symptoms and Signs in Infants, Children and Adolescents, ed 5. WB Saunders, Philadelphia, 1992.
Hay, W, et al: Current Pediatric Diagnosis & Treatment, ed 12. Appleton & Lange, Norwalk, Conn, 1995.
Johnson, K: Primary pediatric care. In Hoekelman, R (ed): The Harriet Lane Handbook. Mosby, St. Louis, 1994.
Parish, L, and Gschnait, F: Sexually transmitted diseases: A guide for clinicians. Springer-Verlag, New York, 1989.
Peter, G, et al: The 1994 Red Book: Report of the Committee on Infectious Diseases. American Academy of Pediatrics, Elk Grove Village, Ill, 1994.
Steele, R: Clinical Handbook of Pediatric Infectious Diseases. Parthenon, New York, 1994.
Summitt, R: Comprehensive Pediatrics. Mosby, St. Louis, 1992.
Uphold, C, and Graham, M: Clinical Guidelines in Family Practice, ed 2. Barrarrae Books, Gainesville, Fla, 1994.
Yen, S, and Jaffee, R: Reproductive Endocrinology. WB Saunders, Philadelphia, 1991.

Amenorrhea

D'ambro, M: Amenorrhea: Griffith's 5 minute clinical consults. Clin Rev 6:115, 1996.
Webb, T: Evaluation and management of amenorrhea. Adv Nurse Pract 3(6):28, 1995.

Cryptorchidism

Hawtney, C: Undescended testes and orchiopexy: Recent observations. Pediatr Rev 11:305, 1990.
Neely, E: The undescended testicle: When and how to intervene. Contemp Pediatr 7:87, 1987.

Dysmenorrhea

Cholst, I, and Carlon, I: Oral contraception and dysmenorrhea. J Adolesc Health Care 8:121, 1987.
Neinstein, L: Menstrual problems in the adolescent. Med Clin North Am 7:1187, 1990.
Polaneczhy, M, and Slap, G: Dysmenorrhea and dysfunctional uterine bleeding. Pediatr Rev 13:83, 1992.

Epididymitis

Abramowitz, M: Drugs for sexually transmitted diseases. Med Lett 36(913):1, 1994.
Centers for Disease Control and Prevention: Sexually transmitted diseases treatment guidelines. MMWR 42(14):1, 1993.
Edelman, C: Urinary tract infections and vesicourethral reflux. Pediatr Ann 17:568, 1988.
Friedman, A: Urinalysis: Oft obtained, oft ignored. Contemp Pediatr 8:31, 1991.
Getes, E, and Irwin, C: Sexually transmitted diseases in adolescents. Pediatr Rev 14:180, 1993.

Herpes Simplex Virus Type 2

Alexander, L: Sexually transmitted disease: Perspectives on this growing epidemic. Nurse Pract 17:33, 1992.
Bowie, W, et al: STD's in '94: The new CDC guidelines. Patient Care 17:29, 1994.
Clark, P, and Byrne, M: Clinical issues in long-term pediatric HIV disease. Maternal Child Nurs 14:164, 1993.
Levin, S, et al: The clinical guide to sexually transmitted diseases. Yearbook, St. Louis, 1987.
Nettina, S, and Kaufman, F: Diagnosis and management of sexually transmitted genital lesions. Nurse Pract 15(1):20, 1990.

Parish, L, and Gschnait, F: Sexually transmitted diseases: A guide for clinicians. Springer-Verlag, New York, 1989.

Hydrocele

Clore, E: A guide to testicular self-exam. J Pediatr Health Care 7:264, 1993.

Hypospadias

Duckett, J: Hypospadias. Pediatr Rev 11:37, 1989.

Labial Adhesions

Howard, B: Labial adhesions. In Hoekleman, RA, et al (eds): Primary Pediatric Care. Mosby, St. Louis, 1992.

Pelvic Inflammatory Disease

Apuzzio, J, and Hoegsberg, B: PID: Hard to find, essential to treat. Patient Care 3:30, 1992.
Gettes, E, and Irwin, C: Sexually transmitted diseases in adolescents. Pediatr Rev 14:180, 1993.
McCormack, W: Pelvic inflammatory diseases. N Engl J Med 330:115, 1994.
Ronenfield, W, and Clark, J: Adolescent gynecology and obstetrics. Pediatr Clin North Am 36:489, 1989.
Shafer, M: Sexually transmitted diseases in adolescents: Prevention, diagnosis and treatment in pediatric practice. Pediatr Rev 13:83, 1994.

Phimosis

Ryan, D, and Doody, E: Genital pain. In Dershewitz, RA (ed): Ambulatory Pediatric Care, ed 2. JB Lippincott, Philadelphia, 1993.

Pregnancy

Davis, S: Adolescent gynecology and obstetrics. Pediatr Clin North Am 36:665, 1989.
Jones, M, and Mandy, L: Lessons for prevention and intervention in adolescent pregnancy: A five-year comparison of outcomes for school-age pregnant adolescents. J Pediatr Health Care 8:152, 1994.
Polaneczky, M, and Slap, G: Menstrual disorders in the adolescent. Pediatr Rev 13:43, 1992.

Syphilis

Alexander, L: Sexually transmitted diseases: Perspectives on this growing epidemic. Nurse Pract 17(10):33, 1992.
Bowie, W, et al: STD's in '94: The new CDC guidelines. Patient Care 4:29, 1994.
Johnson, J: Sexually transmitted diseases in adolescents. Primary Care 14:101, 1987.
Shafer, M: Sexually transmitted diseases in adolescents: Prevention, diagnosis and treatment in pediatric practice. Pediatr Rev 13:83, 1994.
Sharp, V: AIDS update. Clin Rev 5:131, 1995.

Vulvovaginitis

Elvik, S: Vaginal discharge in the prepubertal girl. J Pediatr Health Care 4:181, 1990.
Johnson, J: Sexually transmitted diseases in adolescents. Primary Care 14:101, 1987.
Secor, R: Bacterial vaginosis: A common infection with serious sequelae. Adv Nurse Pract 11, 1994.
Shafer, M: Sexually transmitted diseases in adolescents: Prevention, diagnosis and treatment in pediatric practice. Adolesc Health Update 6:1, 1994.
Touchstone, D, and Davis, D: Consider Chlamydia. Office Nurse 16, 1995.
U.S. Department of Health and Human Services, Centers for Disease Control and Prevention: Sexually transmitted diseases treatment guidelines. MMWR 42(14):1, 1993.

CHAPTER 12

MUSCULOSKELETAL

ASSESSMENT

Musculoskeletal assessment should be a part of any routine examination. Techniques of inspection, palpation, passive and active range of motion, muscle strength, and integrated function are used in the assessment process. As a screening examination, the purpose is to discover any abnormalities or dysfunction of the musculoskeletal system.

Inspection of the musculoskeletal system involves first assessing for symmetry. Nodules, masses, and deformities are examples of lesions that may be responsible for asymmetry. Assess for gait and posture, looking for variations in the manner of movement (Fig. 12–1). In assessing posture, review the spine for degree of straightness. Palpation may reveal areas of tenderness and crepitus often associated with inflammatory processes and joint abnormalities. Assess the joints through passive and active range of motion (Fig. 12–2). In passive range of motion, actions are performed when the examiner moves the patient's body; in active range of motion, the patient performs movement of the muscles. Assessment of muscle strength, which is evaluated for all the major muscle groups, is done by evaluating the manner in which the patient moves against the examiner's resistance, starting with the upper extremities. The nurse practitioner (NP) should compare each side with the other and note the degree of muscle tone.

Musculoskeletal disorders are commonly manifested by pain, weakness, deformities, limitation of movement, stiffness, or clicking of joints. Radiographic and laboratory studies, which may be done to confirm the diagnosis, are disorder specific.

Athletics is a part of the American culture; each year 35 million children and young adults aged 6–21 years participate in organized sports (25% of girls and 50% of boys aged 8–16). For the teen-ager participating in sports, including

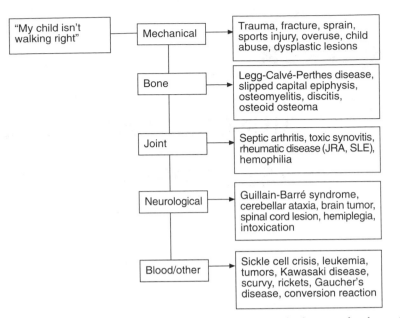

FIGURE 12-1 Classifications of gait disturbance. (JRA = juvenile rheumatoid arthritis; SLE = systemic lupus erythematosus.)

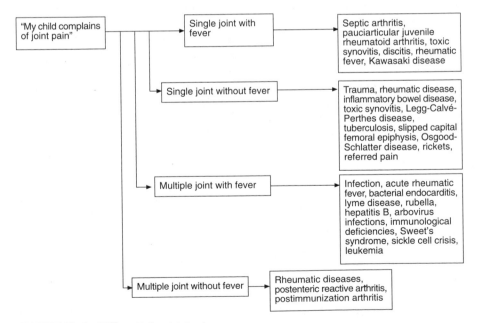

FIGURE 12-2 Differentiating joint pain.

cheerleading, the sport serves as a means to form an identity; this is true for both boys and girls. The NP may serve in the screening process, as a provider of care, and counselor to the adolescent athlete. Boys are 1½ times more likely to be affected than girls; middle and junior high school students have the highest rate of injury, possibly because of skeletal immaturity and inadequate physical conditioning.

Sports injuries have been separated into two main categories: macrotrauma, or a sudden acute trauma from a major force; and microtrauma, or injuries resulting from repetitive tissue trauma. Examples of major trauma are sprains and strains, contusions, fractures, and head injuries. Major injuries most often occur in collision and contact sports, sports with heavy lower extremity involvement, and sports with unreliable playing surfaces. Results of microtrauma are stress fractures, "shin splints," tendinitis, shoulder impingement, and epicondylitis (Fig. 12–3). Sports most responsible for microtrauma include sports requiring endurance or a high level of limb repetition (e.g., distance running), sports with quick stop-start and jumping action (e.g., basketball), sports using a hard surface area, and sports involving repetitive single limb action (e.g., tennis/racquet sports, skiing, swimming, baseball).

Contributing factors identified in sports-related injuries include the following:

Inadequate preparticipation physicals.
Hazardous surfaces in performance or practice areas.
Training and practice errors.
Lack of or improper safety equipment.
Inadequately trained coaches.
Performing while overly tired or injured.
Improper nutrition.
Limited awareness of possible risk or risk factors (Gottlieb, 1994).

The pediatric NP can play an essential role in the health care of adolescent athletes by performing preparticipation health assessments, as well as by adequately assessing and managing injuries.

Preparticipation

SCHEDULING

Ideally, the preparticipation examination should be scheduled 6 weeks before the start of the season. However, many students forget, and either the clinic is deluged with last-minute requests for examinations or the coach schedules a mass screening in the gymnasium at the school. Neither of these options is the best for the NP or the student. The following are some suggested guidelines for optimizing the preparticipation examination:

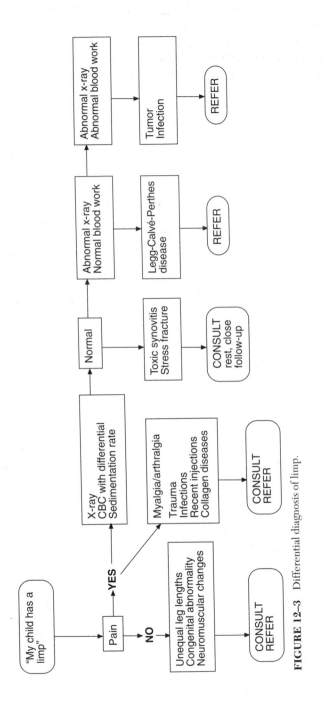

FIGURE 12–3   Differential diagnosis of limp.

Contact the school system to determine the "age" of the physical required. That is, does the examination have to be done just a few days before participation, or can it be done during the summer before the start of the season?

Find out whether the cheerleaders are included as part of the athletic participants.

Find out who reviews the completed forms, or whether they are merely filed for future reference.

Preparticipation Physical Examination, a guide for sports examinations, can be obtained from the American Academy of Family Physicians, P.O. Box 8723, Kansas City, MO 64114 (800-274-2237).

Contact the parents of potential participants at the beginning of the summer to request, at their convenience, a time for a preparticipation examination.

EXAMINATION

Family history: Is there a family history of cardiac problems, particularly sudden death?

Student history: Past health history, including the following questions: Is there a history of chest pains, syncope, or exercise-induced asthma? What is the past history of injuries? What is the anticipated level of sports involvement, and what is the sport? Are there any chronic health problems? What is the nutritional history? Is there a history of substance abuse?

Physical examination: Head to toe, observing particularly height and weight (comparison to monitor growth spurts); vision screening; heart (resting and exercise [85% will have normal ejection-type murmurs]) and lungs; blood pressure (1–3% of teen-agers have hypertension); an orthopedic examination (Table 12–1); Tanner stage (female athletes have onset of menarche 2.3 years later than average with no change in secondary characteristics (see Chapter 11, Table 11–1); and presence or absence of hernias.

Laboratory evaluation: Routine urinalysis and blood counts are usually not necessary. If these tests are performed, be aware of the physiologic changes found in athletes. For example, urinalysis may reveal stress-induced hematuria and albuminuria (particularly if the athlete just came from a practice session), and blood counts may show exercise-induced anemia.

Counseling: Assessment of self-worth. How do the students feel about participating in the sport? How do they feel about themselves? This assessment is particularly important for female athletes, who are particularly susceptible to eating disorders.

Nutrition: Meeting normal guidelines for adolescents, as suggested by the food pyramid, should be stressed.

Body function and health maintenance: Female athletes are vulnerable to menstrual disorders.

Injury risk and prevention: Which sports are played, and what activities do these sports demand (e.g., running, jumping)? Before practice and com-

TABLE 12–1 THE TWO-MINUTE ORTHOPEDIC EXAMINATION

Instructions	Observations
Stand facing observer.	Acromiclavicular joints, general habitus.
Look at ceiling, floor, over both shoulders; touch ears to shoulders.	Cervical spine motion.
Shrug shoulders (examiner resists).	Trapezius strength.
Abduct shoulders 90° (examiner resists at 90°).	Deltoid strength.
Full external rotation of arms.	Shoulder motion.
Flex and extend elbows.	Elbow motion.
Arms at sides, elbows 90° flexed, pronate and supinate wrists.	Elbow and wrist motion.
Spread fingers; make fist.	Hand or finger motion and deformities.
Tighten (contract) quadriceps; relax quadriceps.	Symmetry and knee effusion; ankle effusion.
"Duck walk" (4 steps away from examiner with buttocks on heels).	Hip, knee, and ankle motion.
Back to examiner.	Shoulder symmetry, scoliosis.
Knees straight, touch toes.	Scoliosis, hip motion, hamstring tightness.
Raise up on toes; raise heels.	Calf symmetry, leg strength.

Source: Sports Medicine: Health Care for Young Athletes, American Academy of Pediatrics, Elk Grove Village, Ill, 1991, with permission.

petition, a good warm-up routine helps to prevent injury. The NP can provide information about basic stretching and conditioning exercises (Table 12–2). Review the safety measures being taken, such as types of protective equipment, and what health-care facilities are available.

Parents are often the first to notice possible abnormalities. However, some of these abnormalities are simply developmental variations, depending on the

TABLE 12–2 STRETCHING BASICS

1. Warm up entire body (short, light jog) before *any* stretching.
2. Breathe normally throughout stretching session.
3. Devote 10–15 minutes solely to stretching.
4. Concentrate.
5. Stretch with a partner if possible.
6. Hold each stretch for 20–30 seconds; avoid bouncing.
7. Stretch all muscle groups first; then work specifically on those used most for the chosen sport.
8. Stretch at least 5 minutes after cool down.
9. Lessen stretch if pain occurs.
10. Avoid comparisons to other people.

Source: Adapted from Stretching Principles, Institute for Athletic Medicine, Minneapolis, Minn, 1992, with permission.

age of the child. The NP can respond to these concerns by teaching normal development, counseling the parent, and following up with and/or referring the patient, as appropriate.

Ankle Sprain

Sprain is a stretching of a ligament, whereas a strain is a stretch of a muscle or tendon. Acute ankle sprains may be classified as follows:

Grade I: Caused by low-level activity, such as stepping off a curb.

Grade II: Caused by higher level activity, such as a misstep while running.

Grade III: Caused by vigorous exertion of force during a foot stroke while the ankle is pliantly flexed and internally rotated.

Etiology: Trauma to the ligament, muscle, or tendon and associated ligamental laxity.

Occurrence: Constitutes 5% of all athletic injuries.

Age: All age groups.

Ethnicity: Not significant.

Gender: Occurs equally in males and females.

Contributing Factors: Running, jumping, and other sports activities.

Signs and Symptoms: Child presents to the clinic because of pain or discomfort in the ankle after participating in activities such as walking or running. Have the child describe the circumstances leading to the injury, the site of pain, when the swelling began (immediate swelling may indicate a fracture), and whether weight bearing is possible. Ask what has been done for the injury (e.g., ice, elevation). Ask whether this is a new injury or a reinjury.

Examine ankle for swelling and ecchymosis, crepitus or pain, and limitation of motion. Palpate the ankle, starting with the nontender areas first. Findings in acute ankle sprains vary according to grade:

Grade I: Little functional deficit (can walk with no limp and can hop on ankle; swelling and tenderness localized over the anterior talofibular ligament (ATL), indicative of a possible partial rupture of the ATL.

Grade II: Limping, some functional loss, and localized swelling and tenderness around the ATL, indicating possible rupture of the ATL and tearing of the calcaneofibular ligament.

Grade III: Crutch walking preferred, diffuse pain, and swelling, indicative of complete rupture of the ATL and anterior and bilateral laxity.

Diagnostic Tests: Radiographic studies of affected part: anteroposterior, oblique, and lateral views in neutral and in internal rotation would be negative for fractures, joint incongruity, and degenerative joint disease in cases of uncomplicated ankle sprain. Because edema can mask a fracture, radiographic views will be more satisfactory if done after swelling has subsided. Radiographic studies are often recommended in cases of severe pain, with a history of previous injury, or for a child who is still growing.

Differential Diagnosis

Fracture: Can be seen on radiographic film unless the fracture is cartilaginous; magnetic resonance imaging (MRI) provides more definitive evaluation.

Dislocation: Obvious bony deformity seen on radiographic films.

Ligament tear: External rotation of the foot and tibiofibular compression of the calf causes pain in the ankle.

Tendon tear: Patient has a history of chronic instability that is not responding to treatment (Fig. 12–4).

Treatment

Nonpharmacological

First stage: Treatment is rest, ice, compression (wrapping), and elevation (RICE) to reduce swelling, inflammation, and pain. Grade I and II, partial weight bearing with crutches. Grade III, immobilize with a U-shaped splint, elevate, use ice, and prescribe crutches (prohibit weight bearing).

Second stage: For restoration of function, begin active range-of-motion exercises, while sitting or lying down (using foot, "inscribe" letters [the "alphabet exercises"] in the air) and gait training after swelling has subsided. Weight bearing after 72 hours lessen swelling, reduces pain, and resolves edema.

Third stage: Tape the ankle or use an ankle support or wrap, and begin neuromuscular training and peroneal strengthening. Surgical intervention may be indicated for Grade III injuries.

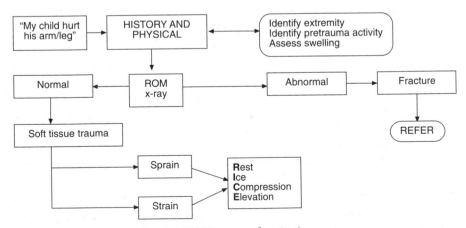

FIGURE 12–4   Sprains and strains. (ROM = range of motion.)

Pharmacology

Acetaminophen, 10–15 mg/kg per dose or 400–480 mg q 4 hours; or ibuprofen, 4–10 mg/kg per dose q 6–8 hours for pain.

Follow-up: Evaluating swelling, inflammation and pain in 24, 48, and 72 hours, and at 2 weeks for evaluation of weight bearing.

Sequelae: Approximately 10–20% of persons with ankle sprains develop chronic functional instability (i.e., episodes in which the ankle "gives way"). Such mechanical instability can predispose these patients to further injury, functional instability, peroneal tendon weakness, or subluxation.

Prevention/Prophylaxis: Properly fitted shoes and proper walking techniques can be preventative.

Referral: Refer to an orthopedist those patients who have gross instability of the ankle or who do not improve within 12 weeks.

Education: Instruct parent and child in the correct use of crutches, if indicated; in proper shoe fit; in correct walking technique; and in exercises that will help an injured ankle. The following are basic guidelines for ankle exercises:

Exercise in stocking or bare feet.

Perform each exercise 10 times and increase by five each day to a maximum of 30 repetitions.

Do not continue any exercise that causes pain.

Perform the exercises three times per day.

Apophyseal Injuries

Apophyseal injuries are characterized by periarticular pain, with inflammation at the site of major tendon insertion at the point of active growth, usually at the heel, knee, hip, and elbow; patients may present with bilateral injuries.

Etiology

Sever's disease (heel): Repetitive microtrauma with inflammatory changes.

Osgood-Schlatter disease: Traumatic induced apophyseal injury to the tibia tuberosity.

Sinding-Larsen-Johansson disease: Multiple episodes of microtrauma to the inferior pole of the patella.

Apophysitis of the hip: Traction on a growing area of bone, usually at the anterior superior and the anterior inferior iliac spine, the iliac crests, and the ischial tuberosities.

Medial epicondylitis: Skeletal immaturity of the medial epicondylar apophysis.

Occurrence: Fairly common.

Age: Occur in 8- to 15-year-old athletes (average age, 11 years).

Sever's disease: Ages 8–13 years.
Osgood-Schlatter disease: Males, 10–15 years; females 8–13 years.
Sinding-Larsen-Johansson disease: Ages 10–13 years.
Apophysitis of the hip: Ages 9–13 years.
Medial epicondylitis: Ages 9–13 years.

Ethnicity: Not significant.

Gender: Occur in males and females (Sever's disease, males; Osgood-Schlatter disease, males and females; Sinding-Larsen-Johansson disease, males; apophysitis of the hip, males; medial epicondylitis, males).

Contributing Factors

Sever's disease: Associated with growth, tight heel cords, or other biomechanical abnormalities; participation in soccer and running.

Osgood-Schlatter disease: Weakened and inflexible quadriceps muscle; participation in sports requiring running.

Sinding-Larsen-Johansson disease: Participation in sports involving running and jumping (e.g., soccer).

Apophysitis of the hip: Associated with muscle-tendon imbalance and growth spurts; implicated activities are distance running and dancing.

Medial epicondylitis: Skeletal immaturity, overuse phenomenon, participation in sports activities requiring repeated overhead arm motion, such as pitching (baseball) and serving (tennis).

Signs and Symptoms: Child is brought to the clinic with pain in one of the following areas: heel, anterior knee, hip (a dull ache), or elbow (tenderness). Physical findings vary by diagnosis:

Sever's disease: Tenderness at the insertion of the Achilles tendon on the calcaneus.

Osgood-Schlatter disease: Pain and swelling over the tibia tubercle with worsening of the pain during running, jumping, and ascending or descending stairs; resisted extension of the knee at 90° of flexion causes pain, whereas resisted straight-leg raising does not. Tenderness and erythema are noted over the tibia tuberosity.

Sinding-Larsen-Johansson disease: Pain over the inferior pole of the patella, worse with running or stair climbing. Palpation of the inferior pole of the patella is positive for tenderness.

Apophysitis of the hip: Dull pain related to activity located near the hip.

Medial epicondylitis: Tenderness over the medial condyle and pain with resisted flexion of the wrist.

Diagnostic Tests: Radiographic studies, when indicated, show the following:

Sever's disease: Partial fragmentation and increased density of the os calcis.

Osgood-Schlatter disease: Enlarged, fragmented, and irregular tibia tuberosity. Bone age is normal.

Sinding-Larsen-Johansson disease: Normal to calcification of the inferior pole of the patella.

Apophysitis of the hip: If the result of a traumatic event with pain, then x-ray.

Medial epicondylitis: Fragmentation of the medial epicondyle.

Differential Diagnosis

Osteosarcoma: Positive radiographic studies; gait disturbances will be noted.

Patellar tendinitis: The child exhibits pain on running and climbing stairs.

Osteomyelitis: Usually affects a single bone, child may experience an acute illness or a subacute illness with fever, severe pain at the affected site, erythema, and swelling. Radiographic studies may be normal in the first 10–14 days of the illness.

Slipped capital femoral epiphysis: Physeal abnormalities and skeletal maturation anomalies.

Treatment

Nonpharmacological

Sever's disease: Activity reduction, RICE, use of heel cups, massage, and stretching of the muscle involved. In rare cases, patient may need crutches for 2–3 weeks.

Osgood-Schlatter disease and Sinding-Larsen-Johansson disease: Wearing of a knee support, and reducing or modifying athletic activity to reach a pain-free level. Initiate a program of stretching and strengthening with resisted straight-leg raises. Patient may need a trial of crutches for 2–3 weeks. Rest, ice for 20 minutes three times per day, compress with ace bandage, and elevate (RICE).

Apophysitis of the hip: Initiate a program of stretching and strengthening of the abdominal and hip muscles; recommend a slow return to activity, as tolerated. Rest, ice for 20 minutes three times per day, compress with ace bandage, and elevate (RICE).

Medial epicondylitis: Initiate a program of stretching and strengthening of the forearm muscles; recommend a slow return to throwing, as tolerated. Rest, ice for 20 minutes three times per day, compress with ace bandage, and elevate (RICE).

Pharmacological

Naproxen, 7.5 mg/kg bid; or ibuprofen, 10 mg/kg qid for relief of pain and inflammation for 2–3 days.

Follow-up: Patient should return every 2 weeks for evaluation of therapeutic response.

Sequelae: None, if properly diagnosed and managed.

Prevention/Prophylaxis: To help prevent these types of injuries from occurring as well as from becoming chronic, a program of stretching and strengthening should be initiated, focusing on the muscles involved in the activity. Proper equipment may also be a factor (e.g., the proper size grip on the tennis racquet, a larger head to produce fewer bad hits, a graphite or composite racquet rather than a wooden or metal one, and a racquet strung less tightly [below 55 lb]).

Referral: Refer patient to orthopedist if there is no improvement after 3 weeks. Refer to a physical therapist for a program of stretching and strengthening exercises.

Education: Increase patient's awareness of overuse injuries and the importance of preparticipation physical conditioning.

Aseptic Necrosis of the Hip (Legg-Calvé-Perthes Disease)

Aspetic necrosis of the hip is an interruption of the vascular supply to the capital femur with necrosis. There are four stages of the disease:

Prenecrosis or vascular occlusion from trauma, hypercoagulation, emboli, or increased intra-articular pressure.

Necrosis accompanied by involvement of the femoral epiphysis, metaphysis, or bone marrow and resulting in fracture or cyst formation (3–6 months from onset).

Revascularization with resorption of dead bone and deformation of the softened femoral head (6–12 months from onset).

Reossification of the deformed femoral head and acetabulum (18–36 months from onset).

Etiology: A disturbance in circulation to the femoral capital epiphysis following trauma or infection.

Occurrence: Unknown.

Age: Occurs at ages 3–12 with peak age of 6–7.

Ethnicity: Occurs most frequently in whites (10 : 1).

Gender: Occurs more frequently in males (5 : 1).

Contributing Factors: Often occurs during periods of rapid growth.

Signs and Symptoms: Child presents with hip pain referred to the knee and thigh, as well as a limp. Examination reveals limitation of movement, disturbance in gait, and thigh atrophy.

Diagnostic Tests: Radiographic studies of the hip demonstrate effusion of the joint and slight widening of the joint space, progressing to decreased bone density and later to alternating areas of rarefaction versus relative density of the epiphysis, decreased bone density, and fractures. Joint aspirates are normal. Bone-age studies reveal a delay in 75% of males and 25% of females.

Differential Diagnosis

Joint aspirate cultures are positive in *septic arthritis.*
Slipped capital femoral epiphysis occurs in adolescent obese males.

Treatment: Protection of the affected joint by maintaining abduction and internal rotation, usually through the use of braces. Surgery may be indicated, particularly when the child's parents or caregivers cannot comply with the requirements of using a brace.

Follow-up: Patient should return for evaluation at least every 3 months.

Sequelae: Sequelae depend on the degree of involvement and the amount of deformity. The prognosis for full return of function is poorer when there is greater involvement of the femoral head and when the disease started later in life.

Prevention/Prophylaxis: None.

Referral: In suspected cases, refer patients to an orthopedist for full evaluation.

Education: Teach parents the importance of the child's wearing the brace. Counsel parents regarding the long-term effects of the disease.

Developmental Dysplasia of the Hip

Developmental dysplasia of the hip, formally called congenital dislocated hip, is a misalignment of the femoral head with the acetabulum. There are three types:

Dislocated: The femoral head is located outside of the acetabulum.
Dislocatable: The femoral head is in the acetabulum, but when displaced by the examiner, the femoral head spontaneously returns to its normal position.
Subluxation: The femoral head can be partially moved out of the acetabulum.

Etiology: Abnormal laxity of the hip joint capsule.

Occurrence: Incidence is 11.7 in 1000 births per year. Occurs more often in siblings of infants who have had the condition.

Age: At birth.

Ethnicity: Less prevalent in African-Americans.

Gender: Females constitute 70% of cases.

Contributing Factors: Hormonal, congenital, and mechanical factors, as well as breech births.

Signs and Symptoms: Child is asymptomatic until older and walking, and then he or she develops a limp. Clinical signs depend on age.

Newborn: Hip instability.
Older infant: Asymmetrical thigh folds, inequality of leg length (Allis sign).
Older child: Gait abnormality (waddling), painful limp, and lurch to affected side (Trendelenburg sign).

Note: In infants aged newborn to 2 years, the thighs can be abducted to touch the examining table; if they cannot be brought to within 25–30° of the table, radiographic studies should be made.

Diagnostic Tests: The following maneuvers should be done during the first 6 months at each well-baby visit to assess hip stability:

Barlow maneuver (dislocation test): Done during the newborn period; positive if the hip is dislocatable.

Ortalani maneuver (reduction test): A maneuver that would be positive at 4–6 weeks of age, but becomes negative by 3–5 months. There is a feeling of slipping (a "clunk") as the femoral head is relocated.

Allis sign: With the hips and knees flexed, the knees are at unequal heights, with the dislocated side lower.

Radiographic studies are negative in the neonatal period but useful after age 6 weeks, when they reveal lateral displacement of the femoral head. It is helpful to have films to compare with later studies. Opinions vary as to whether ultrasound studies are helpful in screening and confirmation studies.

Differential Diagnosis: Congenital short femur, differentiated by radiographic studies.

Treatment

No treatment is required in joint laxity with true dislocation.

Use of double or triple diapers is not effective.

Apply splints such as the Pavlik, Ilfield, or Rosen harness to maintain flexion and abduction of the hip.

Follow-up: Patient should return monthly to clinic for evaluation of progress, at 1 year of age, and then yearly until skeletal maturity is achieved.

Sequelae: Flexion contractures contribute to marked lordosis, resulting in gait problems. Limited abduction results in limp and gluteal muscle weakness. The most serious complication is avascular necrosis of the hip.

Prevention/Prophylaxis: None.

Referral: Refer to orthopedist for confirmation and treatment. Best results are achieved when diagnosis and intervention occur before age 6 months. Ideally, the problem should be identified in the nursery.

Education: Educate the parent in the proper application of the harness and the importance of follow-up evaluations.

Dislocations

Dislocation is the displacement of a bony part from its usual site, usually as a result of trauma.

Etiology

Shoulder: In children, the cause is instability; in adolescents, a tendinitis recurrence or an injury that involves an abduction and external rotation of the shoulder.

Patella: Vigorous quadriceps contraction when the knees are flexed from a valgus position.

Occurrence: Uncommon in children but common in athletes.

Age: Adolescents.

Ethnicity: Not significant.

Gender: Occurs in males, usually athletes; also occurs in females, particularly those with genu valgum.

Contributing Factors: Participation in sports-related activities (e.g., jumping), loose-jointedness, and genu valgum (patellar dislocation). The third factor contributes to the disorder in females, particularly adolescent girls.

Signs and Symptoms: Child presents with the complaint of severe pain in the affected body part. History should include activities preceding the injury, the exact location and distribution of pain, and the quality of the pain. It should also include whether the pain occurs with movement, what limitations or types of weakness there are, and what aggravates and what relieves the pain.
Physical findings depend on type of dislocation:

Patella: The NP will observe slight flexion of the knee and a bony mass lateral to the knee joint, with a flat area over the normal position for the patella.

Shoulder: The NP should inspect for symmetry, swelling, unilateral bony prominences, any changes in skin color, and winging of the scapula. Palpate for tenderness and range of motion, and evaluate the deep tendon reflexes and motor strength.

Diagnostic Tests

Patella: Radiographic studies of the knee for confirmation of dislocation.

Shoulder: Radiographic studies including an anteroposterior, a transthoracic lateral, and an apical oblique film to confirm shoulder instability.

Differential Diagnosis

Patella: None.

Shoulder: If pain radiates below the elbow, suspect some problem in the cervical spine; any tumors found on x-ray produce pain unrelated to movement.

Treatment

Nonpharmacological

Patella: Reduction and immobilization for 3–4 weeks; a physical therapy program to strengthen the quadriceps muscle. Surgery may be necessary to tighten the patellar capsule.

Shoulder: Immobilization with a sling or shoulder brace or spica wrap; isometric exercises (internal and external rotation) with elbow placed at patient's side.

Pharmacological

Nonsteroidal anti-inflammatory drugs (NSAIDs) for relief of pain and inflammation.

Follow-up: In 3 weeks, and then in an additional 3 weeks.

Sequelae

Patella: If there is repeated damage to the cartilage of the joint, the patient is at high risk for premature degenerative arthritis.

Shoulder: Recurrence rate is high in high school athletes.

Prevention/Prophylaxis: None, except preparticipation conditioning for persons involved in sports activities.

Referral: Refer patient to a primary-care physician or orthopedist for reduction and plan of care.

Education: Emphasize the importance of complying with the regimen, as outlined (immobilization, restriction of athletic activity). Emphasize that the strengthening exercises help to reduce the risk of recurrence.

Floppy Infant

The floppy infant displays a decreased resistance to passive movement with abnormal extensibility of the joints and delay in motor milestones. There are two types:

Paralytic group (weakness): Significant lack of movement against gravity.

Nonparalytic group: Floppiness without significant paralysis.

Etiology: Paralytic causes include the following:

Lesion of the lower motor neuron complex: Infantile progressive spinal muscular atrophy is the most common cause (autosomal recessive).

Neuromuscular junction: Causes include botulism (acquired in infants under 1 year) and myasthenia gravis (12% have a mother with myasthenia gravis).

Muscle disease: Includes myotonic dystrophy (autosomal dominant).

Nonparalytic causes are as follows:

Intrauterine or perinatal insults on brain or spinal cord: Constitute 75% of cases.

Hypotonia of central nervous system origin: Trisomy 21, Marfan's syndrome, Turner's syndrome.

Degenerative disorders: Tay-Sachs disease.

Systemic diseases, malnutrition: Cystic fibrosis, celiac disease, deprivation.

Chronic illness: Congenital heart disease, chronic pulmonary disease; metabolic (hypercalcemia) and endocrine (hypothyroid) disorders.
Unknown causes.

Occurrence: Common.

Age: Occurs at birth and in older infants.

Ethnicity: Not significant.

Gender: Occurs equally in males and females.

Contributing Factors: Prematurity, maternal ingestions, and infections such as poliomyelitis.

Signs and Symptoms: The infant is brought to the clinic for an early well-baby visit with the complaint that the "hips are funny." Older infants with the disorder are brought to the clinic when they have not started walking, running, or climbing stairs.

Findings in the newborn nursery include a positive scarf sign (the infant's hands can be pulled across the chest, and the elbows can be pulled past the chin) and a positive hip sign (extended lower extremities can be abducted at the hip more than 160°). Findings in young infants include (1) the classic frog-leg position, with arms limp at the sides; (2) when held horizontally, the infant droops over the hand; (3) when held vertically, it feels as though the infant will slip through the hands; (4) there is marked head lag; and (5) in older infants, there is a delay in achieving motor milestones.

In the paralytic group, the fine-motor, personal/social, and language milestones are normal according to results of the Denver Developmental Screening test. There is weakness in the shoulders and hips, tendon reflexes are absent or depressed, and strength is decreased.

In the nonparalytic group, spasticity is present and reflexes are increased. The Babinski and tonic neck reflexes persist and worsen.

Diagnostic Tests

Blood glucose (hypoglycemia) and calcium (hypercalcemia).
Computed tomographic (CT) scans of the brain to determine the presence of abnormalities.
Spinal fluid examination to rule out meningitis and encephalitis.
Creatine kinase level is normal; elevated creatinine phosphokinase is due to birth trauma, hypoxia, or ischemia.
Electromyography (EMG) is normal. Muscle biopsies show a decrease in voluntary motor activity.

Differential Diagnosis

Hypoglycemia or *hypocalcemia,* excluded on the basis of blood workup.
Sepsis, excluded on the basis of spinal fluid and blood workup.
Weakness, excluded as the child matures.

Treatment: Supportive, based on the ultimate diagnosis.

Follow-up: Monthly to assess growth and development.

Sequelae: In cases secondary to Tay-Sachs disease, the prognosis is death. In other forms, such as floppiness secondary to Marfan's syndrome, the children mature to lead productive lives. Those with paralytic forms (e.g., secondary to congenital muscular dystrophy) may have mental retardation. For those with spinal cord lesions, the result may be a life in a wheelchair.

Prevention/Prophylaxis: Improved prenatal care and delivery techniques as a means of possibly preventing intrauterine and birth problems.

Education: Instruct the family in feeding techniques, because these patients sometimes have problems with chewing and swallowing. For those diseases with a genetic factor, discuss the implications with the family.

Foot Problems

Foot problems are deviations from the normal development of the foot. These problems may be related to *posturing*, the habitual position of the foot; or to *deformity*, which is similar to posturing, except that the foot cannot be manually repositioned. The following are among the most commonly noted problems:

Calcaneovalgus, which occurs as a result of uterine restraint.

Metarsus adductus, which is probably secondary to uterine restraint.

Clubfoot (talipes equinovarus), which in severe cases is attributed to anatomical abnormalities.

Flat foot (pes planus), a condition that occurs as a result of ligamental laxity (Fig. 12–5).

Etiology: Most commonly due to position in utero, but may result from anatomical abnormalities.

Occurrence: Fairly common.

Age: Infancy through early childhood.

Ethnicity: Higher prevalence of pes planus (flat feet) in persons of African descent.

Gender: Occurs equally in males and females.

Contributing Factors: Position of the feet in utero and/or congenital abnormalities.

Signs and Symptoms: Most often noticed in the newborn nursery; however, caregiver may bring infant to clinic with the comment that the feet "turn in" or "turn out."

Calcaneovalgus foot is dorsiflexed at the ankle; bottom of the foot appears convex. May be easily manipulated into normal position.

Clubfoot is a fixed medial deviation of the forefoot, with medial inclination of the heel, and downward point of the foot.

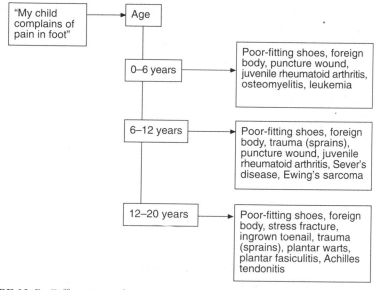

FIGURE 12–5 Differentiating foot pain.

In metatarsus adductus, the heel deviates laterally and the sole of the foot appears to be kidney shaped.

In flat foot, the arch does not develop until between ages 2 and 6; pain usually does not appear before adolescence. To differentiate between flexible flat foot and rigid flat foot (congenital vertical talus), have the child stand on tiptoes and observe the arch. The arch will reappear in cases of flexible flat foot.

Diagnostic Tests: None. Foot problems are manifested on manipulation of the foot; the inability to return the foot to normal alignment is also indicative of problems.

Differential Diagnosis

Differentiate the calcaneovalgus foot from *congenital vertical talus*, which is often associated with neurological disorders.

Deformities associated with *metarsus adductus* include developmental dysplasia of the hip.

Treatment

Metatarsus adductus: Mild, foot exercises; moderate, refer patient for casting when no older than 4 months; after 1 year, surgical intervention is indicated.

Club foot: Newborns should have serial casts applied as soon as possible; patients with severe cases usually require surgery.

Flat foot: Usually a well-fitted tennis shoe.

Follow-up: Monthly until resolution.

Sequelae: Permanent damage to the feet with resulting limited ambulation. Severe cases of clubfoot left untreated can result in a foot that is smaller than the other, a foot that is less mobile, and a leg that is smaller as a result of muscle involvement, resulting in atrophy of the muscle. If not treated, increased stiffening occurs with changes in bone development. The lateral part of the foot has an excess of soft tissue that causes the calf to be thinner.

Prevention/Prophylaxis: None.

Referral: Refer patients who do not respond to foot exercises within 2 months to an orthopedist.

Education: Demonstrate to the parents or caregiver the exercises for remolding the foot. Emphasize the importance of well-fitted shoes for the patient.

Fractures

Fractures are disruptions in bone continuity. There are six types:

Simple: Fracture is straight and in good alignment.
Displaced: Ends of the broken bone are not in good alignment.
Green stick: An incomplete fracture.
Comminuted: Bone is broken into pieces.
Compressed: Ends of the bone are forced or pressed against each other.
Compound: Bone is broken and is piercing the skin.

Etiology: Occurs as a result of birth injury (clavicular), wringing of the limb, or major trauma.

Occurrence: Common.

Age: Any age group.

Ethnicity: Not significant.

Gender: Occurs equally in boys and girls.

Contributing Factors: Sports participation, child abuse, and accidents.

Signs and Symptoms: Child presents with a history of trauma to a body part; often relates that the bone sounded like it "popped."
Findings usually reveal painful swelling with ecchymoses over the affected part. Make careful notation of pulse and sensation. Evaluate range of motion, noting presence of pain and/or crepitus and deformity. Observe for variations in posture (clavicular fractures have a characteristic forward drooping of the affected shoulder) and in gait (the short-stance phase [the time that the extremity bears the body weight] and refusal to walk).

Diagnostic Tests: Radiographic studies of the affected part; in cases of suspected child abuse, review films for evidence of old injuries. If the present injury does not appear on the film, do a repeat x-ray in 10 days to determine the presence of new calcifications, thereby proving the presence of a fracture.
A greenstick fracture, a disruption of the cortex on one side of the bone but cleavage plane of opposite side, is not displaced but angulated as bone ends

are not separated. It is often missed on first radiographic studies. Perform a repeat x-ray in 10 days to determine callus formation.

Stress fractures of the tibia are often missed on the first radiographic film. Do a repeat x-ray in 10 days to determine callus formation.

Clavicular fractures may be angulated but not displaced.

Epiphysial fractures need to be assessed and classified according to the damage of the growth plate (Fig. 12–6).

Spiral fractures of the femur, suggesting a forceful twist of the extremity, are highly suspicious of child abuse.

Differential Diagnosis: None.

Treatment: Because children's bones are less brittle than adults' and because they have greater healing power, most fractures can be treated with closed reduction and casting or splinting. However, complex fractures caused by major trauma require open reduction.

Follow-up

Green stick: Follow up in 7–10 days; do a repeat x-ray to evaluate alignment.

Clavicular: Apply a figure-of-eight dressing that retracts shoulders and brings clavicle into normal alignment. Healing callus will be apparent when consolidation is complete.

For all cases involving casts, patients should return in 48 hours to evaluate status of swelling and cast care, and then every 2 weeks. Perform a repeat x-ray in 1 month to evaluate bone healing.

Sequelae: Deformities due to fracture usually are the result of delayed treatment; however, this occurs less often in children than in adults. The callus formation after clavicular fractures may be noticeable for 1 year postinjury. Damage to the blood supply and innervation can lead to disruption in bone growth.

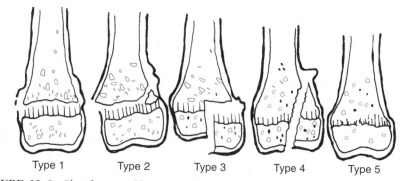

| Type 1 | Type 2 | Type 3 | Type 4 | Type 5 |

FIGURE 12–6 Classification of bone plate injury. The Salter-Harris Classification categorizes physeal injury by morphology. However, to determine a meaningful prognosis using this scale, the site of the injury must be taken into account. For example, a type 1 injury to the distal radius causes less growth disturbances than the same type of fracture at the distal femoral epiphysis. (From Salter, RB, and Harris, WH: Injuries involving the epiphyseal plate. J Bone Joint Surg 45-A:587, 1963, with permission.)

Prevention/Prophylaxis: Prevention of child abuse through parent education in parenting skills; safety measures, including using approved car seats and car seatbelts; use of gates for doorways and stairways, and guards for windows; and doing preconditioning exercises before sports participation.

Referral: Refer patient to a primary-care physician or orthopedist for definitive diagnosis and treatment.

Education: Counseling and instruction of parents in parenting skills. Instruction in safety measures.

Genu Varum/Genu Valgum

Genu varum is a pattern of internal torsion involving the tibia, in which the leg distal to the knee is tilted toward the midline of the body. Bowing is normal until ages 2–3 years. As growth occurs, genus varum changes to genu valgum (knock knee), in which the extremity distal to the knee is tilted away from the midline until ages 8–9 years, when there is a normal straightening with growth.

Etiology: A result of normal intrauterine positioning.

Occurrence: Common.

Age: Occurs at birth to age 8–10 years; by age 10 years, adult alignment occurs.

Ethnicity: Not significant.

Gender: Occurs equally in males and females.

Contributing Factors: Genetic factors: Genu varum is seen in achondroplasia, and genu valgum occurs in Hurler's syndrome. Systemic disease: Anterior bowing of the lower tibia in newborn or later infancy is seen in neurofibromatosis.

Signs and Symptoms: Child is brought to clinic with the complaint that "the legs are bowed." Findings include an internally rotated tibia about the long axis of the leg. Posterior or anterior bowing will occasionally be found.

Diagnostic Tests: If the condition does not show improvement in sequential observations, then radiographic studies are indicated.

Differential Diagnosis: Growth disturbance, as evidenced by changes on x-rays.

Treatment: Bracing may be appropriate; surgical intervention is rarely done, and only children older than 10 are candidates for surgery. The improvement imparted by wearing special shoes or devices is negligible.

Follow-up: Child should return to clinic for regular well-baby visits for serial monitoring.

Sequelae: Risk of permanent misalignment is rare.

Prevention/Prophylaxis: None.

Referral: The criteria for referral to an orthopedist are persistent bowing beyond age 2, bowing that is increasing, bowing in one leg only, and knock knee associated with short stature. Refer patient immediately to a primary-care physician or an orthopedist for posterior or anterior bowing, because these conditions usually require surgical intervention.

Education: Teach parents about normal growth and development. Provide reassurance that this is a self-limiting condition.

Growing Pains

Growing pains are characterized by recurrent, intermittent limb pain, usually in the calf or thigh, behind the knee, and occasionally the arms, lasting at least 3 months, that is nonarticular, and is severe enough to interrupt normal activities. Pain varies in intensity, but it is usually in the form of a deep ache or a sense of restlessness in the limb.

Etiology: Unknown.

Occurrence: May occur in as high as 15–18% of children aged 3–12 years.

Age: Occurs in children aged 3–5 or 8–12.

Ethnicity: Not significant.

Gender: More common in females.

Contributing Factors: Fatigue, infection, emotional factors, and excessive muscle use.

Signs and Symptoms: Child presents with a 3-month history of intermittent pain lasting no more than 2 hours. Pain occurs late in the day or awakens child at night. Pain is not specifically related to joints but interrupts normal activities, such as sleep. Physical findings are negative.

Diagnostic Tests

Radiographic studies are negative.
Laboratory workup is normal.
The erythrocyte sedimentation rate is normal (most useful test), indicating no infectious process.

Differential Diagnosis

Osteoid osteoma: Bone pain at night, relieved by aspirin. The pain is characterized as boring and aching.
Patellofemoral pain syndrome: Occurs in adolescents, affects the knee, and is associated with exercise.
Benign hypermobility syndrome: Complaint of leg pain following exercise.

Fibromyalgia: Most frequently occurs in adolescent females; characterized by aches and pains, multiple points of tenderness, stiffness, and chronic fatigue.

Treatment

   Nonpharmacological

Reassurance, warm baths, and gentle massage. Ask the child to walk during an attack to demonstrate the absence of a limp.

   Pharmacological

If analgesics are necessary for pain, give acetaminophen, 10–15 mg/kg per dose or 400–480 mg q 4 hours; or ibuprofen, 4–10 mg/kg per dose q 6–8 hours.

Follow-up: None.

Sequelae: None.

Prevention/Prophylaxis: None.

Referral: None.

Education: Parents should take child's temperature and check the joints and muscles for redness and swelling.

   Parents often make the diagnosis before bringing the child in to be examined; therefore they come for validation and reassurance that this is indeed a benign and self-limiting condition.

Juvenile Rheumatoid Arthritis

Juvenile rheumatoid arthritis (JRA) is characterized by persistent joint pain lasting at least 6 weeks; it occurs in children under age 16. There are three types, listed from

   Polyarticular JRA (50%): Five or more joints are affected (symmetrical pattern of involvement): small joints of hands and feet, large joints, cervical spine, and temporomandibular, sternoclavicular, and distal interphalangeal joints.

   Pauciarticular JRA (40%): Four or fewer joints are involved: large joints such as knees, ankles, and elbows. May be classified based on function, as follows:

   • Class I: Patient can perform all activities.
   • Class II: Patient performs activities adequately, but with some limitations.
   • Class III: Patient's activities are very limited; can perform self-care only.
   • Class IV: Patient is wheelchair-bound or bedridden.

   Systemic-onset JRA (10%): Number of joints is not relevant; there is remission within 1 year.

Etiology: Unknown.

Occurrence: Affects 100,000 to 250,000 children in the United States.

Age: Occurs in children aged 1–3 years and in young teen-agers.

Ethnicity: Not significant.

Gender: Gender differs as to type:

Polyarticular JRA: Females outnumber males.

Pauciarticular JRA: Young onset and associated with chronic insidious uveitis in female patients; older onset and associated with spondyloarthropathy in male patients.

Systemic-onset JRA: Occurs equally in males and females.

Contributing Factors: Family history of arthritis.

Signs and Symptoms: Evaluation of symptoms is done over a 6-month period. Child presents with complaints of joint pain.

The child with systemic-onset JRA is usually younger, and may present with a history of initial temperature variations greater than 103°F for 2 weeks. There is usually a small, salmon-colored, macular, pruritic rash, usually on the trunk and extremities, that waxes and wanes with the fluctuations in body temperature.

The younger child (about 2) with pauciarticular JRA is usually female; there is a history of asymptomatic swelling of a joint. The older child (usually over 8) is usually male. Systemic signs (e.g., weight loss, anorexia, malaise, diffuse arthralgia) may be present.

The patient with polyarticular JRA presents with no fever or a low-grade fever. Five or more joints are affected (small joints of hands and feet; large joints, cervical spine, temporomandibular joint, sternoclavicular joint, and distal interphalangeal joint).

Physical findings vary according to JRA type:

Polyarticular JRA: There is a symmetrical pattern of joint involvement. Small joints of hands and feet, large joints, cervical spine, temporomandibular joint, sternoclavicular, and distal interphalangeal are involved. Radiographic changes occur within 1 year of onset. There may be hepatosplenomegaly and chronic uveitis.

Pauciarticular JRA: There is slow development of contractures, and nodules over tendons. Joints of the lower extremity (hips, knees, ankles) are usually involved with an asymmetrical pattern. Uveitis, when it occurs, is acute; signs are redness and decreased visual acuity. There is decreased exercise capacity.

Systemic-onset JRA: The number of affected joints is not relevant. There is splenomegaly and lymphadenopathy.

Diagnostic Tests

Polyarticular JRA

Mild anemia.

Leukocytosis.

Rheumatoid factor: 35% seronegative, 5% seropositive.

ANAs: 75% seropositive, 25% seronegative.

Pauciarticular JRA

In young children, laboratory tests are normal. In 50% of cases, ANAs are positive.

In older children, laboratory tests are normal. Rheumatoid factors and ANAs are negative.

Iridocyclitis may occur in up to 30% of cases, especially in girls.

Systemic-Onset JRA

Normocytic/normochromic anemia.

White blood cell (WBC) count elevated, with a shift to the left.

Platelet count elevated.

Erythrocyte sedimentation rate extremely high.

Rheumatoid factors and antinuclear antibodies (ANAs) are negative.

Other

Obtain baseline data on growth and development; obtain midarm circumference in children in whom inadequate weight gain is observed; less than the 10th percentile is suspected of inadequate weight gain.

Obtain triceps skinfold measurements to assess deficits in fat stores.

Differential Diagnosis

Rheumatic fever arthritis: History of streptococcal infection, no morning stiffness, and no eye disease; rash is an erythema marginatum. ANA and rheumatoid factor negative.

Leukemia: No morning stiffness, no rash, and no eye disease; ANAs and rheumatoid factors are negative.

Lyme disease: No morning stiffness; rash is an erythema chronicum migrans; no involvement of the small joints, no eye disease, normal WBC count, and increased immune complexes.

Treatment: Object is to restore function, relieve pain, restore mobility, and provide adequate nutrition to maintain and restore growth and development.

Nonpharmacological

Range of motion and muscle-strengthening program.

Meeting nutritional needs (to address problems ranging from lack of growth to obesity).

Pharmacological

First-line: Naproxen, 7.5 mg/kg bid *or*
               Ibuprofen, 10 mg/kg qid *or*
               Tolmetin sodium, 10 mg/kg tid

Second-line: Methotrexate 5–10 mg/m^2 per week

Uveitis: Steroid eyedrops and dilating agents.

Follow-up: Complete blood count and liver function studies every 1–2 months to evaluate decreased hepatofunction related to medication use; a routine ophthalmological examination with slit lamp every 6 months for 4 years to evaluate ocular complications.

Sequelae: Growth retardation (systemic-onset and pauciarticular JRA), pericarditis and myocarditis (systemic-onset JRA), and residual joint damage destructive symmetric rheumatoid nodules (polyarticular JRA). Those most apt to have problems are those with unremitting synovitis, hip involvement, or positive rheumatoid factor tests.

Prevention/Prophylaxis: None.

Referral: Refer patient to an orthopedist or a rheumatologist to delineate plan of care. If there are any ocular problems, refer patient to an ophthalmologist for testing and intervention. Referral to a nutritionist/dietitian may be necessary.

Education: Assist parents and child in coping with chronic illness. Talk with the child and parents about their "feelings" regarding the illness. The degree to which the child will have to modify activities of daily living depends on his or her functional classification. Use the patient's self-report of functional status. Assist the family in meeting the child's nutritional needs.

Osgood-Schlatter Disease

Osgood-Schlatter disease is defined as a painful prominence (osteochondrosis) of the tibia tubercle.

Etiology: Chronic trauma to the tibia tuberosity by quadriceps overuse.

Occurrence: Common.

Age: Adolescence.

Ethnicity: Not significant.

Gender: More common in males.

Contributing Factors: Participation in strenuous athletic activities such as football, soccer, or basketball; participation in ballet or gymnastics; or the adolescent growth spurt.

Signs and Symptoms: Child presents with a complaint of pain in the knee that worsens with activity and is relieved by rest. Findings include pain and swelling over the tibia tuberosity aggravated by extension of the knee.

Diagnostic Tests: X-ray of the knee shows changes in the tibia tuberosity.

Differential Diagnosis

Osteosarcoma: Radiographic studies are positive, and gait disturbances are noted.

Patellar tendinitis: The child exhibits pain on running and climbing stairs.

Osteomyelitis: Usually affects a single bone; the child may experience an acute illness or a subacute illness with fever, severe pain at the affected site, erythema, and swelling. Radiographic studies may be normal in the first 10–14 days of the illness.

Treatment: Reduce athletic activity and avoid any activity that requires deep knee bending. Give NSAIDs for pain: acetaminophen, 10–15 mg/kg per dose or 400–480 mg q 4 hours; or ibuprofen, 4–10 mg/kg per dose q 6–8 hours. Rest, ice for 20 minutes three times per day, compress with ace bandage, and elevate (RICE). Bracing may be done if patient fails to improve.

Follow-up: Patient should return at 2-month intervals for evaluation.

Sequelae: If disease is not treated, secondary degenerative arthritis may develop.

Prevention/Prophylaxis: Physical therapy to strengthen leg.

Referral: Refer patient to an orthopedist if there is no improvement within 2 months.

Education: Educate parents as to the value of decreasing the child's level of activity. In most cases, the problem resolves spontaneously.

Scoliosis

Scoliosis is a lateral curvature of the spine classified by anatomical location (usually thoracic or lumbar); the curvature is accompanied by a secondary curvature to balance the spine. The posterior vertebral elements rotate toward the concavity of the curve, causing the attached ribs on the convex side to rotate posteriorly. Although in most cases the scoliosis stabilizes spontaneously (as demonstrated by the lower incidence in adults), if detected and treated early, the prognosis is excellent. There are three main types: congenital, neuromuscular, and idiopathic. Classification is made on the basis of the degree of the curvature:

Mild: Less than 20%.
Moderate: Between 20% and 40%.
Severe: Greater than 40%.

Rate of progression is approximately 1° per month.

Etiology: Scoliosis may be due to congenital vertebral anomalies, such as hemivertebra; however, the most common form is idiopathic.

Occurrence: Clinically apparent scoliosis (curve of 5%) occurs in 4% of adolescents.

Age: Usually begins between ages 8 and 10 and may progress into adulthood. Rarely seen in infants, but may occur in children aged 2–4 (more common in Great Britain).

Ethnicity: Not significant.

Gender: Scoliosis is more common in females, the ratio ranging from 4–5 : 1 to 7 : 1.

Contributing Factors: Family history is positive in 30% of cases of idiopathic scoliosis. Neuromuscular scoliosis is often associated with cerebral palsy and spina bifida. Congenital scoliosis is associated with a high incidence of renal problems. Of no value in predicting the prognosis is the presence of lumbar lordosis or thoracic kyphosis. Females whose scoliosis was noted before the onset of menses are at higher risk for progression.

Signs and Symptoms: Adolescents are often asymptomatic, but some may complain of low-back pain.

Findings reveal a noticeable curvature of the spine when anteriorly flexed from the trunk (forward-bending or Adams test). There may be an inequality in hip height, as noted by a difference in the levels of the iliac crests, as well as elevation of one shoulder with asymmetry in the prominence of the scapula.

Diagnostic Tests

Total spinal x-rays (anteroposterior and lateral), performed with arms extended over the head, reveal the location and extent of the curvature.

Platelet calmodulin level is measured as a predictor of progression and severity (e.g., 3.83 ng/μg of protein in children with more than 10° of progression versus 0.06 ng/μg of protein in children with stable curves of less than 5° progression in the previous 12 months).

Differential Diagnosis: Postural compensation due to unequal length of leg, which resolves when treated (Fig. 12–7).

Treatment: The long-range goal is to halt progression of the curvature. Treatment options include the following: for mild scoliosis, none; for moderate, Milwaukee brace or Boston thoracolumbosacral orthosis (TSLO); and for severe, surgical procedure for insertion of Herrington or Luque spinal rods. Compliance with the braces seems to decrease with age: younger children are more compliant and teen-agers less compliant.

Follow-up: For curvatures of less than 10°, evaluate yearly; for curvatures of 10–20° evaluate every 6 months until skeletal maturity to assess progression of the curvature, as progression often occurs during the growth spurt; and for curvatures of 20–30°, evaluate every 4 months.

Sequelae: Severe curvatures may result in diminished lung capacity and low-back pain. Thoracic curvatures may progress into adult life. Lumbar curvatures may lead to subluxation of the vertebrae and to premature arthritic degeneration of the spine in adulthood.

Prevention/Prophylaxis: Routine screening for all children in the preadolescent and adolescent years. Implementation of appropriate treatment is recommended. Many states mandate screening as a means of early detection. Par-

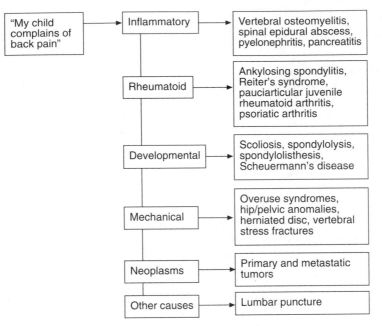

FIGURE 12–7 Differentiating back pain.

ents should receive counseling about genetic transmission and the need for early and periodic screening of children at risk.

Referral: Consult for curvatures of 5–7%; refer for curvatures greater than 20% or in cases where the client is experiencing symptoms.

Education: Inform parents and school health personnel of the importance of screening and follow-up. If the child is to wear a brace, advise the parents in ways to assist the child to use clothing to mask the brace. This will help the child retain his or her self-esteem and positive self-image.

Shin Splints

Shin splints are microtears at the origins of the anterior and posterior tibia muscles resulting in pain and inflammation along the midshaft or distal third of the tibia.

Etiology: An overuse injury involving microtears at the origins of the anterior and posterior tibia muscles.

Occurrence: Common.

Age: Usually does not occur in children under 10.

Ethnicity: Not significant.

Gender: Occurs equally in males and females.

Contributing Factors: Participation in sports that involve running; inadequate preparticipation conditioning.

Signs and Symptoms: Child gives a history of pain along the anterior tibia that increases with activity as well as recent involvement in a sports activity.

The anterior surface of the tibia, which is tender to palpation, may be warm to the touch.

Diagnostic Tests: None.

Differential Diagnosis: None.

Treatment

Nonpharmacological

Rest, elevation, warm compresses, and heel cups may offer relief. Initiate a program of stretching and warm-up exercises that should be done before participation in running or jogging activities.

Pharmacological

If analgesics are necessary for pain, the NP may give acetaminophen, 10–15 mg/kg per dose or 400–480 mg q 4 hours; or ibuprofen, 4–10 mg/kg per dose q 6–8 hours.

Follow-up: Patient should return in 2 weeks to evaluate progress.

Sequelae: None

Prevention/Prophylaxis: Initiate a program of preactivity conditioning exercises.

Referral: None.

Education: Instruct children, caregivers, and coaches in the importance of preactivity conditioning. Reassure parents that this condition is self-limiting.

Tendinitis

Tendinitis is characterized by swelling, pain, and tenderness over the insertion of a tendon, most often involving the Achilles tendon, the patellar inferior pole, or the shoulder.

Etiology: Repetitive mild trauma resulting in inflammation. A shallow bicipital groove allows subluxation of the bicipital tendon (knee); irritation of the avascular portion of the supraspinatus tendon progresses to an inflammatory response (shoulder).

Occurrence: Uncommon in children, but common in athletes.

Age: Usually not before the age 10 and not before participation in sports.

Ethnicity: Not significant.

Gender: Occurs equally in males and females.

Contributing Factors: Participation in sports such as basketball and volleyball (knees); running sports and excessive walking (Achilles tendons); and swimming and tennis (shoulders).

Signs and Symptoms: Obtain a history of the location and distribution of pain. Note whether the pain is related to movement, whether there is a limitation with movement, what aggravates the tenderness, and what relieves it. Physical findings included vary by affected site:

Achilles tendon: Pain on flexion of the foot.
Patella tendon: Localized tenderness at the inferior pole of the patella.
Shoulder: Direct tenderness over the involved structure.

Diagnostic Tests

Achilles tendon: Radiographic studies to rule out fracture; pain on range of motion and perhaps tightened heel cords.
Patella tendon: None.
Shoulder: Radiographic studies that include anteroposterior, transthoracic lateral, and apical oblique (reveals shoulder instability) views. The examiner will be able to elicit a painful arc sign and a Newer impingement sign.

Differential Diagnosis

Achilles tendon: None.
Patella tendon: In Osgood-Schlatter disease, the pain is related to the tubercle of the tibia rather than the inferior pole of the patella.
Shoulder: Torn rotator cuff is indicated by no improvement in 6 weeks and by radiographic appearance.

Treatment

Pharmacological

NSAIDs (usually ibuprofen or acetaminophen) to decrease the inflammatory process in and around the joint capsule.

Nonpharmacological

Achilles tendon: Prescribe rest and elevation; in severe cases, casting may be necessary.
Patella tendon: Prescribe rest, elevation, and restriction of athletic activity.
Shoulder: Instruct patient to position the shoulder to avoid pain and maintain motion (keeping arms close to body, elbow in, palms up). Teach patient to externally rotate arm before reaching, to "work low," and to avoid work or sport-related activities. Prescribe a sling, but do not immobilize the arm. Initiate Codman (pendulum) exercises; later, have the patient "walk" up a wall with his or her fingers.

Follow-up: Patient should return in 3 weeks for evaluation of progress and again in 3 weeks.

Sequelae

Achilles tendon: If associated with plantar fasciitis, there may be a rheumatoid variant. Episodes that last for 2–3 days and are associated with tenosynovitis may be an early indication of familial hyperlipoproteinemia type II.

Shoulder: If there is no improvement in 6 weeks, order imaging studies to determine presence of a rotator cuff tear.

Prevention/Prophylaxis: Proper conditioning before participating in sports that involve running, jumping, and extension of the arm overhead. Patients must learn to pay attention to their bodies and to stop activity before damage occurs.

Referral: If there is no improvement in 6 weeks, refer patient to a primary-care physician or an orthopedist. Refer patient to a physical therapist for strengthening the rotator cuff and scapular rotators.

Education

Achilles tendon: Wear proper shoes when walking. Use heel cups.

Patella tendon: During rehabilitation, patient must comply with the plan of care.

Supraspinatus: During rehabilitation, patient must not do overhead work and must restrict sports activity.

Tibial Torsion

Persistent (past age 16 months) rotation of the leg between the ankle and the knee. A growth disturbance of the proximal tibia growth plate is called Blount disease.

Etiology: Laxity of the knee ligaments, early or excessive weight bearing; may be due to excessive pressure across the medial aspect of the tibia growth plate.

Occurrence: Common.

Age: Most cases occur between ages 2 and 4 years. Can occur from birth to age 18 months, and may also occur in middle childhood and adolescence.

Ethnicity: Occurs more often in dark-skinned races.

Gender: Occurs equally in males and females.

Contributing Factors: Precocious walking and African ancestry.

Signs and Symptoms: Child presents with the complaint of "toeing in." Findings depend on age: At birth to 16 months, the angulation is 20° but decreases to neutral rotation by 16 months. Findings of an angulation greater than expected for age should be investigated. In severe bowing, the varus angulation is greater than 20°.

Diagnostic Tests: Radiographic studies to assess the medial tibia growth plate reveal a characteristic angular deformity at the proximal tibia. MRI has some advantages over radiographs: There is no ionizing radiation and the shape of the ossified and cartilaginous epiphysis is clearly defined, as are the meniscal and physeal abnormalities.

Differential Diagnosis: None.

Treatment: For the most part, no treatment is needed, and rarely are braces prescribed. In some more severe cases, an external rotation splint worn at night or a Brown brace may reverse the process and restore growth.

Follow-up: Patient should return at 2-month intervals for evaluation of bowing.

Sequelae: Without treatment, irreversible damage to the tibia growth plate can occur.

Prevention/Prophylaxis: Children usually outgrow the condition by age 16 months.

Referral: Refer patient to an orthopedist if condition continues after age 16 months.

Education: Teach parents the parameters of normal growth and development. Reassure parents that this condition is usually self-limiting but needs regular monitoring.

REFERENCES

General

Behrman, R, and Kliegman, R (eds): Nelson Essentials of Pediatrics. WB Saunders, Philadelphia, 1990.
Doenges, M, and Moorhouse, M: Nursing Diagnoses with Interventions, ed 4. FA Davis, Philadelphia, 1993.
Green, M: Pediatric Diagnosis: Interpretation of Symptoms & Signs in Infants, Children and Adolescents, ed 5. WB Saunders, Philadelphia, 1992.
Hay, W (ed): Current Pediatric Diagnosis & Treatment, ed 12. Appleton & Lange, Norwalk, Conn, 1995.
Stockman, J: Difficult Diagnosis in Pediatrics. WB Saunders, Philadelphia, 1990.

Assessment

Bratton, R, and Agerter, A: Preparticipation sports examination: Efficient risk assessment in children and adolescents. Postgrad Med 98(2):123, 1995.
Castiglia, P: Sports injuries in children. J Pediatr Health Care 9:32, 1995.
Dyment, P: The triple-threat sports exam. Patient Care 26:97, 1992.
Gottlieb, A: Cheerleaders are athletes too. Pediatr Nurs 20(6):630, 1994.
Overbaugh, K, and Allen, JG: The adolescent athlete, Part I: Preseason preparation and examination. J Pediatr Health Care 8:146, 1994.

Ankle Sprain

Baker, C, and Todd, J: Intervening in acute ankle sprain and chronic instability. J Musculoskel Med 12:51, 1995.
Birrer, R, et al: Ankle: Don't dismiss a sprain. Patient Care 26:6, 1992.

Apophyseal Injuries

Drillings, G, et al: Common tennis injuries. Hosp Med 31:20, 1995.
Galea, A, and Albers, J: Patellofemoral pain: Beyond empirical diagnosis. Phys Sports Med 22(4):48, 1994.

Leach, R, and Zecher, S: Tennis injuries: Helping players get back on the court. Consultant 35:1657, 1995.

Peck, D: Apophyseal injuries in the young athlete. Am Fam Phys 51:1891, 1995.

Quashnick, M: The diagnosis and management of plantar fasciitis. Nurse Pract 21(4):50, 1996.

Roland, GC, and Beagley, M: Management of acute knee injuries. Fam Pract Recert 13(8):52, 1991.

Developmental Dysplasia of the Hip

Aaronsson, DD, et al: Developmental displasia of the hip. Pediatrics 94:201, 1994.

Curry, L, and Gibson, L: Congenital hip dysplasia: The importance of early detection and comprehensive treatment. Nurse Pract 17:49, 1992.

Rudy, C: Developmental displasia of the hip: What's new in the 1990's? J Pediatr Health Care 10:85, 1996.

Speers, A, and Speers, M: Care of the infant in a Pavlik harness. Pediatr Nurs 18:229, 1992.

Dislocations

Bronstein, R: On-field management of football injuries. J Musculoskel Med 12:14, 1995.

Onieal, M: Problems of the shoulder. J Am Acad Nurse Pract 6:283, 1994.

Tibone, J, and Shaffer, B: A functional approach to managing shoulder impingement. J Musculoskel Med 12:37, 1995.

Floppy Infant

David, WS, and Jones, JR: Electromyography and biopsy correlation with suggested protocol for evaluation of the floppy infant. Muscle Nerves 17:424, 1994.

Foot Problems

Churgay, CA: Diagnosis and treatment of pediatric foot deformities. Am Fam Phys 47:883, 1993.

Fractures

Leventhal, J, et al: Fractures in young children: Distinguishing child abuse from unintentional injuries. Amer J Dis Child 147(1):87, 1993.

Growing Pains

Henrickson, M, and Passo, M: Recognizing patterns in chronic limb pain. Contemp Pediatr 11:33, 1994.

Juvenile Rheumatoid Arthritis

Purred, K, et al: You are what you eat: Healthy food choices, nutrition, and the child with juvenile rheumatoid arthritis. Pediatr Nurs 22:391, 1996.

Wright, FV, et al: Development of a self-report functional status index for juvenile rheumatoid arthritis. J Rheumatol 21:536, 1994.

Osgood-Schlatter Disease

American Academy of Family Physicians: Osgood-Schlatter disease: A cause of knee pain in children. Am Fam Phys 51, 1995.

Yashar, A, et al: Determination of skeletal age in children with Osgood-Schlatter disease by using radiographs of the knee. J Pediatr Orthopedics 15:298, 1995.

Scoliosis

Ascion, J: Understanding curvature of the spine (scoliosis). Fam Pract Recert 13:67, 1991.

Jonides, L: Congenital scoliosis: A case presentation. J Pediatr Health Care 9:139, 1995.

Kindsfater, K, et al: Levels of platelet calmodulin for the prediction of progression and severity of adolescent idiopathic scoliosis. J Bone Joint Surg 76:1186, 1994.

Renshaw, T: Diagnosis and management of idiopathic scoliosis. Fam Pract Recert 13:47, 1991.

US Preventative Services Task Force: Screening for adolescent idiopathic scoliosis policy statement. JAMA 269:2664, 1993.
US Preventative Services Task Force: Screening for adolescent idiopathic scoliosis policy statement. JAMA 269:2667, 1993.
Winter, R, et al: Letters to the editor: Screening for scoliosis. JAMA 273:185, 1995.

Shin Splints

Batt, ME: Shin splints—A review of terminology. Clin J Sports Med 5(1):53, 1995.

Tendinitis

Latimer, H, and Taft, T: Shoulder disorders: Six questions and a hands-on examination are keys to diagnosis. Consultant 34:1304, 1994.
Stevens, M: Heel pain. Physician and Sports Medicine 20(4):87, 1992.

Tibial Torsion

deSanctis, N, et al: Infantile type of Blount's disease: Considerations concerning etiopathogenesis and treatment. J Pediatr Orthoped 4:200, 1995.
Ducou le Pointe, H, et al: Blount's disease: Magnetic resonance imaging. Pediatr Radiol 25:12, 1995

CHAPTER **13**

CENTRAL AND

PERIPHERAL

NERVOUS SYSTEM

ASSESSMENT

During assessment of the neurological system, a complete history is the most critical component. Careful documentation of the onset of symptoms within the developmental context is important, along with a detailed accounting of the chief complaint. If a congenital disorder is suspected, a careful review of pregnancy, labor, delivery, and newborn status is indicated. Also, a careful developmental assessment of the child should be obtained. A variety of assessment tools can be used; currently, the Neonatal Behavioral Assessment Scale provides more information regarding assessment of behavior than a traditional neurological examination. Familiarity with neurological development is also essential (see Chapter 1, Table 1–4).

Family history should be obtained, and gross-motor, fine-motor, social, and language skills (see Chapter 1, Table 1–2) should be evaluated.

The examination should be performed in a safe, nonthreatening environment. The child should be made as comfortable as possible. Child and parent behavior should be observed at the outset and throughout the examination. The child's mental status, cognitive function, and level of alertness should be evaluated. If a traumatic injury has occurred, the pediatric trauma scale (see Chapter 7, Table 7–3) should be used for assessment.

The size and shape of the head should be documented. The anterior and posterior fontanel should be examined. Cranial nerve function, motility, locomotion, and deep tendon and primitive reflexes should be evaluated. The sensory examination should not be used for diagnostic purposes in small children because it is often unreliable. Gait and stature may provide insight into the diagnosis of disorders such as cerebral palsy (CP) and muscular dystrophy.

Soft neurological signs should be evaluated but may be misleading. Soft neurological signs are a deviant performance on a motor or sensory test. Although the presence of two or more signs can be used in the diagnosis of a particular neurological problem, it is more appropriate to use these signs as an indicator that this child should be monitored closely to exclude other disorders in the differential diagnosis. The following are among the special diagnostic procedures that may be indicated:

Lumbar puncture and cerebrospinal fluid (CSF) examination.
Computed tomography (CT) scan.
Electroencephalography (EEG).
Magnetic resonance imaging (MRI).
Electromyelography (EMG).

Examination of the neurological system includes the history as well as a hands-on examination. The history should include present illness and questions regarding the onset of the problem, whether pain is involved, pain location, any sensory defects (e.g., hearing loss, visual disturbances, pain, vertigo), any type of injury sustained either recently or in the past, any reflexive responses (e.g., vomiting, coughing, tics), any behavioral changes, or any changes in motor or balance. Past medical history, particularly the birth history, should be investigated with an emphasis on any problems, resuscitation efforts, feeding problems, and maternal substance abuse or infections during the pregnancy. Any injuries or infections sustained by the child (e.g., meningitis, encephalitis, head injuries [mild or major], cardiovascular and respiratory problems, environmental exposure to toxins [especially lead], or drug exposure) should be documented. Another area to assess is metabolic problems (e.g., diabetes) and thyroid problems, whose symptoms can often be confused with central nervous system (CNS) problems. The nurse practitioner (NP) should ask about past neurological problems and about any psychiatric problems. The family history should be discussed further to identify any relatives with similar problems, migraine headaches, or any other neurological problems that have a genetic component.

Next, the child's developmental history should be evaluated, including when the developmental milestones were met; language, gross-motor, and fine-motor skills; and social and school performance.

The examination should include close observation of the child during the initial phase of the examination; that is, during the history taking. Often the astute observer can learn much by watching children walk or play. Next, cerebral function, cranial nerve function, motor function, sensory function, and finally reflexes should be tested.

Behavior and mental status should provide insight into cortical function, which includes responsiveness, judgment, memory, general knowledge, mood, and affect. Depending on the age of the child, speech, voice, and organization of the thought process should be assessed.

During the motor examination, muscle size, tone, and strength should be checked. The child should be asked to stand from a prone position to assess for Gower's sign, which is present when patients use their arms to push off from their bent knees and gradually straighten the rest of their body in order to assume the upright position. A positive sign may indicate muscular dystrophy. Denver Developmental Screening will also help to assess fine- and gross-motor skills and social and behavioral attributes. Deep-tendon, superficial, and primitive reflexes should be evaluated. Superficial reflexes include abdominal and lower abdominal, gluteal, cremastic, and plantar reflexes. Primitive reflexes include sucking, rooting, Moro, grasp, neck, stepping, plantar, palmar, asymmetrical tonic neck, and Landau.

The cranium, including the head circumference, should be examined. Plot the results to see whether the circumference falls within two standard deviations of normal. The symmetry and shape of the skull should also be evaluated. When the sutures are too wide, as in the case of increased intracranial pressure when the sutures become separated, auscultation over the skull or above the eyes can elicit a bruit; and percussion of the skull can produce a "cracked pot" sound. The skull should be transilluminated in infants: When there is an absence of cortical tissue, transillumination across the skull will be visualized.

Because infants operate on a subcortical level, their examination is more limited. Measurement, transillumination, and primitive reflexes should all be measured. Motor testing includes observation for symmetry of movement, fisting of hands (asymmetry), opisthotonos, scissoring, abnormal cry, and tremors, which can all be negative indicators. Cranial nerves are tested by observing a variety of physiological functions:

Blinking: Cranial nerve II.
Tracking through certain visual fields: Cranial nerves III, IV, and VI.
Facial grimaces, hearing (tested with a bell): Cranial nerves V and VII.
Gag reflex: Cranial nerves IX and X.

Cerebral Palsy

CP is an acquired, nonprogressive neurological problem manifested as a disorder of movement and position resulting from an insult or anomaly of the CNS. CP results in a number of handicaps related to motor function. Depending on the affected area, the handicap can include mental retardation (75%), seizures (33%), neurosensory disorder, hyperkinesis, speech and learning problems, and emotional problems for both the child and family. There are three main types: spastic, athetoid, and ataxic.

Spastic CP is a severe form of the disease. It has marked motor impairment, which is most often accompanied by mental retardation and a seizure disorder. Athetoid CP is a rare form of the disease that is identified by hypotonia and poor head control, feeding problems, and tongue thrust. Ataxic CP is characterized by ataxic movements, tremors, nystagmus, and abnormalities of voluntary movements.

Etiology: In many cases, the etiology of CP is known. A cerebral insult resulting in a period of anoxia may be the underlying cause. About 85% result from an intrauterine or delivery problem. The condition is known to result from an injury to the pyramidal or extrapyramidal tract, but the cause is not always discovered.

Occurrence: Occurs in 1–3 in 1000 live births per year in the United States.

Age: Most frequently identified in the newborn or toddler ages.

Ethnicity: Not significant.

Gender: Occurs equally in males and females.

Contributing Factors: A maternal trauma (e.g., head trauma, motor vehicle accident, fall), resulting in cerebral anoxia; toxemia and preeclampsia; and fetal problems (e.g., difficult or prolonged deliveries, umbilical cord knots, abnormal presentations, postmaturity, fetal distress).

Signs and Symptoms: The parents will relate that there were prenatal risk factors or delivery complications and that the infant had a floppy or "rag doll" musculature up to age 6 months. The child may have a history of seizures and feeding problems. Growth is less than expected, developmental milestones are delayed, and there is a persistence of primitive reflexes. Parents may relate that they had difficulty diapering due to scissoring of legs; they may also report that the child has a history of head injury or meningitis. On inspection, the child will be small for age with hypotonia (especially if under 6 months), or hypertonia (over 6 months). Asymmetrical movement will be noted in the arms and legs. Hearing and visual problems (strabismus, nystagmus) may exist. Hydrocephaly and microcephaly are also common. Poor muscle tone (under 6 months) and difficult movement (e.g., contractures, scoliosis, hip dislocations) are noted. Deep-tendon reflexes are increased. Persistent primitive reflexes are easily elicited. Skin should be checked for dermatological signs of other syndromes, such as neurofibromatosis. Oromotor dysfunctions and communication and learning disorders also need to be assessed.

Diagnostic Tests

CT of the head to identify brain malformations.
Chromosomal and metabolic studies to identify single-gene disorders.
Denver Developmental Screening Test II to evaluate delays.
Hearing and vision tests to reveal abnormalities.
EEG to evaluate whether a seizure disorder is present.

Differential Diagnosis

Prematurity is differentiated by neurological delays that are not permanent. Milestones are generally met more quickly in premature children than in CP children.

Erb's palsy relates to muscle/nerve compression and affects only one arm.

Spinal cord lesion produces similar symptoms, but in CP the "lesion" is on the brain, not the spinal cord.

Progressive encephalopathy is differentiated by progressive deterioration of neurological signs.

Muscular dystrophy is a progressive neuromuscular disorder, whereas CP is a nonprogressive disorder.

Treatment: There is no specific treatment plan for CP. Rather, treatment should be done as a team, including a primary health-care provider, social worker, dentist, physical and occupational therapists, ophthalmologist, developmental psychologist, and educators. This team should develop an overall plan of care. Treatment is directed toward maximizing function and preventing further handicaps.

Although no specific drugs can alter the disease process when severe spasticity is found, baclofen, dentrolene sodium, and diazepam (Valium) may be useful. Surgical intervention, specifically heel cord release, may also be appropriate.

Follow-up: Regularly scheduled health-care visits should be maintained. Pneumonia and flu vaccine should be given in addition to routine immunizations. When needed and appropriate, speech, physical, and occupational therapy should be available. A yearly eye and hearing examination should also be offered.

Sequelae: Besides their multiple health problems related to the disease process, children with CP may also have learning disorders, low self-esteem, and family problems.

Prevention/Prophylaxis: As the cause often remains obscure, currently the best prevention would be early prenatal care and regular health maintenance. Also, early, aggressive intervention for all problems associated with CP should be instituted.

Referral: Refer children with CP to speech, physical, and occupational therapists, as well as a pediatric neurologist, dentist, and ophthalmologist, when first diagnosed and as needed. A regular health-care provider can serve as the gatekeeper for these services. Refer child to a social worker, who can assist the family with obtaining services and benefits, such as Supplemental Security Income (SSI). A nutritionist should also be a part of the team.

Education: Teach parents that children who have CP have a variety of needs and that CP is a nonprogressive, lifelong condition. Assure them that although there are sometimes limitations in potential secondary to the disease, many children with CP do experience success in their lives. Inform parents of potential problems such as reflux, which can cause pneumonia; the appearance of seizure symptoms; or other problems that may cause complications. Encourage the family to have a close relationship with the primary health-care provider.

Encephalitis

Encephalitis is an inflammation of the brain; diagnosis is made on the basis of neurological manifestations and epidemiological information without the assistance of histological information. True identification of this pathogen can be established only by examination of the brain tissue. Generally, the disease is the sequela of another viral illness. Its insidious onset often progresses rapidly to coma and sometimes even death.

Etiology: Although only about 25% of all reported cases have established etiologic agents, it is known that enteroviruses or arboviruses, herpesviruses, and occasionally nonviral agents cause the majority of cases. Some other known causes include mumps, measles, rubella, the pox group, rabies, parvovirus, influenza types A and B, and adenovirus. Nonviral causes include *Rickettsia*, *Mycoplasma pneumoniae*, bacterial meningitis, tuberculosis, spirochetes, fungal agents, and certain protozoans.

Occurrence: The majority of cases occur in summer and fall.

Age: Any age.

Ethnicity: Not significant.

Gender: Occurs equally in males and females.

Signs and Symptoms: The history varies from child to child: There is a broad spectrum of clinical manifestations, and the predictability of the pattern of this disease is uncertain. The parent or child may report any or all of the following in the history of this illness:

Acute onset of illness accompanied by fever, headache, or screaming or inconsolability in infants.
Abdominal pain, nausea, and vomiting.
A mild nasopharyngitis.
Increasing fever accompanied by mental confusion, rigidity of the body, seizures, and occasionally incontinence of both bladder and bowel.
Unprovoked emotional outbursts.

The NP should be careful to inquire about recent contact with any persons, animals (specifically horses), or ticks that may have transmitted the causative organism. Exposure to heavy metals, environmental substances, or pesticides should also be considered.

During inspection, the child appears ill. The skin feels warm or hot and the abdomen is tender to touch. During the examination, the patient may have difficulty cooperating or following the requests made by the NP. There may be occasional emotional outbursts. Some photosensitivity may be noted.

If the patient has a concomitant disease, such as mumps or chickenpox, findings are similar to those of that disease.

The abdomen may have hyperactive bowel sounds when vomiting is present, and there may be some tenderness upon percussion of the abdomen. If there is a preceding or concomitant upper respiratory disease, adventitious lung sounds may be heard.

Diagnostic Tests

A lumbar puncture is mandatory when encephalitis is suspected.

Smears for bacteria and appropriate rapid-antigen identification tests on the CSF should also be done.

If warranted by the history, an acid-fast bacillus stain and culture for microbacteria should be performed.

In viral encephalitis, the CSF is clear, the leukocyte count may vary from zero to several thousand, the percentage of polymorphonuclear cells is increased, protein levels are either not elevated or moderately elevated, and glucose concentration is normal.

Blood cultures to identify specific pathogens.

Swabs should be used to collect pathological material from the oral and rectal mucosa for the purpose of identifying specific pathogens.

Differential Diagnosis

Exposure to noxious substances (e.g., heavy metals, pesticides), differentiated by history and blood screening.

Neurological neoplasm, differentiated by examination.

Brain tumor, differentiated by CT or MRI of the head.

Seizure disorder, differentiated by an EEG.

Treatment: If encephalitis is suspected, a physician should dictate and institute all treatment regimens. Child should be admitted to a tertiary-care setting with an intensive care unit (ICU) and available neurological physicians to oversee his or her care.

Follow-up: Closely supervise the child for months postinfection because the sequelae often require supportive services and rehabilitation.

Sequelae: CNS problems including intellectual, motor, psychiatric, visual, and auditory impairment may result. There may also be cardiovascular, hepatic, and pulmonary problems. The young infant who contracts encephalitis has a grave prognosis, as does the child with herpes simplex viral encephalitis, who would have the worst prognosis.

Referral: Refer child immediately to a physician for admittance to a hospital.

Prevention/Prophylaxis: Encephalitis secondary to measles, mumps, and rubella has been well controlled since the advent of immunizations for those diseases. For those cases of encephalitis caused by arboviruses, there has been less success because of the lack of a vaccine. Control of insect vectors via spraying and the use of pesticides can somewhat control the problem, but eradication has not yet been achieved.

Education: Teach parents the importance of children receiving their immunizations on time.

Headache

Headache, a common presenting symptom in the older pediatric group and in febrile children, is simply described as a pain in one or more regions of the head. Because a headache may represent a severe underlying pathology, all headaches should be carefully assessed. Children are poor historians and often respond unpredictably to a headache. Therefore the NP should obtain a history including family history and symptomology, perform a careful examination, and refer when a severe underlying pathology is suspected. Several types of headaches are known, including the following:

Vascular (classic) migraine headache.
Muscular contraction (tension or psychogenic) headache.
Cluster headache.

The migraine headache is usually unilateral, but does not always occur on the same side. It is generally preceded by an aura (subjective sensations preceding a migraine), which may be followed by neurological signs such as tingling and weakness in an extremity. Temporary paralysis may follow a migraine headache. Throbbing gradually increases in intensity to a peak in 1 hour and then the headache pain may gradually diminish in anywhere from a few hours to several days. Eighty percent of migraine patients have a family history of migraines.

Tension headaches are characterized by a dull, aching pain accompanied by occipital pain and tightness across the scalp. Tension headaches are more commonly seen in middle age. These headaches can persist for a long period of time, with pain often described as a vicelike grip on the head. Tension headaches do not have any associated nausea or vomiting, but may often be associated with a period of high tension or emotional distress. There is no aura or neurological deficit, although patients often state that their scalp is sore during and after a tension headache. Along with that discomfort, the muscles in the posterior neck may be tense and sore.

Cluster headaches are characterized by intense pain associated with rhinorrhea, lacrimation, and flushed skin. These headaches occur at night, are generally localized to one orbit, and last approximately 1 hour. The pain tends to occur in clusters over a period of a few nights to weeks and then usually disappears.

Etiology: The specific etiology of vascular (classic) migraines, muscle contraction (tension or psychogenic) headaches, and cluster headache is unknown.

Occurrence: Headaches occur in 5–20% of the pediatric population; prevalence increases proportionally with age.

Age: Headaches have been documented in the literature in children as young as 1 year, but they are more common in adolescents.

Gender: During adolescence, headaches occur more in females. In males, onset is generally before age 10.

Ethnicity: Not significant.

Contributing Factors: Familial history, environmental irritants, hormonal changes, food allergies, type A personalities, stress, and bright lights may contribute to the occurrence of these three classes of headaches.

Signs and Symptoms: A detailed family history, review of symptoms, and a detailed account of the headache needs to be obtained from the patient. The presence or absence of a migraine aura and the frequency, intensity, duration, and location of the pain should be obtained. Age of onset and subsequent course of the headaches should be documented. Treatments that are used to decrease discomfort should be given. Possible environmental stimulants should be identified (Figs. 13–1 and 13–2).

Inspection may reveal photophobia or phonophobia; if the headache is a migraine, there may be accompanying vomiting or nausea. With a cluster headache, rhinorrhea may be observed. The optic fundus should be observed when the source or type of headache is unknown to rule out eye changes associated with elevated blood pressure, hemorrhage, or glaucoma.

Percussion and palpation of the head will not reveal any significant findings. With a tension headache, there may be some increased sensitivity in the head. There may also be a rise in blood pressure or pulse in response to the pain. Auscultation may reveal cranial bruits.

Diagnostic Test: The actual diagnosis of a headache, which is really a symptom rather than a disease, is often made by history alone, because there are no tests or findings that can document a headache. To rule out organic pathology, however, a CT scan of the head, an EEG, and a myelogram are often performed.

Differential Diagnosis

Sinus headache is differentiated by the location of the pain, which is generally over the antrum or around the eyes and most frequently associated with sinus congestion. There is also an accompanying diagnosis of bacterial sinusi-

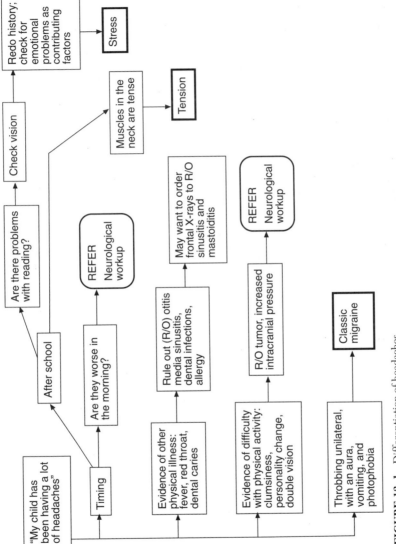

FIGURE 13-1 Differentiation of headaches.

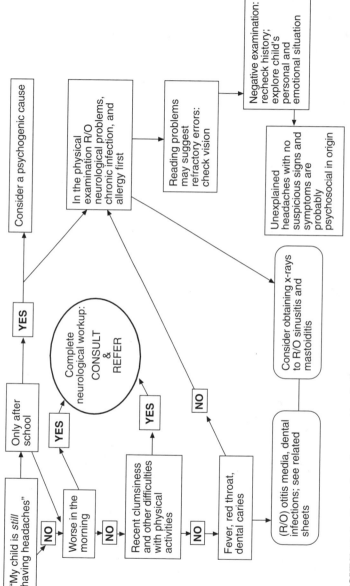

FIGURE 13–2 Evaluation of repeated headaches.

tis. The sinuses may be tender, and the overlying skin may be sensitive. The headaches often begin at night and intensify with changes in position.

Hypertension headache is differentiated by an accompanying diagnosis of hypertension and the fact that the headaches are generally seen first thing in the morning and are mild to moderate in intensity.

Glaucoma can also cause headaches; the pain is located around the orbits and may be associated with nausea and vomiting. The pupils are fixed and semi-dilated, and the sclerae are injected.

Brain tumor–associated headache does not have a specific characteristic, but tends to be a severer, more deep-seated pain that may come and go and tends to worsen at night. It may even awaken the patient. Occasionally, it may occur in the very early morning hours, also awakening the patient. Usually vomiting accompanies the headache.

Congenital malformations of the head and cervical vertebrae are differentiated by CT scans of those areas.

Lead encephalopathy is differentiated by a lead level greater than 50.

Dental abscesses are differentiated by signs and symptoms of infection and pain: fever, swelling, and an elevated white blood cell (WBC) count.

Severe anemia is differentiated by a hemoglobin of less than 7.

Treatment: Specific causes, if known, and identification of exacerbating agents dictate the treatment regimen. Cautious use of medication is mandated in the pediatric population. Management of an acute headache includes analgesics and antiemetics. Acetaminophen (5–10 mg/kg q 4–6 hours) is used if the headache is mild, infrequent, and of short duration. A variety of medications can be given for both analgesic and abortive therapy (Tables 13–1 and 13–2).

TABLE 13–1 ANALGESIC DRUGS FOR BOTH MIGRAINE AND TENSION HEADACHES

Drug	Dosage
Acetaminophen	10–15 mg/kg; not to exceed 90
NSAIDs	
Ibuprofen	5–10 mg/kg per dose (200–800 mg/dose q 6–8 hours; maximum 40 mg/kg per day)
Naprosyn	10 mg/kg per day (250–500 mg bid)
Anaprox	220–550 mg 1st dose; maximum dose 825 mg/day
Aleve	220 mg bid
Stadol*	1 spray in one nostril only

*Not recommended for children under age 18 years.
NSAIDs = nonsteroidal anti-inflammatory drugs.

TABLE 13–2 ABORTIVE PHARMACOLOGICAL PROPHYLAXIS FOR MIGRAINE HEADACHES

Drug	Dosage
Ergotamine tartrate	SL 2 mg
or	
Cafergot	1 mg ergotamine with 100 mg caffeine
Dihydroergotamine (DHE)	0.5–1.0 mg IM; can be repeated in 1 hour
Metoclopramide (Reglan)	Up to 1 mg/kg
Prochlorperazine (Compazine)	2.5–5.0 mg*
Promethazine	0.25–1.0 mg/kg q 4 hours
Sumatriptan	6 mg SC or 100 mg PO

*For young children up to 0.1 mg/kg.
IM = intramuscularly; PO = by mouth; SC – subcutaneously.

Follow-up: Follow-up is generally done about 2 weeks after initiation of treatment regimen; however, the patient should be instructed to come to the office or the emergency room immediately if there is severe pain, paresthesia, or other symptoms. Thereafter, follow-up is done on a semiregular basis (e.g., every 3–6 months) or as symptoms dictate.

Sequelae: Recurrent migraine headaches often result in poor school performance, days missed from school or work, behavioral problems, and depres-

TABLE 13–3 PHARMACOLOGICAL PROPHYLAXIS FOR MIGRAINE HEADACHES

Drug	Dosage	Contraindications
Propranolol	1–2 mg/kg per day bid or tid	Asthma, cardiac arrhythmia, depression, diabetes
Methysergide	Adolescents: 2 mg bid or tid after meals (not to be used longer than 3 months)	*Not* recommended for children. Use is restricted to *severe* headaches
Amitriptyline	Adolescents: 0.1 mg/kg at bed time (HS) (may be increased every 2 weeks) Children: 0.5–2 mg/kg	*Not* approved for children under 12
Cyproheptadine	Children: 0.2–0.4 mg/kg per day in two to three divided doses Adolescents: 4–10 mg/day	None
Nortriptyline	10 mg/day HS	None

sion. Poor self-esteem, difficult peer relationships, and high stress levels may also occur.

Prevention/Prophylaxis: Avoidance of known irritants or stimuli is the most effective nonpharmacological prophylaxis. Table 13–3 outlines the drugs used for pharmacological prophylaxis.

Referral: If the diagnosis is uncertain or the headaches are not controlled with treatment regimens, refer the child to a pediatric neurologist or headache clinic.

Education: Educate children and parents regarding stimuli that are suspected to trigger headaches. Also, teach them to recognize the worsening of signs and symptoms. Children can often be taught relaxation techniques to decrease the severity of the headache symptoms. Stress the use and proper timing of headache medications. Teach children and parents to pay careful attention to the signs and symptoms of depression.

Meningitis

Meningitis is a CNS infection characterized by an inflammation of the brain, specifically the meninges. Early diagnosis and treatment of bacterial meningitis is critical because all cases of *untreated* meningitis result in death. Delayed treatment results in serious, permanent neurological sequelae.

Etiology: Bacterial meningitis is most commonly caused by *Haemophilus influenzae* type B (HIB), *Neisseria meningitidis*, or *Streptococcus pneumoniae*. β-Streptococcus, *Escherichia coli*, and *Listeria monocytogenes* are the most common of the organisms that cause meningitis before age 1 month. Aseptic meningitis is caused by an enterovirus. Other rarer forms of meningitis are the sequelae of diseases such as Lyme disease and herpes.

Occurrence: Aseptic meningitis occurs in 1.5–4 in 100,000 children per year in the United States, with younger children having the greater incidence. Bacterial meningitis in the neonatal period occurs in 100 in 100,000 live births. The incidence decreases to 45 in 100,000 children at age 2 months, again peaking to 75–80 in 100,000 at age 8 months.

Age: Occurs at any age between the neonatal period and adulthood, with a greater incidence in the very young infant.

Ethnicity: Not significant.

Gender: Occurs equally in males and females.

Contributing Factors: A head trauma involving a fracture of the paranasal sinus or congenital sinus increases the risk of meningitis. These fractures allow bacteria to enter the meninges more easily. Meningitis can occur postoperatively (especially after neurosurgical surgery) if a shunt has been implanted.

Signs and Symptoms: The parent may report a recent bout of fever, irritability, lethargy, and poor feeding. Restlessness is reported in all children. If old enough, the child will complain of a headache. Sometimes, if the auditory nerve is involved, hearing alterations may be noted. The older child has a recent history of vomiting, along with a variety of other symptoms (e.g., fever, nausea, listlessness, irritability, photophobia, nuchal rigidity, seizures). In the very young child, the parent reports that the "soft spot" seems enlarged and protruding (bulging fontanel).

A positive Kernig and Brudzinski sign can also be elicited. The Kernig sign is elicited by flexing the hip and then extending the leg at the knee. If this produces pain in the hamstring, the sign is considered positive. The Brudzinski sign is accomplished by laying the patient down and flexing the neck. If there is an involuntary flexing of the hip, the sign is positive. A raised red rash (a potential sign of septic shock) may be seen and palpated. Children may also report pain (arthralgia or myalgia) when muscles and joints are palpated. Tachycardia and tachypnea will be evident.

Diagnostic Tests

Complete blood count (CBC) shows an elevated WBC count (greater than 20,000).

Blood and urine cultures are positive for bacteria.

EEG demonstrates increased intracranial pressure.

Lumbar puncture demonstrates a turbid or purulent fluid and elevated WBC count in the CSF.

Counterimmunoelectrophoresis (CIE) and latex-particle agglutination test of the CSF, blood, and urine can facilitate rapid diagnosis of *H. influenzae, S. pneumoniae, N. meningitidis* and Group B streptococcus infections.

Differential Diagnosis

Influenza, bacteremia, Kawasaki disease, Rocky Mountain spotted fever, brain tumor, cat-scratch fever, and *toxic ingestion* (all of which may mimic the signs and symptoms of meningitis), differentiated by a lumbar puncture.

Brain tumor, differentiated by CT scan of the head along with an MRI.

Treatment: Meningitis is a medical emergency; all treatment should be initiated in a tertiary-care setting. As soon as all cultures are obtained, intravenous access should be established and antibiotics initiated. These may include the following:

Ampicillin: Under age 7 days, 50 mg/kg q 12 hours; over age 7 days, 50 mg/kg q 6 hours.

Amikar: Under age 7 days, 10 mg/kg q 12 hours; over age 7 days, 10 mg/kg q 8 hours.

Gentamycin: Under age 7 days, 2.5 mg/kg q 12 hours; over age 7 days, q 8 hours.

Cefotaxime: Under age 7 days, 59 mg/kg q 12 hours; over age 7 days, 50 mg/kg q 8 hours.

Ceftriaxone: 50 mg/kg q 24 hours.

Children's acetaminophen (Tylenol) and/or ibuprophen (Advil) can be used for fever and headache (see Chapter 8, Table 8–6a and 8–6b). Appropriate anticonvulsants should be given for seizures (see seizures section in this chapter). Phenobarbital is used for seizures. Dexamethasone is also used for bacterial meningitis, specifically *H. influenzae* or pneumococcal meningitis.

Follow-up: Careful audiologic evaluation (yearly) and regularly scheduled check-ups should be done to evaluate attainment of developmental milestones. If there are problems with intelligence, development, or seizures, the patient needs to be monitored regularly.

Sequelae: Meningitis can cause serious, irreversible neurological problems, such as seizures, brain damage (irreversible), and intellectual, motor, visual, and auditory impairment. The severity of these sequelae will vary from patient to patient. Damage to the cardiac system and even death are other possible sequelae.

Prevention/Prophylaxis: Increased use of the HIB series of immunizations for infections has dramatically decreased the incidence of bacterial meningitis in children.

Referral: Refer patient to a physician as soon as meningitis is suspected. Arrange for immediate admission to a tertiary-care setting.

Education: Inform parents that although the sequelae vary, many children survive meningitis with few, if any, subsequent problems. Some children do have long-term problems, so continued regular health-care visits and maintenance of a normal immunization schedule are important parts of their health care. When motor and cognitive impairment has occurred, parents need to stay in close contact with PTs, OTs, developmentalists, teachers, and other support personnel as needed.

Reye's Syndrome

Reye's syndrome is an acute noninflammatory encephalopathy that includes one of the following criteria:

Fatty changes of the liver confirmed by either biopsy or, in the case of death, autopsy.

Aspartate transaminase (AST), alanine transaminase (ALT), or serum ammonia values three times normal.

Greater than 8 WBCs/mm^3 in the CSF.

No other reasonable explanation for neurological or hepatic changes.

Etiology: Reye's syndrome is associated with *H. influenzae* type A and B infection and is also a sequela of chickenpox. Generally, however, the etiology is unknown. There is a clear indication that ingestion of aspirin or aspirin-containing drugs may elicit or exacerbate the syndrome.

Occurrence: Incidence is 0.15 in 100,000 children per year in the United States; 16–28% of cases are preceded by chickenpox.

Age: Peak incidence is at age 6 years; most cases occur in children between ages 4 and 14.

Ethnicity: Ninety percent of all cases occur in whites, 4% in African-Americans, and 6% in other ethnic groups.

Gender: Occurs equally in males and females.

Contributing Factors: A history of a recent case of chickenpox or other viral illness.

Signs and Symptoms: Parent reports that the child was recovering from an upper respiratory illness, chickenpox, or gastroenteritis when he or she suddenly became acutely ill. Child presents with a history of nausea and vomiting as well as altered behavior (e.g., irritable, combative, confused, less responsive, lethargic). Child has no focal neurological signs. Hyperpnea, irregular respirations, and dilated and sluggish pupils are seen. Palpation and percussion reveal mild hepatomegaly. Auscultation reveals increased bowel sounds and hyperventilation. Seizures may be present. In the late stages, stupor, loss of deep-tendon reflexes, decerebrate posturing, and possibly even coma may occur.

In infants, the signs and symptoms are slightly different: The infant typically presents with an acute onset of respiratory disease (with tachypnea and apnea), followed by seizures and coma.

Diagnostic Tests

Serum transaminase, ammonia, prothrombin, creatine, and amino acid levels are increased.
Blood glucose level (especially in children under 4) is decreased.
EEG shows slow wave abnormalities.

Differential Diagnosis

Meningitis, differentiated by a lumbar puncture showing a WBC count greater than 8/mm^3 in the CSF; Reye's syndrome does not have this finding.
Septicemia, differentiated by a blood culture.
Salicylate poisoning, differentiated by a salicylate level greater than 25.
Acute hepatitis, differentiated by a hepatitis screen.

Treatment: Immediate referral for admission to a tertiary-care setting is critical. The illness should be staged (Table 13–4). In stages I and II, supportive, symptomatic care is given. Intravenous fluids (10% dextrose solution) are instituted to decrease lipolysis. Children at later stages are managed in the ICU; treatment may include the administration of mannitol to reduce cerebral edema, vitamin K to alter clotting abnormalities, neomycin sulfate enemas to

TABLE 13–4 STAGING OF REYE'S SYNDROME

Stage	Symptoms and Signs
I	Subtle central nervous system changes are present. These may include confusion, lethargy, and apathy. No abnormalities are noted in posture, pain response, or pupillary reaction.
II	Delusion, irritability, restlessness, combativeness, and disorientation are all noted. There is normal posture, but pupillary reaction is sluggish.
III	Decerebrate posture is seen. There is deep coma and sluggish pupils.
IV	Coma, decerebrate posture, sluggish pupils, and inconsistent or absent doll's head phenomenon.
V	Coma, flaccidity, nonreactive pupils, and absent doll's head phenomenon.

decrease serum ammonia levels, and plasma in cases of disseminated intravascular coagulation.

Arterial blood gases, glucose, blood urea nitrogen, and hematocrit should be closely monitored to identify problems as they occur. Other treatments may also be given, but they are clearly beyond the scope of the NP.

Follow-up: Nonspecific. In children over 2 years who have had Reye's syndrome, psychological testing should be done, because they frequently have resultant learning problems. Otherwise no other follow-up is necessary.

Sequelae: The mortality rate is approximately 30%; 10% of survivors have severe CNS problems.

Prevention/Prophylaxis: Early identification and aggressive treatment often result in a better prognosis. Avoidance of aspirin and aspirin-containing products during the course of a viral illness has greatly reduced the incidence of Reye's syndrome.

Referral: Refer patient to a physician, preferably a pediatric neurologist, as soon as the diagnosis is suspected.

Education: Teach parents not to use aspirin or aspirin-containing products when treating fever and/or pain in children. Fever-reducing agents such as acetaminophen or ibuprophen should be substituted. Encourage parents *not* to be overprotective after the illness, but to be alert for both subtle and overt signs of brain damage, such as learning, communication, school, or behavioral changes and difficulties.

Seizure Disorder

A seizure is a misfiring of the neurons resulting in an involuntary paroxysmal disturbance of the brain. This misfiring results in an altered or total loss of consciousness accompanied by abnormal motor behavior and sensory or autonomic dysfunction. Epilepsy can be defined as a condition in which the patient has recurrent seizures not related to any other organic or traumatic causes. Table 13–5 lists three different types of seizures along with more specific information. Seizures are classified as partial or generalized:

- Partial seizures include simple partial, motor, sensory, autonomic, psychic, complex partial, or partial seizures with secondary generalization.
- Generalized seizures include absence, generalized tonic-clonic, tonic, clonic, myotonic, and atonic seizures, as well as infantile spasms.

TABLE 13–5 CLASSIFICATION OF SEIZURES

Seizure Type	Age	Associated Symptoms
Partial seizure	All ages	Consciousness is not impaired. Seizure begins locally and can affect any part of the body. Causes include trauma, infection, and tumor. Patient exhibits asynchronous clonic or tonic movements and may have an aura. Seizure lasts 10–20 seconds (simple) or 1–2 minutes (complex partial). EEG is characterized by spikes or sharp waves. Movements tend to involve the face, neck, and extremities (simple); may be accompanying autonomic behaviors (complex).
Generalized seizures (absence)	Ages 4–8 most common	Lasts 5–30 seconds. Patient may have lapses of consciousness. There is no aura or falling, but patient may have hyperventilation preceding the seizure. More common in girls.
Infantile spasms	Infancy	Head drops suddenly or there is flexing of the body during the spasm. EEG is abnormal; condition is very difficult to treat.
Clonic, tonic, tonic-clonic	Any age	Most common seizure types. Grand mal seizures begin with aura and loss of consciousness; 15% of patients are incontinent during the seizure. Characterized by rhythmic clonic contractions alternating with relaxation of all muscle groups. Child may bite tongue during the seizure. Followed by a postictal period lasting from 30 minutes to 2 hours, often accompanied by vomiting and severe frontal headache.

Etiology: The specific etiology of seizures is unclear; however, anatomical lesions, developmental and genetic factors, pharmacological agents, and cellular malfunction may be causative factors. Immaturity of the brain is often an underlying cause. Other potential causes are trauma, infections, and biochemical or metabolic alterations.

Occurrence: Two percent of all children have experienced a type of seizure.

Age: Seventy-five percent of all seizures occur before age 18 years.

Ethnicity: Not significant.

Gender: Seizures occur more frequently in males than females.

Contributing Factors: Head trauma, meningitis, and a family history of seizures.

Signs and Symptoms: The patient's age, type and frequency of the seizure, the presence or absence of specific neurological symptoms, and any events preceding the seizure should be ascertained in the history. Parents should be questioned regarding any underlying disease, such as diabetes, renal disease, or cardiovascular disorder. The parents should be asked whether the child has had any CNS infections or trauma, or whether they suspect drug use; the family history must be obtained.

Seizures may be observed along with either of two possible neuromuscular responses: lip smacking or eye blinking. Focal abnormalities and weakness may also be present. The health-care provider should observe for neurocutaneous diseases when the patient presents with café au lait spots, facial hemangioma (Sturge-Webber syndrome), ash leaf spots, or adenoma sebacium (tuberous sclerosis).

Blood pressure may be elevated in cases of concomitant renal disease, and subtle cardiac signs may be found when there is an accompanying cardiovascular disorder (Fig. 13–3).

Diagnostic Tests

An abnormal EEG supports the diagnosis of epilepsy; however, the EEG can be normal in seizure patients. If seizure disorder is still the primary diagnosis, a CT scan of the head should be done.

CT may reveal a tumor, abscess, or atrioventricular abnormality.

A fasting glucose test should be done to rule out diabetes.

Differential Diagnosis

Behaviors such as daydreaming, breathholding spells, temper tantrums, and inattentiveness are differentiated by the absence of any neurologic findings.

Syncope is differentiated by changes in blood pressure not associated with seizures and by a normal EEG or CT scan.

Sleep disturbances and apnea are differentiated by sleep studies and a pneumogram, which are negative in seizure disorders.

Migraine headaches are differentiated by the patient's history and by a normal CT or EEG.

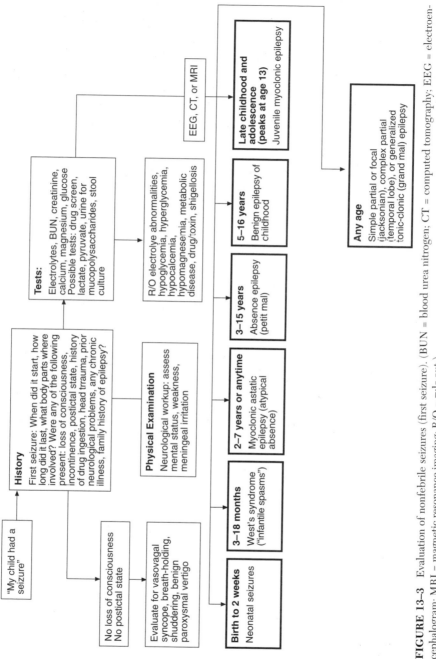

FIGURE 13-3 Evaluation of nonfebrile seizures (first seizure). (BUN = blood urea nitrogen; CT = computed tomography; EEG = electroencephalogram; MRI = magnetic resonance imaging; R/O = rule out.)

Intoxication is differentiated by positive blood and/or urine drug and alcohol screening.

In *tics*, the movements can be suppressed, whereas in seizures they cannot.

Treatment: Table 13–6 lists the most common agents used for treatment, the type of seizure for which the agent is used, and the dose. Other treatment regimens include corticotropin (ACTH) as the preferred agent for infantile spasms, but this regimen is out of the NP's scope of practice. Oral prednisone may also be used in place of intramuscular corticotropin.

A ketogenic diet may be used in severe cases of seizures, particularly complex myoclonic epilepsy. This diet restricts carbohydrates and protein and is very high in fat. Although the exact mechanism of the diet regimen is unknown, it is suspected that it may inhibit neurotransmission in the brain, thereby decreasing or in some reported cases eliminating seizures.

Follow-up: Children with seizure disorders should be followed closely when first put on medication. Symptoms and blood levels of the medications should be evaluated at least monthly; once the medication level is therapeutic and there are no further seizures, the child can be followed on a regular schedule, with the parents calling or bringing the child in if they suspect that the medication is

TABLE 13–6 ANTICONVULSANTS OF CHOICE—MAINTENANCE DRUGS

Drug	Absence Seizure	Tonic-Clonic Seizure	Simple Partial Seizure	Complex Partial Seizure
Phenobarbital: 3–5 mg/kg per day		†	†	†
Phenytoin: 5–10 mg/kg per day		*	*	*
Carbamazepine: 15–30 mg/kg per day		*	*	*
Ethosuximide: 20–30 mg/kg per day	*			
Valproic acid: 15–60 mg/kg per day	*	*	†	†
Primidone: 10–25 mg/kg per day		*		†

*First-line medication.
†Second-line medication.

no longer therapeutic. Remember that as a child's body weight increases, medication doses must be increased. Routine examinations should also be performed and immunizations administered. There is, however, a slight disagreement among neurologists with regard to the diphtheria, pertussis, and tetanus (DPT) immunization: Some feel that pertussis should not be included for seizure patients, whereas others feel that its inclusion is still appropriate.

Sequelae: Epilepsy, when poorly controlled, can alter a child's growth and development potential. If well controlled, children have few problems overall. If a grand mal seizure lasts longer than 30 minutes, the patient is at increased risk for brain damage. Overall, the mortality rate of seizures is 10% in the United States.

Prevention/Prophylaxis: Avoidance of environmental triggers such as pharmacological or photic stimuli (e.g., flashing lights, such as those found in discotheques) can prevent the occurrence of seizures. Obtaining adequate rest, as well as guarding against emotional stress, may deter the occurrence of a seizure.

Referral: The diagnosis of the specific type of seizure should be performed by a pediatric neurologist. If there is specific cause to suspect a seizure disorder, or results of an EEG or CT scan are abnormal, obtain a neurological consultation.

Education: Teach families the importance of taking the seizure medications on a regular schedule and maintaining a close relationship with a primary-care provider. In addition, teach the parents safety precautions in the event of a seizure. Emphasize the importance of precautionary measures such as avoiding certain stimuli, getting adequate rest, and developing strategies to cope with stress.

Bell's Palsy

Bell's palsy is an acute unilateral facial nerve (cranial nerve VII) paralysis not associated with any underlying cranial neuropathy or brain stem dysfunction. This common disorder occurs as early as infancy. Most cases resolve in 2 weeks, but some take up to 6–8 weeks to resolve. Only about 5% of patients have long-term residual weakness.

Etiology: Bell's palsy is thought to be a postinfectious neuritis that usually develops abruptly within 2 weeks after a systemic viral infection. In about 20% of all reported cases, the preceding infection was caused by Epstein-Barr virus.

Occurrence: Common in childhood.

Age: Can occur at any age between infancy and adulthood.

Ethnicity: Not significant.

Gender: More frequent in females.

Contributing Factors: Infection with a virus, particularly Epstein-Barr.

Signs and Symptoms: The patient reports an abrupt loss of sensation on the affected side of the face. The patient is unable to close the eye or mouth, wrinkle the forehead, or puff out the cheek on the affected side. The corner of the mouth droops, and the upper and lower face are paretic. Additionally, taste on the anterior two-thirds of the tongue is lost on the affected side. Occasionally ear pain is reported. The patient will have an open, sometimes tearing eye, drooping of one side of the mouth, and loss of muscle tone on one side of the face. Palpation reveals lack of sensory response on the affected side of the face.

Diagnostic Tests: Assessment of the cranial nerve VII (facial nerve) should be done. This can be accomplished by checking the patient's sense of taste of salt and sugar and by asking the patient to smile, grimace, puff cheeks, and raise eyebrows.

Differential Diagnosis

Facial nerve tremors, differentiated by a CT scan of the head.
Brain stem infarction, differentiated by an arteriogram of the head.
Trauma of the facial nerve, differentiated by bruising, swelling, or other signs of trauma.

Treatment: Treatment is symptomatic. Protection of the cornea with eye drops, such as an ocular lubricant, is especially important. Other treatment regimens, such as steroids and surgical decompression of the facial canal, have not proved helpful. Comfort measures such as using a straw to drink and taping the eye closed at night are also helpful.

Follow-up: Initial follow-up should take place 2 weeks after the paralysis. Symptoms should resolve between 6–8 weeks. Further follow-up is unnecessary in about 85% of all cases.

Sequelae: Eighty-five percent of all cases recover completely and spontaneously. Less than 5% of all patients are left with permanent, severe facial weakness.

Prevention/Prophylaxis: None.

Referral: If facial weakness has neither improved nor resolved within 2 weeks, refer the patient to a neurologist.

Education: Instruct the patient and family that care needs to be taken to prevent eye keratoses. Teach measures for taking care of the eye, including the use of lubricants and taping at night. Reassure the patient and family that nearly all cases resolve spontaneously.

REFERENCES

General

American Academy of Pediatrics: The 1994 Red Book: Report of the Committee on Infectious Diseases. American Academy of Pediatrics, Elk Grove, Ill, 1995.
Behrman, R: Nelson Textbook of Pediatrics, ed 14. WB Saunders, Philadelphia, 1992.
Burg, F, et al: Treatment of Infants, Children, and Adolescents. WB Saunders, Philadelphia, 1990.

Burns, C, et al: Pediatric Primary Care. WB Saunders, Philadelphia, 1996.
Krugman, S, et al: Infectious Diseases of Children. CV Mosby, St. Louis, 1992.
Menkes, J: Textbook of Neurology. Lea & Febiger, Philadelphia, 1980.
Rosenstein, B, and Fosarelli, P: Pediatric Pearls: The Handbook of Practical Pediatrics. Mosby, New York, 1993.
Samuels, M: Manual of Neurogenic Therapeutics. Tuile, Broome & Co, Boston, 1987.
Urion, D, et al: Neurological problems. In Avery, ME, and First, LR (eds): Pediatric Medicine, ed 2. Williams & Wilkins, Baltimore, MD, 1994, pp 770–783.

Bell's Palsy

Cohen, M: Perspectives on craniofacial asymmetry. Int J Maxillofacial Surg 24:127, 1995.
Katz, J, et al: Bell's palsy as a sign of Burkitt's lymphoma in children. Blood 86:2052, 1995.
Manfre, L, et al: Bell's palsy and visualization of the facial nerve by MRI. Rev Laryngol Otol Rhinol 116:91, 1995.
Murahani, S, et al: Bell's palsy and herpes simplex virus. Ann Intern Med 27:124, 30, 1996.

Cerebral Palsy

American Academy of Pediatrics, Committee on Children with Disabilities: Pediatric services for infants and children with special health care needs. Pediatrics 92:163, 1993.
American Academy of Pediatrics, Committee on Children with Disabilities: Screening infants and young children for developmental disabilities. Pediatrics 93:863, 1994.
Barabas, G, and Taft, L: The early signs and differential diagnosis of cerebral palsy. Pediatr Ann 15:205, 1986.
Coplan, J: Evaluation of the child with delayed speech or language. Pediatr Ann 14:203, 1985.
Eicher, P, and Batshaw, M: Cerebral palsy. Pediatr Clin North Am 40:537, 1993.
Krauss, J, and Nourjah, P: Epidemiology of uncomplicated brain injury. J Trauma 28:1627, 1988.
Montgomery, T: When "not talking" is the chief complaint. Contemp Pediatr 11:49, 1994.
Torfs, C: Prenatal and perinatal factors in the etiology of cerebral palsy. J Pediatr 116:615, 1990.

Encephalitis

Johnson, R: The pathogenesis of acute viral encephalitis and post infectious encephalomyelitis. J Infect Dis 155, 1987.

Headache

Altemer, W: A pediatrician's view: Headache and the primary care pediatrician. Pediatr Ann 24:446, 1995.
Barlow, C: Headaches and migraines in childhood. Clinics in Developmental Medicine, 91, JB Lippincott, Philadelphia, 1984.
Frenichel, G: Migraines in children. Neurol Clin North Am 3:77, 1985.
Maytal, H, et al: The value of brain imaging in children with headaches. Pediatrics 96:413, 1995.
Prensky, A: Diagnosis and treatment of migraine in children. Neurology 29:506, 1979.

Meningitis

Centers for Disease Control and Prevention: Recommended childhood immunization schedule—United States, January–June, 1996. MMWR 43:959, 1996.
Epstein, S, and Reilly, J: Sensorineural hearing loss. Pediatr Clin North Am 36:1501, 1989.
Hoekelmann, R: A pediatrician's view: HIB vaccination now! Pediatr Ann 19:683, 1990.
Jadavji, T: Sequelae of acute bacterial meningitis in children treated for 7 days. Pediatrics 78:21, 1986.

Reye's Syndrome

Barrett, M, et al: Changing epidemiology of Reye's syndrome in the United States. Pediatrics 77:598, 1986.

Mitchell, R, et al: Hepatic and encephalopathic components of Reye syndrome: Analysis of admission data from 209 patients. Neurology 35:1236, 1985.

Shaywitz, B, et al: What is the best treatment for Reye's syndrome? Arch Neurol 43:729, 1986.

Trauner, D: Reye's syndrome. Curr Probl Pediatr 12:75, 1982.

Seizures

Isselbacher, K, et al: Harrison's Principles of Internal Medicine. McGraw-Hill, New York, 1995.

Samuels, M: Manual of Neurologic Therapeutics. Little, Brown, & Co, Boston, 1987.

Shantz, D, and Spitz, M: What you need to know about seizures. Nursing 23(11):34, 1993.

Sagraves, R: Antiepileptic drug therapy for pediatric generalized tonic-clonic seizures. J Pediatr Health Care 4:314, 1990.

Gardner, S, and Hagedorn, M: Physiologic sequelae of prematurity: The nurse practitioner's role, part VII: Neurologic conditions. J Pediatr Health Care 6:263, 1992.

Roddy, S, and McBride, M: Seizure disorders. In Hoekelmann, R (ed): Primary Health Care, ed 2. Mosby-Year Book, St. Louis, 1992, pp 1484–1490.

CHAPTER 14

ENDOCRINE,

METABOLIC, AND

NUTRITIONAL

ASSESSMENT

Much of the physical assessment of the endocrine and metabolic systems and nutritional status is integrated into the physical examination. Of the endocrine glands, the thyroid is the only one that can be palpated. Inspection of the skin, hair, nails, facial appearance, reflexes, and musculoskeletal system can provide other clues to identifying endocrine and metabolic disorders and nutritional status.

The endocrine system affects a variety of organs, including the pituitary gland, thyroid, adrenals, gonads; and can have a significant impact on growth and sexual development.

Galactosemia, phenylketonuria (PKU), and diabetes mellitus are the most common endocrine and metabolic problems seen in children in the primary-care setting. Menstrual irregularities in prepubertal and pubertal girls and gynecomastia in boys may indicate an endocrine problem.

Children with nutritional and metabolic disorders may exhibit similar symptoms: Either they are not receiving adequate nutrition or they cannot effectively metabolize the food they are eating. In infants, failure to thrive may indicate an endocrine, metabolic, cardiac, neurological, or renal disorder, or it may be caused by parental detachment, lack of adequate nutritional knowledge, or deficiency in infant care.

A complete history is essential for determining the underlying cause of any of these symptoms. Feeding schedules and amounts of foods in the child's normal diet should be determined, as well as the social environment during feedings or meals. To help determine the growth of the child in the last year both in height and size, the caregiver should be asked how the size of the child's clothing has changed. If short stature is a concern, the height of the family members should be noted. The patient's short height may be genetic and not clinically significant. The child's normal elimination patterns should be assessed. Chronic diarrhea may indicate a metabolic problem.

If the child or parent has concerns regarding sexual development and gonadal function, they should be asked gender-specific questions: for example, whether any signs of sexual development are evident, such as hair (pubic, axillary, and/or facial), scrotal, or testicular growth; or whether and when menses began. A review of past growth is essential, as is the necessity of plotting growth at each visit. The patient or caregiver should *always* be questioned about the use of any medications, such as steroids, that can alter growth.

If thyroid disease is suspected though uncommon in children, associated conditions should be investigated, such as diabetes mellitus, Turner's syndrome or trisomy 21. Maternal intake of iodine-based medications during pregnancy should also be determined.

Either acute or chronic problems with vomiting, dehydration, weakness, fatigue, or pallor may be subtle clues to adrenal hypofunction. Symptoms of adrenal hyperfunction include sexual developmental problems, significant electrolyte imbalances, a "moon face," truncal adiposity, and muscle weakness or wasting (Figs. 14–1 and 14–2).

During the physical examination, stature should always be measured and plotted; the child's appearance, overall proportions, and any outward signs of sexual development noted; thyroid palpated; and genitalia carefully examined (Fig. 14–3).

Because of the nature of most endocrine and metabolic disorders, genetic counseling is usually needed. In certain diseases (e.g., PKU), special dietary needs must be met; therefore, the patient should be referred for dietary counseling when appropriate. The long-term implications of these disorders require provision of as much education and support for the patient as possible.

Proper nutrition should be emphasized at every visit, particularly when the child is overweight or underweight and no organic cause is identified. Discuss the importance of behaviors that foster mother-infant bonding during feedings.

Cystic Fibrosis

Cystic fibrosis (CF), an autosomal-recessive genetic disorder, is found in infants and young children. Characterized by chronic lung problems, pancreatic insuffi-

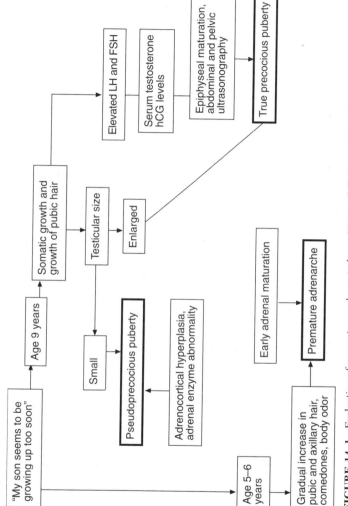

FIGURE 14-1 Evaluation of precocious puberty in boys. (FSH = follicle-stimulating hormone; hCG = human chorionic gonadotropin; LH = luteinizing hormone.)

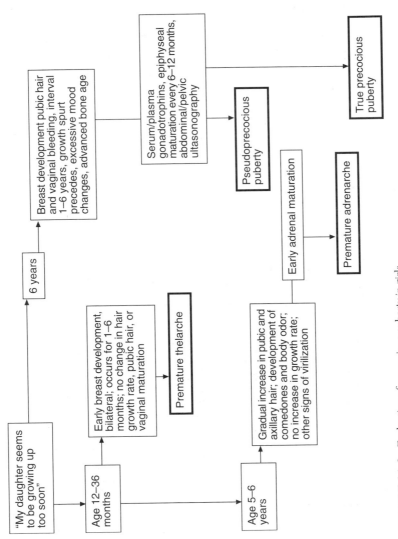

FIGURE 14-2 Evaluation of precocious puberty in girls.

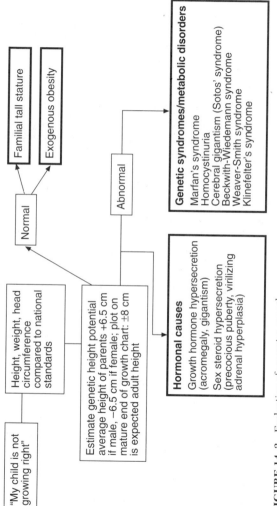

FIGURE 14–3 Evaluation of excessive growth.

ciency, and abnormally high levels of electrolytes (specifically sodium chloride) in the sweat, the disease is caused by the dysfunction of the exocrine glands. The disease affects the pulmonary, gastrointestinal, endocrine/metabolic, and reproductive systems. Transmitted on the seventh chromosome, it is the most common lethal, genetically transferred disease.

Age: Present at birth, but diagnosis can be made at any age; the oldest recorded age of diagnosis of CF is 65 years.

Ethnicity: CF is more common in whites (1 in 2000); it occurs at a very significantly lower rate in African-Americans.

Gender: Occurs equally in males and females.

Contributing Factors: Genetically transmitted.

Signs and Symptoms: The parent may report that the child sweats heavily and that the skin tastes salty when kissed. The child also has a history of chronic lung infections or recurrent bouts of pneumonia or bronchitis caused by unusual organisms such as *Pseudomonas*, *Klebsiella* and *Staphylococcus*. These infections are accompanied by wheezing, coughing, tachypnea, and cyanotic episodes. Chronic constipation may also be reported; the stool is foul-smelling, frothy, and pale. The child may have delayed weight gain (compared to failure to thrive in the infant) and delayed growth, and the older child may have delayed appearance of secondary sexual characteristics.

The following questions may help in obtaining a thorough history when CF is suspected:

Does the child have chronic constipation or has there been a need for regular use of suppositories to enable the child to have regular bowel movements?
What does the child's stool look like? Does it have a foul odor?
What is the child's appetite like? Has the child grown as expected?
How often does the child get respiratory infections or have other respiratory problems?
Does anyone else in the family have cystic fibrosis, or has anyone had similar complaints?

The child, who appears small for his or her age, may have a barrel chest and cyanosis. There may be a cough and other signs of respiratory problems, such as tachypnea and dyspnea. Distal clubbing may be noted. Stool may be palpated in the abdomen, and a prolapsed rectum may be noted. A significant delay of secondary sexual characteristics in the adolescent may be expected. Bone age is retarded. The skin may be sweaty and the parent may report with a salty taste to it. If a fever is present or if the child has become overheated, there will be signs of dehydration. Nasal polyps may be visualized on inspection of the nares. The abdomen is distended, is dull to percussion, and has decreased bowel sounds. The liver is palpable. Decreased sounds at the bases of the lungs are noted when pneumonia is present. Wheezing may be heard on auscultation of the lungs, and the lungs are hyperinflated.

Diagnostic Tests

The main diagnostic test used is quantitative pilocarpine iontophoresis (sweat chloride test). In the very young infant (under age 3 months), use a test for stool trypsinogen.

If results of the sweat chloride test are inadequate, genetic screening is done. A CF screen can be done in certain reference laboratories.

Stool analysis demonstrates absent or diminished trypsin and chymotrypsin.

A 72-hour fecal fat excretion test may be done to demonstrate increased fat in the stool. Fat-soluble vitamins and albumin are decreased in the blood.

Respiratory excretions should be analyzed for the presence of *Pseudomonas,* which is highly suspicious for CF when other symptoms are present.

Differential Diagnosis

Malabsorption syndrome is differentiated by a negative sweat chloride test or genetic screen for CF.

Recurrent reactive airway disease by negative sweat chloride test and genetic screen for CF.

Infants with *failure to thrive (nonorganic)* respond to changes in nutritional intake.

Congenital lung malformation is differentiated by x-ray of the lungs.

Immune deficiency disease is differentiated by laboratory tests; those children will have a negative sweat chloride test or genetic screen for CF.

Treatment: Treatment often centers around providing adequate nutritional supervision to foster the child's normal growth and development within his or her limitations. Treatment also concentrates on improving pancreatic function and decreasing the frequency and severity of pulmonary diseases.

For the most part, children with CF are treated on an outpatient basis and are hospitalized only when either their respiratory system is severely compromised or they have a severe infection. The approach should be multidisciplinary, including a specialist with advanced knowledge in the management of CF; a primary health-care provider; a nutritionist; a physical therapist, when needed; a social worker, who can assist the family in meeting the needs brought on by a chronic illness; and a respiratory therapist.

Postural drainage accompanied by chest physiotherapy should be a part of the child's everyday routine. Pancreatic enzyme replacement, prescribed by the specialist, should also be administered on a daily or regular basis. The child should be encouraged to engage in regular exercise and to practice good nutrition. The diet should allow liberal use of salt; intake of high-protein, high-calorie (1.5 times greater than the recommended allowance for age), and high-fat foods; and daily vitamin supplements. Oxygen for home use should be available. Antibiotics should be given immediately in the presence of an infection to allay exacerbation of the disease (Table 14–1). Human recombinant deoxyribonuclease (DNase), a new aerosolized mucolytic agent, may be used to

TABLE 14–1 ANTIMICROBIAL AGENTS FOR
LUNG INFECTION IN CYSTIC FIBROSIS

Route	Organisms	Agents	Dosage (mg/kg per 24 hr)	Doses/24 hr
Oral	Staphylococcus aureus	Cloxacillin	50–100	3–4
		Cefaclor	40–60	3
		Clindamycin	20	3–4
		Erythromycin	50–100	3–4
		Amoxicillin/clavulanate	40	3
	Haemophilus influenzae	Amoxicillin	50–100	3
		Trimethoprim-sulfamethoxazole	20*	2–4
		Chloramphenicol	50–100	3–4
	P. aeruginosa	Ciprofloxacin	15–30	3
	Empirical	Tetracycline	50–100	3–4
Intravenous	S. aureus	Oxacillin	150–200	4
	P. aeruginosa	Gentamicin or tobramycin	8–20	1–3
		Amikacin	15–30	2–3
		Netilmicin	6–12	2–3
		Carbenicillin		
		Ticarcillin		
		Piperacillin		
		Mezlocillin or		
		Azlocillin	250–450	4–6
		Ticarcillin/clavulanate	250–450	4–6
		Imipenem/cilastatin	45–90	3–4
	P. aeruginosa and cepacia	Ceftazidime	150	3
Aerosol	P. aeruginosa	Gentamicin	40–80†	2–4
		Tobramycin	40–80†	
		Carbenicillin	500–1000†	

Source: Behrman, R: Nelson's Textbook of Pediatrics. WB Saunders, Philadelphia, 1992.
*Quantity of trimethoprim.
†mg/dose.

decrease the viscosity of mucus and improve airway clearance. Enemas may be needed to improve evacuation of the bowel, and at times, a bowel-cleaning solution such as GoLYTLEY may also be needed. Although not readily available, transplants for the lung, pancreas, and liver may be done.

Although the early use of antibiotics, antivirals, mucolytics, and bronchodilators can reduce the progression of respiratory symptoms, these measures cannot stop the overall progression of the disease. Currently, the development of effective antipseudomonal therapy can improve the overall prognosis of the disease, but it should not be presented to parents as a cure for the disease because no known cure exists.

Follow-up: Follow-up for the child with CF is continuous. The team should maintain a well-formulated plan in order for the child to achieve the optimal outcome. Ideally, the child should be monitored at a CF center at least three times per year. Early intervention for all real or suspected infections should be stressed; routine immunizations should be given along with specialized immunizations.

Sequelae: Common sequelae include chronic lung infections, bronchitis, bacterial or viral pneumonia, and *Pseudomonas* infections. Other complications include pneumothorax, hemoptysis, right-sided heart failure, diabetes mellitus, metabolic alkalosis, malnutrition, growth retardation, sterility, intestinal obstructions, biliary cirrhosis, and bleeding esophageal varices. Ultimately, death occurs; the life expectancy of CF patients is a median of 29 years.

Prevention/Prophylaxis: Parents should be given adequate genetic counseling so that they can make informed choices as to future pregnancies. Early intervention is always important. Yearly influenza immunization should be provided. The child also needs adequate protection against measles and pertussis. The child should not receive general anesthesia: Epidural, local, or spinal anesthesia should be used for all surgical procedures. Most important for the child and the family is the maintenance of good team work and support for the management of both acute and long-term problems associated with the disease.

Referral: When CF is suspected, and certainly as soon as the diagnosis is confirmed, refer the patient to a pediatrician and a pediatric endocrinologist, preferably one who specializes in CF.

Education: Teach parents the dietary management of CF. Train them to provide early intervention for infections or other complications. Inform parents and children regarding all of the treatments, therapies, and implications of the disease. Teach them the techniques of chest physiotherapy and respiratory care, and help them recognize the signs of a compromised respiratory system.

Hypothyroidism

Hypothyroidism, a deficiency in the production of thyroid hormone or a defect in the receptor, can be an acquired or congenital problem. Establishment of national neonatal screening programs can be credited for the early detection of this potentially fatal disorder.

Etiology: Congenital hypothyroidism (CH) is due to thyroid dysgenesis. Acquired hypothyroidism (AH) is most commonly caused by lymphocytic thyroiditis.

Occurrence: Congenital hypothyroidism occurs in 1 in 3500 live births. Acquired hypothyroidism occurs in 1 in 500–1000 school-age children.

Age: CH, at birth; AH, any age beyond the newborn period.

Ethnicity: Not significant.

Gender: More prevalent in females (2 : 1 congenital); (4 : 1 acquired).

Contributing Factors

Acquired: If the child has had a thyroidectomy, has been exposed to a goitrogen (e.g., iodides, antithyroid drugs or other medications), has an iodine deficiency, or has been exposed to irradiation of the thyroid tissue, there is an increased risk of thyroid disease.

Congenital: Genetic predisposition, Down's syndrome.

Signs and Symptoms: In CH, there is a family history of the disease, prolonged gestation, increased birth weight, delayed first stool, feeding difficulties, constipation, and general lethargy. Physical examination reveals a distended abdomen, a yellow tinge to skin, peripheral cyanosis, macroglossia, and hypotonia. There is delayed closure of the posterior fontanel; cool, dry, scaly skin; poor capillary refill; an umbilical hernia; and possible signs of respiratory distress (e.g., retractions, wheezing, coarse breathing sounds).

In AH, the history is more vague. Parents sometimes note delayed growth. They may report decreased appetite, lethargy, poor school performance, cold intolerance, and delayed puberty. Physical examination may reveal a goiter, delayed dentition, and dry skin. Muscle weakness, tenderness of the anterior neck, and cool, dry skin are also noted.

There will be an increased need for sleep in both groups.

Diagnostic Tests

CH is diagnosed when on the newborn thyroid screen the thyroxine (T_4) level is low and a follow-up thyroid-stimulating hormone (TSH) is high. If the TSH level is greater than 25 μU/L, a pediatric endocrinology workup is needed.

Skull x-ray demonstrates a large fontanel and wide suture lines.

AH is diagnosed by a low T_4 and a high TSH. A follow-up endocrinology workup is needed to make the final diagnosis.

An electrocardiogram (ECG) may reveal an enlarged heart.

Chest x-ray shows "beaking" of the ribs (curvature and narrowing at ends of ribs resulting in a beaklike appearance).

Differential Diagnosis

Transient hypothyroidism is distinguished from thyroid disease because the T_4 and TSH levels will return to normal, whereas in AH or CH they will not.

Sleep apnea is differentiated by an abnormal pneumogram.

Constipation is a transient condition, but in AH and CH it persists despite changes in diet or the use of medication.

Down's syndrome is differentiated by chromosomal testing.

Congenital cardiac defects are differentiated by abnormal cardiac findings that do not generally accompany hypothyroidism.

Short stature is differentiated by failure of thyroid replacement therapy to cause an increase in height.

Treatment

CH: Give levothyroxine (Synthroid) at 10–15 μg/kg per day to maintain T_4 levels within 10–15 μg/dL range. Improvement is noted in 7–21 days. Height increases and skeletal maturation responds rapidly. Thyroid tests (T_4, TSH, and free T_4) should be done every month for the first 6 months, then every other month for 6–12 months, and then every 3 months. Bone age needs to be determined at the start of therapy and at age 1 year.

AH: Give levothyroxine sodium at 3–5 μg/kg up to a maximum of 100–150 μg once per day at least 30 minutes before eating. Treatment should start at the lowest levels; TSH levels should be monitored every 2–3 months or more often when there are dosage changes or signs of increased hypothyroidism or hyperthyroidism.

Follow-up: The child should keep regularly scheduled health-care maintenance appointments besides having TSH level checked every 2–3 months.

Sequelae: Children's growth expectations are met when hypothyroidism is treated early; however, children with long-standing hypothyroidism may lose up to 7 cm of predicted adult height.

Prevention/Prophylaxis: Congenital, none; acquired: avoidance of goitrogens, adequate iodine in diet, and follow-up after radiation treatment to ensure early detection of a problem.

Referral: If hypothyroidism is suspected, refer patient to a pediatric endocrinologist immediately for confirmation of the diagnosis. Afterward, manage the patient's follow-up.

Education: Teach the parents to give medications each day at the same time to maintain an adequate thyroid level. Signs that the child's levels may be too low include increased fatigue, weight gain, skin and voice changes, and dryness of the skin or hair. Note any of these changes and order an immediate TSH level.

Acromegaly (Giantism)

Acromegaly is a condition related to hypersecretion of pituitary hormones (primarily growth hormone [GH]), resulting in abnormal growth mainly of the distal parts of the body. Often this oversecretion affects all portions of the body. The oversecretion of GH results in hyperplasia of the somatotrophs.

Etiology: Acromegaly is most often caused by a pituitary adenoma, but other causes include hypothalamic or pancreatic tumors.

Occurrence: Rare (1 in 4000).

Age: Although it may occur as early as age 2, it is most evident at puberty.

Ethnicity: Not significant.

Gender: Occurs equally in males and females.

Contributing Factors: Pituitary or hypothalamic disease, embryological defects, tumor, or exposure to radiation.

Signs and Symptoms: When the tumor occurs in very young children, before epiphyseal fission occurs, parents voice concern at the extreme height of the child and report at least one significant growth spurt. Children may also complain of visual changes or problems related to compression of the optic nerve. In older children, the history may include delayed sexual changes and a sudden onset of menses. The older child may have coarse facial features, protruding jaw, height beyond the norm for age, enlarged hands and feet, and thickened skin. Often the teeth are separated, and dorsal kyphosis is evident. Percussion and palpation may reveal a tumor of the pancreas.

Diagnostic Tests

Growth hormone levels are elevated (greater than 10 μg/mL).

Serial height and head circumference measurements are taken to document abnormal growth spurts.

Skull x-ray, along with computed tomography (CT) or magnetic resonance imaging (MRI) of the head, may reveal a pituitary adenoma or hypothalamic tumor. A CT of the abdomen may reveal a tumor of the pancreas.

Differential Diagnosis

Hereditary tall stature is differentiated by family history.

Precocious puberty is different because the epiphysis closes early and stature is ultimately short.

Marfan's syndrome and *homocystinuria* are differentiated by normal growth hormone levels.

Central nervous system mass is differentiated by a CT or MRI of the head.

Treatment: The goal of treatment is to reduce the GH level or, if a tumor is present, to shrink the size of the tumor. Pharmacological management is accomplished with bromocriptine to decrease the size of the tumor. Generally, surgery is performed or radiation therapy instituted and should be done by a pediatric endocrinologist. Counseling, both psychological and genetic, should be initiated for the child and parents.

Follow-up: Patient should maintain regular health-care visits. If medications are used, follow-up is as frequent as weekly or monthly.

Sequelae: Dental problems related to the increased size of the mandible, delayed sexual development, and perhaps arrested development.

Prevention/Prophylaxis: Regular screening and health-care visits that include a meticulous measurement of height and head circumference should be done. Otherwise, there is no way to prevent acromegaly from occurring.

Referral: As soon as this condition is suspected, refer the patient to a pediatric endocrinologist.

Education: Educate the parents and children as to the nature of this rare disorder. Inform parents of the course of the disease and the treatment regimen; offer counseling. Because these children have difficulty with activities that require coordination, parents should be prepared to assist them with these activities and to provide them with safety measures.

Short Stature

Constitutional (familial) short stature, the most common cause of short stature in children, is an abnormally short stature relative to the age of the child. Pituitary dwarfism is related to insufficient GH. Congenital short stature is caused by hypothyroidism. Primordial short stature is caused by intrauterine growth retardation.

Etiology: No causative agent is noted in constitutional short stature; rather, it is caused by constitutionally delayed growth. Pituitary dwarfism is caused by insufficient levels of GH. Thyroid insufficiency may cause congenital short stature. Intrauterine growth retardation is the cause of primordial short stature.

Occurrence: Rare (1 in 4000).

Age: Present from birth.

Ethnicity: Not significant.

Gender: Occurs equally in males and females.

Contributing Factors: Family history of short stature.

Signs and Symptoms: A family history of delayed growth, short stature, and related skeletal and pubertal delays is given by the parent. In the cases of pituitary dwarfism, hypothyroid-induced short stature, and primordial short stature, the patient usually has no prior history. In pituitary dwarfism, the birth weight is normal, but there is decreased height at birth with small hands and feet (Fig. 14–4).

Hypothyroid-induced short stature: Patient may report persistent constipation.

Constitutional short stature: Growth curve is at about the third to fifth percentile.

Pituitary dwarfism: Patient has cherublike or infantile facial features with persistent infantile fat distribution, the norm being a loss of infantile fat and elongating of face with approaching puberty.

Hypothyroid-induced and primordial short stature reveal no significant findings by inspection except short stature.

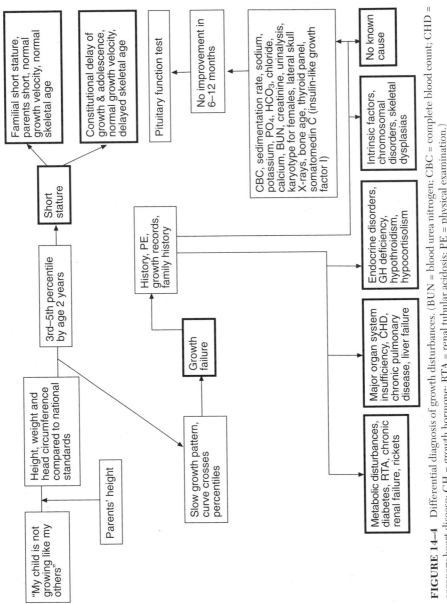
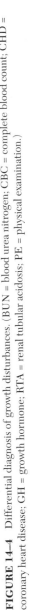

FIGURE 14–4 Differential diagnosis of growth disturbances. (BUN = blood urea nitrogen; CBC = complete blood count; CHD = coronary heart disease; GH = growth hormone; RTA = renal tubular acidosis; PE = physical examination.)

Diagnostic Tests

No abnormalities in laboratory tests are found in constitutional short stature. In primary dwarfism, GH levels are reduced.

Sonograms done during pregnancy revealed intrauterine growth retardation in cases of primordial short stature.

Altered thyroid function tests (TSH, T_4) are present in hypothyroid-induced short stature.

Prolonged hyperbilirubinemia is present in hypothyroid-induced short stature.

X-ray in pituitary dwarfism shows delayed epiphyseal maturation.

Bone age is delayed in all cases except constitutional short stature (i.e., greater than two standard deviations).

Serial height and head circumference measurements are taken for comparison to the norm.

Differential Diagnosis

Hypothyroidism, differentiated by bilirubin test and by abnormal TSH and T_4 levels.

Treatment: Pharmacological treatment, if indicated, includes testosterone for boys starting at age 14 years. The dose is typically 50–100 mg intramuscularly per month for 3–6 months. For girls, low-dose estradiol is administered by 12–13½ years.

When GH insufficiency is the problem, GH is also administered at a rate of 0.043 mg/kg per day beginning very early in life (under 10 years). The goal of therapy is to improve growth rates.

Parents and children should receive reassurance and support regarding height expectations. Although some improvement in height is likely, the child will probably continue to be somewhat shorter than his or her classmates. Psychological counseling, when indicated, should be available.

Follow-up: Serial height and head circumference measurements should be taken about every 1–3 months.

Sequelae: Short stature is associated with psychological or emotional problems, poor learning and school performance, delayed sexual maturation, and developmental delays.

Prevention/Prophylaxis: None.

Referral: As soon as a problem related to stature is suspected, refer the patient to a pediatric endocrinologist.

Education: Counsel families regarding the emotional problems often encountered with significant short stature (third to fifth percentile). Care should be taken when explaining therapies so that neither the child nor the parent has unrealistic expectations regarding the outcomes.

Insulin-Dependent Diabetes Mellitus

Insulin-dependent diabetes mellitus (IDDM) is a common childhood illness. Although its etiology is not completely understood, it is known that this disorder of immune function leads to the destruction of pancreatic islet (β) cells, resulting in an inappropriate utilization of carbohydrates due to insulin deficiency. Adequate management of nutritional, medical, behavioral, and emotional aspects of diabetes are important in improving the quality of life and the overall prognosis.

Etiology: Marked lipolysis, proteolysis, and ketone-body formation results from decreased synthesis of glycogen, protein, and fat. Serum glucose and ketone levels are elevated, increasing the osmotic level in the kidneys; consequently the kidneys are affected by increased urinary loss and loss of potassium, sodium, and ammonium.

Occurrence: IDDM constitutes 97% cases of childhood diabetes, occurring in 15 in 100,000 children in the United States.

Age: Peak onset is between ages 7 and 13 years.

Ethnicity: Incidence ranges from country to country: The lowest rate is in Korea (0.6 in 100,000) and the highest in Finland (35 in 100,000).

Gender: Occurs equally in males and females.

Contributing Factors: Genetic predisposition is the most significant predictor of IDDM in children, although the process of inheritance is not understood.

Signs and Symptoms: Child presents with a recent history of polyuria, polydipsia, and polyphagia accompanied by weight loss. Usually there are no significant findings. There will be an increased urinary frequency along with nighttime polyuria and enuresis.

Changes in appetite and thirst are also apparent to the parents. Weight loss may be noted. The child may appear dehydrated and may have Kussmaul respirations.

Diagnostic Tests

Serum glucose (fasting) levels greater than 130 mg/dL or random serum glucose levels greater than 200 are found.

Urine should be checked for presence of ketones.

In children, oral glucose tolerance tests are rarely necessary to confirm the diagnosis.

Differential Diagnosis

Polydipsia, polyuria, and impaired urinary concentration sometimes occur with *hypercalcemia* and *potassium deficiency,* differentiated by serum levels, which reveal increased calcium and decreased potassium in the blood.

Primary renal diseases, differentiated by isotonic urine. In diabetics, hypotonic urine is present.

Psychogenic polydipsia, differentiated by the patient's withholding fluids but failing to produce concentrated urine.

Treatment: Early treatment and aggressive management are the keys to the successful treatment of IDDM. Long-term goals of treatment include maintaining normal growth and development, regulating glucose metabolism, preventing acute complications, and promoting the patient's acceptance of the disease.

Treatment should involve a multidisciplinary team including a diabetes educator, nurse or nurse practitioner, dietitian, social worker, psychologist or therapist, primary health-care provider, and pediatric endocrinologist.

Growth should be monitored and growth curves plotted at intervals of 3–6 months, depending on the child's age.

Insulin, the primary agent used in the treatment of IDDM, is initially given at 0.6–0.8 units/kg per day in two divided doses: half given before breakfast and half given before dinner. Each dose should be made up of regular (immediate-acting) and NPH (short-acting) insulin (2 : 1). After approximately 3–4 months, most children experience a "honeymoon phase," requiring significantly less insulin. Conversely, illness, anxiety, and the onset of puberty increase the requirement for insulin. All changes in insulin should be instituted by a physician. Ever-changing brand names have slight differences; thus a switch in brand may alter the patient's typical reaction to the insulin dose.

If the dawn phenomenon (AM hyperglycemia) or Somogyi phenomenon (AM hypoglycemia resulting from PM hypoglycemia) occurs, adjustments need to be made in the scheduling of doses. For the dawn phenomenon, the PM dose of intermediate-acting insulin needs to be increased. For the Somogyi phenomenon, the PM dose of intermediate-acting insulin needs to be decreased or it may be managed by increasing the carbohydrate content of evening snacks.

For adolescents, changes brought on by puberty may change requirements, so 1.5–2 units/kg per day should be the dose schedule adhered to in the teenage years.

External infusion pumps are not generally used in young children but should be considered with unstable diabetes or severe, chronic illness.

A protocol acceptable to both the child and the health-care provider should be established for glucose monitoring. At least an AM blood glucose reading is needed. A range of 80–160 is considered acceptable. When there are readings above or below this range, the health-care provider should be contacted. If the reading is greater than 240, urine should be tested for the presence of ketones.

Glycosylated hemoglobin (HbA_{1c}) should be measured by the health-care provider because it indicates degree of adherence to the regimen of medication for a 2–3 month period *preceding* the examination. Results of 4–6% are normal; 9–13% indicates very good to good control, and greater than 15% indicates poor control. HbA_{1c} should be measured every 3 months or in cases of stress or illness.

Nutritional regimens suggest that the child's diet should consist of 50–60% carbohydrates, 12–20% protein, and less than 30% fat. Three snacks per day are recommended for children.

Exercise should be regular and moderate; when strenuous exercise is expected, adjustments should be made for the possibility of hypoglycemia.

Follow-up: Routine health-care visits should be maintained. Changes in blood glucose levels should be reported to health-care providers as they occur.

Sequelae: Diabetes mellitus is a complex disease that has far-reaching consequences when poorly controlled. Problems frequently seen in diabetic children include blindness, learning disorders, emotional problems, and renal and neurological consequences. Puberty and the development of secondary sexual characteristics are often delayed. Depression and rebellion are commonly seen in adolescent patients, for which quick, effective intervention is required. Long-term complications include peripheral and autonomic neurological changes, early onset of heart problems, and retinal changes.

Prevention/Prophylaxis: Because there is an inherited predisposition to the disease, it cannot be prevented. Onset may be delayed by good nutrition and weight management. However, exacerbations can be treated and prevented by anticipation of changes in insulin dosage during the honeymoon phase and during illness, stress, exercise, and adolescence. Also, regular measurement of the HgA_{1c} can help validate the child's reports of having been compliant with the medication regimen and can help determine an appropriate plan for the child.

Referral: When diabetes is suspected, the child should be referred to a pediatric endocrinologist or diabetes specialist. The team should then be contacted to assist in developing a comprehensive, efficacious plan to foster the best outcomes for the child.

Education: With the assistance of a diabetes educator, teach parents, children, and other interested family members the disease process, the signs and symptoms of hyperglycemia and hypoglycemia, and the proper action to take when there are complications. Over time, long-term strategies need to be discussed with the family to decrease complications that may arise.

Milk Protein Sensitivity and Lactose Intolerance

Milk sensitivity is an allergic response to whey proteins and casein and is characterized by an intolerance to cow's milk–based products. There may also be a crossover allergic response to soy protein products.

Lactose intolerance is the inability to digest carbohydrates (disaccharides, glucose, and galactose).

Etiology

Milk protein sensitivity: Unknown, but thought to be some form of mediated immunologic process.

Lactose intolerance: The most common cause is lactase deficiency: Primary lactose intolerance is a decline in intestinal lactase activity that is genetically determined; secondary lactose intolerance, the most common form, has been associated with infectious processes such as AIDS, rotavirus and other infections of the small bowel, as well as damage to the small bowel as noted in celiac disease (gluten sensitivity).

Occurrence: Common. Milk protein sensitivity is estimated to be present in 0.5–1.0% of infants. An estimated 30% of milk protein sensitive persons will also be soy-sensitive.

Mexican-Americans (70% by the age 18) and African Americans (50% of 4- to 5-year-olds) are lactose intolerant.

Age: Milk protein sensitivity usually occurs within the first month of life and resolves during the first year. Lactose intolerance occurs in older age groups, usually after the age of 5 years.

Ethnicity: African-Americans and Mexican-Americans have a higher incidence of lactose intolerance. Other minority groups affected are Indians of North, South, and Central America, and people of Mediterranean descent. Asian children seem to have a history of earlier onset than do other groups.

Gender: Occurs in girls and boys.

Contributing Factors

Milk protein sensitivity: Family history of allergies may contribute to infant-feeding difficulties.

Lactose intolerance: Infections of the gastrointestinal tract, other illness such as celiac disease ("short gut"), which reduces the surface area required for absorption of lactose.

Signs and Symptoms

History

Milk protein sensitivity: Infant is brought to the clinic with the complaint that the baby is not tolerating the present formula. Caregiver relates a history of fussiness, crying, colicky abdominal pain, excessive gas, vomiting, and diarrhea with streaks of blood in the stools. The history may include the presence of skin rashes, clear runny nose and congestion.

Lactose intolerance: Child is brought to the clinic because of watery diarrhea, complaints of feeling bloated, flatulence, vomiting, and abdominal cramping.

Physical Examination

Milk protein sensitivity: Findings reveal an infant that is not gaining weight appropriately for age. There may be skin rashes and the diaper area may be more irritated than usual, due to increased number of stools. There will be clear drainage from the nose and some nasal "stuffiness." Blood-streaked stools are consistent with milk protein intolerance in infants.

Lactose intolerance: The findings of the physical examination will vary, depending on the severity of the symptoms. Long-term symptoms can lead to dehydration, electrolyte imbalance, and metabolic acidosis.

Diagnostic Tests

Milk protein sensitivity: Diagnostic criteria include cessation of symptoms after elimination of the milk products from the diet and the recurrence within 48 hours of rechallenge. Skin test for milk sensitivity will confirm diagnosis if the test is positive. Obtain a CBC, a total protein, and albumin. Obtain a stool to examine for occult blood and fecal leukocytes. In extreme cases a small bowel biopsy will demonstrate partial villous atrophy and eosinophilic infiltrates. A barium swallow may be useful to evaluate for pyloric stenosis.

Lactose intolerance: Breath hydrogen test: An increase in expired hydrogen of 20 ppm over the baseline, which is the lowest value obtained, is a positive text. Exclude products containing lactose from the diet.

Differential Diagnosis

Cystic fibrosis will have a positive sweat chloride test.

Pyloric stenosis will have a positive radiograph and the characteristic projectile vomiting.

Nonorganic failure to thrive. Observe the mother-infant interaction and the feeding technique if neglect and abuse are suspected.

Secondary formula protein intolerance due to mucosal injury following a rotavirus infection, a viral antigen in the stool as measured by enzyme-linked immunosorbent assay (ELISA) is confirmatory. Usually resolves in a month.

Primary carbohydrate malabsorption due to congenital disaccharide deficiency is rare in infancy. The stool contains excessive quantities of carbohydrates.

Treatment: Eliminate the suspected food from the diet. Infants are often placed initially on Enfamil or Similac with Iron; the iron may be a cause of the gastric upset. Try the new formula for a week; if it is not tolerated well, try a different one. Examples of some of the substitutions are: ProsoBee or Isomil (soy-based), Nutramigen or Progestimil (also used with malabsorption disorders), and Alimentum (for infants who cannot tolerate other formulas.

Try Lacto-free formula if you suspect a lactose intolerance. Improvement of symptoms may occur with the use of milk containing lactase-producing microorganisms as well as milk pretreated with microbial-derived lactase, such as Dairy Ease (Sterling Health Division of Sterling Winthrop, New York, NY), Lactaid (McNeil Consumer Products Co., Fort Washington, PA) and Lactrase (Schwarz Pharma, Kremeres Urban Co., Milwaukee, WI).

Follow-up: Reevaluate weekly for weight, feeding pattern, and alleviation of symptoms on the new formula. When formula tolerance has stabilized, resume regularly scheduled visits.

Sequelae: Infants who have extreme milk protein sensitivity and lactose intolerance are at risk for developing failure to thrive and associated growth retardation.

Prevention/Prophylaxis

Milk protein sensitivity: The best method of prevention is for the infant to be breast-fed. Diarrhea in breast-fed infants may be relieved by the elimination of milk from the diet of the mother.

Lactose intolerance: None.

Referral: Normally none; in severe cases, refer to a pediatric gastroenterologist. The Women's Infant and Children's program is helpful for families who need assistance for special formulas. A written prescription is required for eligible mothers to obtain special formulas.

Education: Instruct patents in proper bottle-feeding techniques and how to read food labels to identify offending substances such as whey, casein, or lactose. Let them know that lactose is frequently used as a filler substance in capsules and tablets; choose medication accordingly.

Obesity

Obesity is a condition in which the body weight is 20% above the desired weight for age, gender, height, and body build. Obesity can be related to increased adipose tissue that is typed as either hypertrophy, an increase in the size of the fat cells; or hyperplasia, an increase in the number of fat cells. Although the size of a fat cell can be reduced, the number is not very easily decreased; therefore obesity due to hyperplasia is a more difficult form of obesity to treat.

Etiology: Inadequate activity levels or psychosocial factors that result in a child's turning to food for comfort can contribute to obesity in children. The intake of calories beyond the recommended number, coupled with a decreased level of activity or slowed metabolism, can also result in obesity. There is an interplay between genetic and environmental factors, but this is not clearly understood.

Occurrence: Twenty-seven percent of all children and 21% of teenagers in the United States are obese. Of these, it is estimated that one third to one half of the children and up to 80% of the teenagers who are obese will remain obese into adulthood.

Age: Can occur at any age.

Ethnicity: Not significant.

Gender: Occurs equally in males and females.

Contributing Factors: Up to 50% of children diagnosed with Prader-Willi syndrome, Down's syndrome, or spina bifida will be obese. In general, any disorder that reduces energy output, limits mobility, or impinges on the body's metabolism can increase the risk of obesity at any age.

Signs and Symptoms: The parent may relate a diagnosis of a disorder or disability that has caused a decreased activity level for the child. They may also relate that many members of the family are obese. The child presents with a history of decreased level of activity, intake of an increased amount of calories, and a sense of being "always hungry." Previous attempts at weight reduction may have been unsuccessful. The child's level of activity—time spent in aerobic sports or exercise, time spent reading or watching television, and sleep history—should be evaluated. The pattern of eating and the quality of food consumed in a day should also be reviewed.

Height and weight, body frame, and muscle mass should be evaluated. In uncomplicated obesity, the only significant finding is weight greater than expected for the height and age of the child. Obesity is diagnosed when triceps skin fold is greater than 85%, and weight for height is greater than the 75th percentile.

In extremely obese patients it may be difficult to palpate or percuss any organs. Blood pressure should be monitored because it is sometimes elevated in obese persons (Fig. 14–5).

Diagnostic Tests: None for uncomplicated obesity.

Differential Diagnosis

Diabetes mellitus is differentiated by elevated blood glucose levels when fasting.

Hypothyroidism is differentiated by TSH level, which is normal in obesity but decreased in thyroid disease.

Hypoparathyroidism is differentiated by laboratory tests to assess the function of the parathyroid gland. The results will show decreased levels in this disease, but not in obesity.

Inborn errors of metabolism are differentiated by a positive PKU test and by routine tests for galactosemia or maple syrup urine disease.

Treatment: Although a reduction in the child's caloric intake should be stressed, a "diet" is not an effective approach to the problem of obesity. Rather, the child should be encouraged to increase physical activity and eat well-balanced meals. Diets often encourage eating disorders, so they may actually interfere with normal growth and development.

Evaluate the relationship between the parent and child as well as the parents' attitudes about eating and food. Positive behavioral techniques centered around improving self-esteem, attitudes, and body image should be taught. The child, parent, and health-care provider should set realistic goals to decrease weight.

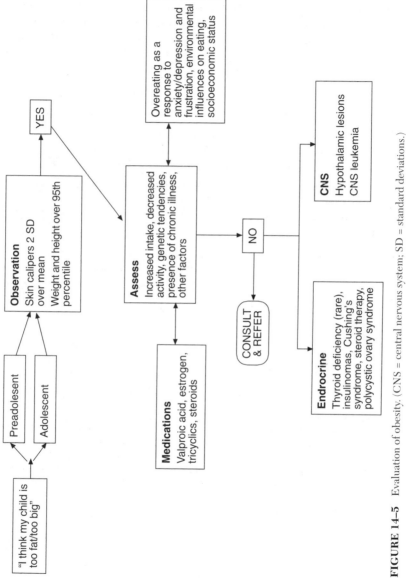

FIGURE 14–5 Evaluation of obesity. (CNS = central nervous system; SD = standard deviations.)

Children should be taught that they should eat only until they are full and that the old adage of "clean your plate" often leads to obesity. Daily exercise should be stressed, decreased television viewing time enforced (less than 4 hours per day), and positive feedback and praise given to the child. Rewards should be incorporated into positive behavioral strategies: All weight loss, improved dietary habits, and increased physical activity should be acknowledged.

Follow-up: Weekly weight and monthly height measurements are recommended until optimal weight is achieved.

Sequelae: Obesity increases the likelihood of hypertension, impaired glucose tolerance, low self-esteem, depression, social isolation, and orthopedic problems.

Prevention/Prophylaxis: Good nutritional strategies should be employed in every family. Balanced meals, low-calorie nutritional snacks, and an exercise program should be started early and become part of a family's regular practices.

Referral: If a metabolic disorder is suspected, immediately refer the patient to a pediatric endocrinologist. To assist the child and parent in sound meal and snack planning, refer the child to a nutritionist in conjunction with medical supervision.

Education: Encourage parents to set the example for good nutritional patterns. Although dieting in children is not usually a good method of controlling obesity, teach families to change their eating patterns. Institute positive reinforcement strategies.

REFERENCES

Behrman, R: Nelson's Textbook of Pediatrics, ed 14. WB Saunders, Philadelphia, 1992.

Bernard, J, et al: Pediatric Endocrinology, ed 2. Williams & Wilkins, Baltimore, 1993.

Doenges, M, and Moorhouse, M: Nursing Diagnoses with Interventions, ed 4. FA Davis, Philadelphia, 1993.

Green, M: Pediatric Diagnosis: Interpretation of Symptoms & Signs in Infants, Children and Adolescents, ed 5. WB Saunders, Philadelphia, 1992.

Hay, W, et al: Current Pediatric Diagnosis and Treatment, ed 12. Appleton & Lange, Norwalk, Conn, 1995.

Lifshitz, F: Pediatric Endocrinology: A Clinical Guide, ed 2. Marcel Dekker, New York, 1990.

Peter, G, et al: The 1994 Red Book: Report of the Committee on Infectious Diseases. American Academy of Pediatrics, Elk Grove Village, Ill, 1994.

Rosenstein, B, and Fosarelli, P: Pediatric Pearls: The Handbook of Practical Pediatrics, ed 2. Mosby, St. Louis, 1993.

Acromegaly

Connaughty, S: Accelerated growth in children. J Pediatr Health Care 6:316, 1992.

Melmed, S: Acromegaly. N Engl J Med 322:966, 1990.

Short Stature

Allen, D, et al: Therapeutic controversies: Growth hormone treatment in non–growth hormone deficient subjects. J Clin Endocrinol Metab 79:1239, 1994.

Johnson, A, and Blizzard, R: Growth hormone treatment. In Pediatric Endocrinology. Marcel Dekker, New York, 1992.

Cystic Fibrosis

Lemen, R: Pediatric lung disease. Chest 102:2326, 1992.

Ramsey, B, et al: Nutritional assessment and management in cystic fibrosis. Am J Clin Nutr 5:108, 1992.

Schidlow, D, et al: Cystic fibrosis foundation conference report on pulmonary complications of cystic fibrosis. Pediatr Pulmonol 15:187, 1993.

Stern, R: The primary care physician and the patient with cystic fibrosis. J Pediatr 114:31, 1989.

Taussig, L: Cystic Fibrosis. Thieme-Stratton, New York, 1984.

Tizzano, F, and Buchwald, M: Cystic Fibrosis: Beyond the gene to therapy. J Pediatr 120:337, 1992.

Tizzano, F, and Buchwald, M: Recent advances in cystic fibrosis research. J Pediatr 122:985, 1993.

Diabetes

Allen, D, and MacDonald, M: Pancreas and islet cell transplantation for type I diabetes mellitus: Does it have a role for children? Adv Pediatr 37:391, 1990.

Drash, A, and Arslania, S: Can insulin dependent diabetes mellitus be cured or prevented? Pediatr Clin North Am 37:1467, 1990.

Dunger, D: Diabetes in puberty. Arch Disabled Child 67:569, 1992.

Erick, L: The newly diagnosed child with diabetes. Adv Nurse Pract 4(9):14, 1996.

Kawonen, M: A review of recent epidemiologic data on the incidence of type I diabetes mellitus. Diabetologia 36:883, 1993.

Hypothyroidism

American Academy of Pediatrics, American Thyroid Association: Newborn screening for congenital hypothyroidism: Recommended guidelines. Pediatrics 80:745, 1987.

Bellesario, R, et al: Newborn screening for hypothyroidism in New York state. In Advances in Neonatology, Exerpta Medica, Amsterdam, 1987.

Milk Protein Sensitivity and Lactose Intolerance

Behrman, R, and Kliegman, R (eds): Nelson, Essentials of Pediatrics. WB Saunders, Philadelphia; 1990.

Castiglia, P: Lactose intolerance. J Pediatr Health Care 8:36, 1994.

Green, M: Pediatric Diagnosis: Interpretation of Symptoms & Signs in Infants, Children, and Adolescents, ed 5. WB Saunders, Philadelphia: 1992.

Hay, W, et al (eds): Current Pediatric Diagnosis & Treatment, ed 12. Appleton and Lange, Norwalk, Conn, 1995.

Stockman, J: Difficult Diagnosis in Pediatrics. WB Saunders, Philadelphia, 1990.

Obesity

Albertson, A, et al: Nutrient intake of 2 to 10 year old American children. J Am Dietetic Assoc 92:1492, 1992.

Ekvall, S, et al: Dealing with nutritional problems in children with developmental disorders: prevention, assessment and treatment. Topics Clin Nutr 8:51, 1993.

Gortmaker, S, et al: Inactivity, diet, and the fattening of America. J Am Diet Assoc 90:1247, 1990.

Mellin, L, and Frost, L: Child and adolescent obesity: The nurse practitioner's use of the shapedown method. J Pediatr Health Care 6:187, 1992.

Satter, E: How to get your kids to eat . . . but not too much. Bull, Palo Alto, Calif, 1987.

CHAPTER 15

PSYCHOSOCIAL

ASSESSMENT

Psychosocial disturbances constitute nearly 50% of children's visits to the health-care provider's office. Familiarity with age-appropriate variations will assist in determining the level of and concerns related to psychosocial issues (Table 15–1).

Effective interviewing and discussions with the child and caregivers facilitate the raising of relevant issues and early recognition of problems. During the first encounter with the child and caregiver, the appearance, behavior, cognition, and thought processes (ABCT) should be evaluated.

Deviations in *appearance* in children can be more difficult to determine than in adults. During assessment of posture and body movements, the child's relationship with the provider should be observed. Children who are anxious about visiting the office often "hang back" and look at the floor, or obsessively cling to the caregiver at an age when this is not developmentally appropriate.

In adolescents, appropriate dress is a function of their social group—to look the same as their peers, or even to look different than the rest, is a social statement. Uncleanliness of the clothing and the body may be the first clue to self-neglect, parental neglect, or depression in adolescents. However, children are often brought from the playground or from school at the end of the day without a chance to "freshen up." Therefore, serial observations are necessary in order to determine how dress and grooming reflect a child's mental status.

Behavior is interpreted on the basis of what is to be expected for that age group: It is normal for a curious child to want to explore the examining room, but such behavior is considered abnormal in an adolescent or adult. Mood and affect can be observed during conversation with the child. It is helpful to validate concerns about the child's behavior, mood, and affect by asking the caregiver what the child is like at home, school, or day care.

TABLE 15–1 RELATIONSHIP AMONG TASKS, CONCERNS, AND CONDITIONS

Infant (birth to 1 year)	Toddler (1–3 years)	Preschooler (3–6 years)	School-age Child (6–11 years)	Adolescent (11–20 years)
		Tasks		
Emotional attachment	Beginning of the separation-individuation process	Taming of the internal world of fantasy	Skills development	Identity formation
		Concerns		
Temperament variations	Sleep disturbances, breath holding, temper tantrums	Childhood fears: bedtime, darkness, ghosts, monsters, learning disabilities, nightmares	Childhood fears, school avoidance, primary nocturnal enuresis	Turmoil, sexuality, concerns as to whether the young adult will "make it" in society
		Conditions		
Failure to thrive	Night terrors, breath holding, autistic spectrum disorder, anxiety	Enuresis, encopresis, schizophrenia, anxiety, exaggerated temper tantrums	Attention-deficit/hyper-activity disorder, autism, depression, anxiety	Anorexia, bulimia, depression, substance abuse, anxiety, self-injurious behavior

Cognition can be ascertained by the child's history of school functioning. It should be determined whether the child is in the grade appropriate for his or her age. Adolescents can be tested much like adults; for example, they can be asked direct questions about how they feel and how today is different from yesterday. Children under 6 should take the Denver Developmental Screening test: Any failure to achieve particular developmental milestones should be noted.

The *thought processes* of adolescents can be considered much like those of adults; for example, questions are asked about long-term goals and how they see and relate to the world around them, family, peers, and school. The behavioral checklist developed by Jellinek, Evans, and Knight in 1979 is a quick screening tool for school-age children. This checklist, which covers mood, play, school, friends, and family relations, can be completed in about 5 minutes, while the parent waits. Areas to explore during the interview process include the following:

The loss of significant others.
Parents' work and child-care arrangements.
Persons who live in the home.
Any family crises.
Sleeping arrangements.
Social support.
Family, school, and peer relationships.

Parents as well as children often do not recognize the symptoms they describe as being associated with psychological problems. Therefore, the responsibility of the primary caregiver is to be alert to the history, appearance, symptoms, and affect of patients suspected to have such problems.

Anorexia

Anorexia is a serious eating disorder characterized by failure to maintain an adequate amount of weight appropriate for age and height (i.e., weight 15% below expected). Anorexia is due to a pervasive fear of becoming fat or gaining weight despite current underweight status, and to a significant distortion of perceived body size or body shape. Amenorrhea (non–pregnancy related) of at least three consecutive cycles can occur secondary to anorexia.

Etiology: Unknown, but there seems to be a familial pattern.

Occurrence: Occurs in 1% of teen-agers.

Age: Age distribution shows a bimodal distribution of onset at 12–14 years and at 17–18 years.

Ethnicity: Occurs more commonly in Western civilization, particularly in middle- to upper-class white females.

Gender: The female-to-male ratio is 20 : 1; 90–95% of anorexics are female.

Contributing Factors: Major transitions, such as entering high school or college or marrying; "finicky" eating in childhood; and perfectionist behavior appear to be factors. Seventy-five percent of girls ages 9–12 diet three to five times in a year, thus setting the pattern for disordered eating.

Signs and Symptoms: Caregiver complains that the child "plays with her food and is losing weight." Child contradicts the caregiver about her food intake, but is concerned that she is "too fat." During the history, the girl should be asked what she considers the perfect weight, whether she is on a diet, what she does to maintain her weight (anorexic girls have a history of excessive exercise), and what she thinks of her current weight. It would be helpful to obtain a weight history to determine her growth pattern. Postmenarchal females should be asked about the frequency of periods and amount of the flow. Past diet history should be noted. The Eating Attitudes Test and the Eating Disorder Inventory are useful assessment tools.

The physical examination may be normal. Loss of subcutaneous fat may not be evident until the patient disrobes. Bradycardia or hypotension may be present. There may be dry skin, cold extremities, limpness and loss of sheen of the hair, prominent ribs, and a scaphoid abdomen. Growth charts are abnormal in prepubertal and pubertal children with signs of anorexia nervosa of 6 months' duration or longer. Projected heights should be calculated as well as the ideal weight (Fig. 15–1).

Diagnostic Tests

Complete blood count (CBC) to assess nutritional status.
Erythrocyte sedimentation rate to exclude inflammatory bowel disease or collagen vascular disease.
Electrolyte studies to determine hypochloremic alkalosis and hypocalcemia due to vomiting.
Urinalysis to demonstrate concentration of urine; however, urine is not concentrated in the late stages of anorexia.
Serum total protein and albumin, which are usually normal.

Differential Diagnosis

In patients with *cancer, diabetes mellitus, hyperthyroidism,* or *chronic renal disease,* there is weight loss, but no fear of obesity or disturbance of body image.
Patients with *depression* may present with loss of appetite and weight loss.

Treatment: Treatment is multidisciplinary, involving a primary-care provider, mental health professional, and dietitian. The first goal is for the patient to increase caloric intake in order to gain weight. The dietitian plans a diet sufficient for weight gain. If there are no severe metabolic disturbances, the patient can be treated on an outpatient basis, with weekly visits to members of the treatment team. Mental health counseling includes not just the patient, but the entire family.

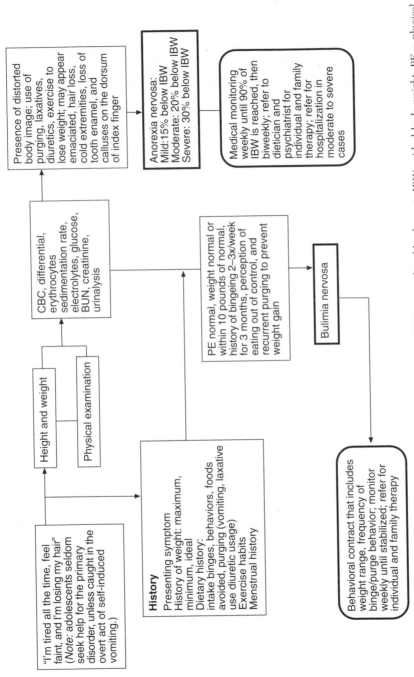

FIGURE 15–1 Evaluation of eating disorders. (BUN = blood urea nitrogen; CBC = complete blood count; IBW = ideal body weight; PE = physical examination.)

Contracting has been found to be a useful strategy. The contract should include long-term weight goals, rate of weight gain, amount of allowable exercise, frequency of visits, and the minimum weight that requires hospitalization (25–30% of ideal body weight).

Follow-up: Height, weight, and subcutaneous fat are measured weekly; chest and abdominal examinations are also done weekly.

Sequelae: Complications, which are many, involve all body systems. Among the complications are amenorrhea or irregular menses, decreased triiodothyronine (T_3) and increased reverse triiodothyronine (rT_3), (thyroxine [T_4] and thyroid-stimulating hormone [TSH] levels are normal), dehydration, osteoporosis, bradycardia, congestive heart failure, dental erosion (if anorexia is accompanied by vomiting), pancreatitis, constipation, hematuria, leukopenia, anemia, and stunted growth. The mortality rate is 10%, with 2–5% committing suicide.

Prevention/Prophylaxis: Reduce the messages children get about the "perfect" weight. Assist girls in forming a positive self-image.

Referral: Consult with or refer patient to a primary-care physician for definitive diagnosis and admission to the hospital, if necessary. Refer patient to a mental health counselor for family therapy, to a dietitian for appropriate meal planning, and to a support group.

Education: Instruct patient and family about the illness. Provide factual knowledge, not myths. Teach patient about eating and appropriate eating patterns; many have lost sight of what constitutes a normal eating pattern.

Anxiety

Anxiety is a vague, uneasy feeling whose source is unknown or nonspecific. Normal developmental anxiety is categorized as follows:

Stranger anxiety (5 months to 1½ years, with a peak at 6–12 months)
Separation anxiety (7 months to 4 years, with a peak at 18–36 months)
Anxiety from or even phobia of the dark and "monsters" (3–6 years)

"Appropriate" anxiety is a feeling that occurs, when anticipating a painful or frightening experience, when avoiding the memory of such an experience, and in instances of child abuse. There are three major anxiety disorders:

1. Anxiety states
2. Phobic anxiety
3. Posttraumatic stress disorder

Anxiety is different from fear: Fear is a response to a known, external, real threat.

Etiology: Unknown. Possible disruption of parent-infant relationship and a history of a stressful event, situational change, or chronic illness.

Occurrence: Occurs in 10% of school-age children and adolescents.

Age: Any age. Age-normal fears or anxieties can develop into anxiety disorders.

Ethnicity: Not significant.

Gender: Occurs equally in males and females.

Contributing Factors: Environmental factors such as emotional overstimulation, family discord and/or violence, and harsh disciplinary methods.

Signs and Symptoms: Child may present with a history of increased dependence on home and parents, avoidance of social interaction outside the family, avoidance of anxiety-producing stimuli, decreased school performance, increased self-doubt and irritability, and ritualistic behaviors (e.g., washing, counting). Caregivers may have observed increased fear and worries, uneasiness and apprehension, and frightening themes in play and fantasy. They may also have noted decreased concentration, hyperactivity, dizziness and light-headedness, shortness of breath, panic, and sleep disturbances. Child may also complain of heart palpitations, nausea and vomiting, fatigue, and headaches or stomachaches.

Physical findings may be negative. Findings, if seen during an episode, may reveal shortness of breath, flushing, sweating, and dry mouth and/or tachycardia. Effective interviewing to elicit detailed history is important, as is behavioral observation of an episode if possible. Adolescents can complete the Hamilton Anxiety Rating Scale as an adjunct to diagnosis.

Diagnostic Tests: None. To rule out organic/physiological causes, order the following tests:

Drug screen for toxicity.
Thyroid panel for hypothyroidism and hyperthyroidism.
Blood glucose level for hypoglycemia.
CBC for anemia.
Electrocardiogram (ECG) for arrhythmias or mitral valve prolapse.

Differential Diagnosis

Abuse of illicit substances, medications, alcohol, and recreational substances (caffeine, chocolate): Drug history.
Hyperthyroidism: T_4 and T_3 elevation and TSH suppression.
Anemia: Hemoglobin levels less than 11 g/dL.
Hypoglycemia: Fasting blood glucose levels less than 60 mg/dL.
Hypoxemia: Partial pressure of oxygen (PO_2) decreased in pulmonary disease, hypoventilation, anemia, and carbon monoxide poisoning (PO_2 normal in anxiety).
Cardiopathy, such as dysrhythmia, high-output state, and mitral valve prolapse: ECG shows abnormalities.

Treatment

Nonpharmacological

For older children, facilitate identification of precipitating event, development of coping skills, and support systems. Establish an open, trusting relationship with the child. Promote well-being by prescribing a balanced diet and exercise.

Pharmacological

Imipramine, 3–5 mg/kg per day in two divided doses. Start dosage at 1 mg/kg per day and increase to no more than 3 mg/kg per day every 4–5 days, as tolerated. Clinical effectiveness may not be seen until 4–6 weeks after initiation of treatment.

Tricyclic antidepressants appear to have more cardiotoxic effects in children than in adults. Observe for heart rates over 130 beats/min, blood pressure 130/85 mm Hg, and changes in the ECG. Anticholinergic responses are also seen with the use of tricyclic antidepressants.

Follow-up: At each dosage increase, and then every 3–4 months, obtain height, weight, pulse, blood pressure, and ECG readings.

Sequelae: Long-term effects of childhood anxiety problems are unknown.

Prevention/Prophylaxis: Anticipatory guidance for parents to help them deal with their child's normal fears in an appropriate manner.

Referral: Consult or collaborate with a psychiatrist for definitive diagnosis and pharmacological intervention when anxieties exceed developmental norms.

Education: Educate parents regarding normal childhood development. Instruct parents in the dosage, purpose, and side effects of antianxiety medications.

Attention-Deficit/Hyperactivity Disorder

Attention-deficit/hyperactivity disorder (ADHD) is a multifaceted, chronic disorder in which the child exhibits difficulty sustaining attention, controlling impulses, and inhibiting activity level to meet the demands of a given situation. It is a neurologically based problem involving an interference in the brain's ability to procure, store, process, and produce information. Approximately 50% of the behaviors persist into adulthood. The disorder has two forms: (1) impulsivity and hyperactivity and (2) inattention, disorganization, and difficulty completing tasks (Fig. 15–2).

Etiology: There appears to be a pattern of hereditary transmission. It has also been suggested that this disorder may be related to birth complications, or to a disease of or trauma to the central nervous system (CNS). Research has not supported a relationship to food additives. Current theories suggest an imbalance of neurotransmitters, such as dopamine, in the premotor cortex and superior frontal cortex.

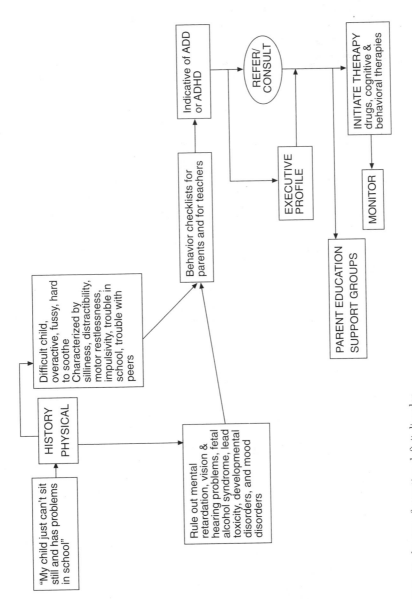

FIGURE 15–2 Evaluation of attention-deficit disorder.

Occurrence: Occurs in an estimated 9–12% of school-age children.

Age: Occurs in children (usually under 7); may persist into adolescence and adulthood.

Ethnicity: Not significant.

Gender: More prevalent in males (3 : 1).

Contributing Factors: Chaotic households; possibly a family history of similar behavior. Maternal smoking during pregnancy may increase risk.

Signs and Symptoms: Child is brought to clinic because of behavior, noted either in the home or in the classroom, consisting of disruption, lack of attention, and/or daydreaming. Physical findings are negative. Data related to birth and developmental history should be gathered, gross and fine motor skills assessed, and a family and home assessment conducted. An in-depth assessment of the behavior requires interviews with parents, the child, and teachers. Impulsive and disruptive behaviors are seen to a greater degree and frequency than what is considered appropriate for developmental age. These behaviors are reported to have been present for at least 6 months, and they are evident in two or more settings, such as home and school. Table 15–2 indicates the diagnostic criteria as delineated by the American Psychiatric Association in the *Diagnostic and Statistical Manual of Mental Disorders, 4th rev.(DSM-IV-R)*.

Diagnostic Tests

Computed tomography (CT), magnetic resonance imaging (MRI), and electroencephalography (EEG) are of no diagnostic use.

Psychological testing is done to rule out mental retardation and to test cerebral function.

The Conners, ACTeRs, or Schnelle test, or the Nursing Evaluation for Attention-Deficit Disorders, is given. Behavior rating scales are disclosed to the parents and teachers.

Vision and hearing screening tests are performed to check for deficits; the child will qualify for interventions under Public Law 94-142 if deficits are found.

Differential Diagnosis

Children with *hearing deficits* may have hyperactivity.

Poor parenting skills may result in a child with impulsive behaviors.

Besides having vocal tics, patients with *Tourette's syndrome* also have motor tics. The disorder may be exacerbated by the stimulant medications used for ADHD.

Mental retardation is usually not seen in cases of ADHD.

Fetal alcohol syndrome is differentiated by family history and facies.

Lead toxicity is differentiated on the basis of laboratory data.

Sleep disturbances (retiring late, arising early) may mimic ADHD.

Absence seizures (history of daydreaming or staring spells) should be ruled out by EEG.

TABLE 15–2 DIAGNOSTIC CRITERIA FOR
ATTENTION-DEFICIT/HYPERACTIVITY DISORDER

A. Either 1. or 2.:
  1. Six (or more) of the following symptoms of **inattention** have persisted for at least 6 months to a degree that is maladaptive and inconsistent with developmental level:
  Inattention
  a. often fails to give close attention to details or makes careless mistakes in schoolwork, work, or other activities
  b. often has difficulty sustaining attention in tasks or play activities
  c. often does not seem to listen when spoken to directly
  d. often does not follow through on instructions and fails to finish schoolwork, chores, or duties in the workplace (not due to oppositional behavior or failure to understand instructions)
  e. often has difficulty organizing tasks and activities
  f. often avoids, dislikes, or is reluctant to engage in tasks that require sustained mental effort (such as schoolwork or homework)
  g. often loses things necessary for tasks or activities (e.g., toys, school assignments, pencils, books, or tools)
  h. is often easily distracted by extraneous stimuli
  i. is often forgetful in daily activities
  2. Six (or more) of the following symptoms of **hyperactivity/impulsivity** have persisted for at least 6 months to a degree that is maladaptive and inconsistent with developmental level:
  Hyperactivity
  a. often fidgets with hands or feet or squirms in seat
  b. often leaves seat in classroom or in other situations in which remaining seated is expected
  c. often runs about or climbs excessively in situations in which it is inappropriate (in adolescents or adults, may be limited to subjective feelings of restlessness)
  d. often has difficulty playing or engaging quietly in leisure activities
  e. is often "on the go" or often acts as if "driven by a motor"
  f. often talks excessively
  Impulsivity
  g. often blurts out answers before questions have been completed
  h. often has difficulty awaiting turn
  i. often interrupts or intrudes on others (e.g., butts into conversations or games)
B. Some hyperactive-impulsive or inattentive symptoms that caused impairment were present before age 7 years.
C. Some impairment from the symptoms is present in two or more settings (e.g., at school [or work] and at home).
D. There must be clear evidence of clinically significant impairment in social, academic, or occupational functioning.
E. The symptoms do not occur exclusively during the course of a Pervasive Developmental Disorder, Schizophrenia, or other Psychotic Disorder and are not better accounted for by another mental disorder (e.g., Mood Disorder, Anxiety Disorder, Dissociative Disorder, or a Personality Disorder).
Code based on type:
314.01 Attention-Deficit/Hyperactivity Disorder, Combined Type: If both Criteria A1 and A2 are met for the past 6 months
314.00 Attention-Deficit/Hyperactivity Disorder, Predominantly Inattentive Type: If criterion A1 is met but Criterion A2 is not met for the past 6 months.
314.01 Attention-Deficit/Hyperactivity Disorder, Predominantly Hyperactive-Impulsive Type: If Criterion A2 is met but Criterion A1 is not met for the past 6 months.
Coding note: For individuals (especially adolescents and adults) who currently have symptoms that no longer meet full criteria, "In Partial Remission" should be specified.

Source: Reprinted with permission from the Diagnostic and Statistical Manual of Mental Disorders, Fourth Edition. Copyright 1994 American Psychiatric Association.

Hypothyroidism is differentiated on the basis of laboratory data.

Treatment

Behavioral Management

Parents should be given the following strategies:

Reduce environmental stimuli.

Focus on the child's positive traits, thereby increasing his or her self-esteem.

Keep things as organized as possible, give the child responsibilities (e.g., list of chores), and reward progress (e.g., with gold stars).

Be specific, make directions simple, and make eye contact with the child.

Use the "time out" method of discipline; a kitchen timer can be useful as a means of increasing the child's sense of time.

Adolescents may benefit from making daily lists of what they want to accomplish, keeping an appointment book or planning calendar, keeping a note pad handy to write down ideas or items they want to remember, breaking down projects into smaller tasks that are more manageable, and posting schedules, plans, or errands. When they achieve their goals, they should reward themselves.

Pharmacological Management

Stimulants

Methylphenidate (Ritalin), 0.2–0.5 mg/kg per dose. Usual dosing is before school and at noon; depending on behavior, a third dose may be given in the late afternoon (approximately 4 PM). Dosage should be titrated upward weekly, to 5–60 mg per day, by the primary-care provider. Peak action is within 2 hours, and the effects dissipate within 6 hours. Children usually have weekends and summers off therapy.

Not recommended for children under age 6. Ritalin is contraindicated in children with a history (personal or familial) of motor tics or Tourette's syndrome, or if family members have untreated substance abuse disorders.

Pemoline tablets (Cylert), 37.5 mg/day single dose. Dosage should be titrated upward weekly to a maximum dose of 112.5 mg/day. Children usually have weekends and summers off therapy. Not recommended for children under age 6.

Dextroamphetamines are similar to methylphenidate in therapeutic onset and duration of action. Usual dosage is 2.5–10 mg/dose before school and at noon. The action of sustained-release spansules may last 8 hours. Not recommended for children under age 3.

Antidepressants

Bupropion (Wellbutrin): Begin with 50 mg AM and at noon. May titrate upward to a maximum dose of 150 mg. Usually not given in the evening because it tends to stimulate the child.

Desipramine (Norpramin) 1–2 mg/kg per day in two divided doses. This drug is contraindicated in children with a family history of cardiac disease, or who have a known seizure disorder.

α-Adrenergic Agonists

Clonidine, in conjunction with methylphenidate, is initiated at 0.05 mg at bed-time. That dose is increased after 3–5 days by giving an additional 0.05 mg in the morning. Dosage can be increased by 0.05 mg alternating morning, noon, and evening until the total daily dose is 0.3 mg in three divided doses (3–5 μm/kg per dose). The benefit of adding clonidine to the treatment regimen is that the dosage of methylphenidate may often be decreased by 30–50%. Clonidine is contraindicated in patients with known renal or cardiovascular disease. Baseline ECG should be obtained before therapy is started.

Follow-up: Monitor patient every 2 weeks until dosage is stable. Monitor for side effects, such as decreased appetite, headache, stomachache, and insomnia. Medications are contraindicated in children with hypertension. Monitor growth and development. Regularly monitor behavior, school achievement, and response to medication. Monitor hepatic function every 6 months.

Sequelae: Without interventions, these children experience increasing problems in school, thus increasing their feelings of failure and worthlessness. Fifty to seventy percent of juvenile crime is estimated to have been perpetrated by children with ADHD and conduct disorders; of these children, 50–60% will continue to have symptoms into adulthood, thus experiencing problems with work and personal relationships.

Prevention/Prophylaxis: None.

Referral: Refer patient to a Children's Developmental Center and/or a mental health center. Refer parents and older children to a support group if possible.

Education: Instruct parents and teachers that the disorder may be inherited and may persist into adulthood, but that treatment is available. Refer parents to support groups. Instruct parents about the dosage, purpose, and side effects of the medications. Ensure that parents understand the importance of a complete evaluation prior to a definitive diagnosis. Some parents nearly demand such a diagnosis and treatment to obtain the related financial benefits.

Autistic Spectrum Disorder

Autistic spectrum disorder is the current term for a group of disorders including autistic disorder; pervasive developmental disorder, not otherwise specified (PDD, NOS); Rett's syndrome; and Asperger's disorder—all of which manifest a common deficit in the ability to relate to others.

Autistic disorder: Severe atypical behavior characterized by severe abnormality of reciprocal social relatedness; severe abnormality of communication development (including language); and restricted, repetitive, and stereotyped patterns of behavior, interests, activities, and imagination (Church & Caplan). This is a lifelong disorder.

Pervasive developmental disorder, NOS: A developmental disorder characterized by impairment of the quality of social interaction and communications, impairment does not meet the full criteria for autistic disorder.

Rett's syndrome: A neurodegenerative disorder that primarily affects females, who present with microcephaly, stereotypical hand movements (handwringing), social withdrawal, and loss of communication skill.

Asperger's disorder: A less severe developmental disorder of autistic-like children with normal intelligence. They have delays in speech and language, abnormal interactions with peers, and tend to be concrete, rote thinkers. Many are able to control their behavior and are thus considered socially acceptable.

Etiology: Unknown; a suggested cause is central nervous system dysfunction or an abnormality occurring at time of fetal brain development.

Occurrence

Autistic disorder: Incidence rate is 0.7–4.5 cases per 10,000.

Pervasive developmental disorder: Occurs in 10–12 per 10,000 children.

Age

Autistic disorder: Onset is prior to 3 years of age.

Pervasive developmental disorder: First year of life.

Rett's syndrome: 5–48 months.

Asperger's disorder: Early childhood.

Ethnicity

Autistic disorder: Ethnicity is not significant.

Gender

Autistic disorder: Occurs more in boys (3–4 : 1) than girls.

Pervasive developmental disorder, NOS: More common in boys (4 : 1).

Rett's disorder: Occurs primarily in girls.

Asperger's disorder: Occurs in boys and girls.

Contributing Factors

Autistic disorder: There seems to be increased incidence in children with perinatal problems such as rubella, phenylketonuria, encephalitis, and fragile X syndrome. One-quarter of families with an autistic child have family members with language-related problems.

Pervasive developmental disorder: Extended time of exposure and reexposure while undergoing treatment for plumbism has been suggested as a contributing factor in PDD. There may be a sibling with PDD.

Signs and Symptoms

History

Autistic disorder: Parents often have noted that this child does not like to be held and comforted and does not talk. In addition, there may be an abnormal response to sensory stimuli, abnormal sensitivity to pain, heat, and cold, a tendency to taste and smell objects, hyperactivity, sleep disturbances, and self-injurious behavior. These are expressed in varying degrees.

Pervasive developmental disorder, NOS: The parent may report a different cry during the child's infancy, feeding problems, colic and sleep problems; in older children, families report aggressive, violent or out-of-control behaviors, tantrums, or problems with speech.

Rett's syndrome: Development of multiple defects after period of normal functioning. Between 5 and 48 months of age, head growth decelerates and there is loss of hand skills. Impairment of gait or trunk movements is noted. There may be a history of periodic apnea during wakefulness, intermittent hyperventilation, breath-holding spells, peripheral vasomotor disturbances, or seizures.

Asperger's disorder: Motor skills are delayed or motor clumsiness is noted. There is no delay in speech, language, cognitive development, or self-help skills.

Physical Examination

Physical findings are not remarkable. However, the developmental assessment reveals delays in meeting milestones, particularly in language and social skills. In Rett's syndrome the lack of head growth is evident and there is impairment of gait and trunk movements. There may be loss of teeth due to bruxism.

Diagnostic Tests

Autistic Disorder

Vision and hearing screening should be normal.

Screening for metabolic disorders (especially for defects of carbohydrate, amino acid, organic acid, fatty acid, lysosomal, purine, and peroxisomes), and fragile X syndrome (cytogenic analysis to identify other abnormalities).

In older children and adolescents use of diagnostic tools such as the Autism Behavior Checklist and the Autism Diagnostic Interview is suggested.

Serotonin levels for appropriate therapeutic management.

Differential Diagnosis: Vision and hearing problems; language development is often delayed, but developmentally delayed children usually are interested in interpersonal interaction.

Mental retardation: 70% have an IQ of less than 70.

Metabolic disorders and fragile X syndrome: Testing may or may not be negative; increased incidence is seen in these disorders.

Treatment

Nonpharmacological

Due to the variability and severity of symptoms as expressed, any treatment considered should be planned for the specific individual. These children may receive occupational therapy, physical therapy, speech therapy, behavioral and social skills training and educational tutoring. Consistency among the care givers as to expectations, rules, and behavioral management is important. Language skills.

Pharmacological

Autistic disorder:

Haloperidol, 0.5–4 mg/day to modify disruptive, hyperactive, and aggressive behavior.

Fenfluramine may be helpful in children with elevated serotonin.

Naltrexone may help control self-injurious behavior.

Use of stimulants may make the symptoms more severe.

Pervasive Developmental Disorder, NOS:

Clinical trials are ongoing for the use of risperidone (optimal dosage range is 0.75–1.5 mg daily, in divided doses) for fidgitiness.

Methylphenidate (Ritalin) may be used if ADHD co-exists.

Fluoxinetine (Prozac), a selective serotonin reuptake inhibitor (SSRI), may be used to reduce rituals or compulsions.

Follow-up: Schedule well-child visits. Monthly for developmental and therapeutic assessments.

Sequelae

Autistic Disorder

Seizure disorders may eventually be seen in approximately 25% of autistic children; ⅙ may become gainfully employed as adults; ⅙ able to function in structured environments; best prognosis is in children of normal intelligence and in those who have symbolic language skills by age 5 years.

Prevention/Prophylaxis: Appropriate prenatal care for the mother.

Referral: Refer any suspected cases to a developmental center for evaluation and multidisciplinary management. Refer parents to a support group.

Education: Educate parents in effective coping methods and behavioral management techniques.

Encourage the parents to develop a strong support system.

Instruct parents about the medication's dosage, purpose, and side effects.

Breath Holding

Breath holding is a paroxysmal, spontaneous, reflexive event occurring during expiration in healthy children that resolves in time. The child is provoked, cries, becomes noiseless, may have a change in skin color, and may lose consciousness. Cyanotic changes are usually noted as a response to anger, whereas acyanotic changes occur in spells related to an injury. Rarely does a spell proceed to asystole or a seizure.

Etiology: Unknown, but appears to be a learned behavior in response to anger, frustration, or injury.

Occurrence: Occurs in 0.1–5% of children under age 6.

Age: Occurs in children aged 6 months to 6 years.

Ethnicity: Not significant.

Gender: Occurs equally in males and females.

Contributing Factors: Trigger events that upset or frustrate the child. May be associated with pica and iron deficiency anemia.

Signs and Symptoms: Child presents with a history of breath-holding spells. Physical examination is negative.

Diagnostic Tests: None. If frequency increases, test for the following:

EEG to rule out seizure disorders.
Blood studies to rule out anemia.
Other disorders, which would be differentiated by history.

Differential Diagnosis

In *seizures*, the EEG results are abnormal.
In *sleep apnea*, the history reveals that episodes occur while child is asleep.
Rett's syndrome is a neurodegenerative disorder that affects females, who present with microcephaly, stereotypical hand movements, social withdrawal, and loss of communication skills that are related to a psychological disorder.

Treatment

Behavioral

Parents should do the following:

Monitor the event but treat it in a matter-of-fact manner, because it is impossible to protect the child from all upsetting events.
Help the child to control his or her responses to upsetting events.
Prevent self-injurious behavior.

As in temper tantrums, the child's demands that precipitated the "spell" should not be granted. In the case of syncope, the parent should place the child in the lateral supine position to protect the head and prevent aspiration. Parents should maintain a patent airway, but not do cardiopulmonary resuscitation (CPR) unless true respiratory arrest has occurred.

Pharmacological

None.

Follow-up: None.

Sequelae: None.

Prevention/Prophylaxis: For spells accompanied by bradycardia or asystole, atropine 0.01 mg/kg per dose has been used to prevent spells. Help the young child to learn more appropriate measures to deal with the frustrations of growing up.

Referral: None.

Education: Educate parents in techniques to assist the child in dealing with frustrations. Be supportive to parents, and reassure them that their child will outgrow this behavior.

Bulimia

Bulimia is a serious eating disorder characterized by the following:

Recurrent episodes of secretive binge eating (two times per week for 3 months), followed by self-induced vomiting (90%) and the use of laxatives (50–75%) or diuretics (10–34%) to compensate for the eating.

Excessive exercise and concern about weight or body shape.

Lack of control over the eating.

Use of restrictive diets.

Other impulsive behaviors.

Binge eating is defined as rapid consumption of large amounts of food (5000–20,000 calories of high-carbohydrate food at a time).

Etiology: Unknown.

Occurrence: Occurs in 3–5% of the general population.

Age: Primarily occurs in the older adolescent.

Ethnicity: Not significant.

Gender: Females account for 90% of the bulimic population; 10% are males. History may reveal gender differences: Males tend to be concerned with sexual identity and maintaining body shape and muscle tone; females are concerned with perception of body image and tend to exercise less.

Contributing Factors: Low self-esteem and personalities characterized by overachievement and perfectionism seem to be implicated. Additionally, 60% of female bulimia patients have been sexually abused. Bulimia, in both men and women, may be a form of self-medication for depression, anxiety, and loneliness. Coaches who encourage dehydration before weigh-ins and before games or matches may play a role in the subsequent binge eating among players.

Signs and Symptoms: Child is brought to clinic usually because the caregiver has noticed the self-induced vomiting after meals. Bulimia may be suspected during the history taking for an initial complaint of depression. Ask the following questions:

What does she consider the perfect weight?

Is she on a diet?

What does she do to maintain her weight (these girls have a history of excessive exercise)?

What does she think of her current weight?

It would be helpful to obtain a weight history to determine the patient's growth pattern. Postmenarchal females should be asked about the frequency of periods and the amount of blood flow. Inquire as to her past diet behavior. The Eating Attitudes Test and the Eating Disorder Inventory are useful assessment tools.

The physical findings may include weight that is normal or slightly above normal; salivary gland enlargement, esophagitis, callus formation on knuckles of first and second fingers from inducing vomiting; and erosion of dental enamel on posterior surface of the front teeth from constant contact with the stomach acid (see Fig. 15–1).

Diagnostic Tests

CBC to assess nutritional status.

Erythrocyte sedimentation rate to exclude inflammatory bowel disease or collagen vascular disease.

Electrolyte studies to determine hypochloremic alkalosis and hypocalcemia due to vomiting.

Metabolic acidosis due to laxative abuse.

Urinalysis to determine concentration of urine.

Serum total protein and albumin are usually normal.

Differential Diagnosis: The disorders that cause vomiting are many; bulimia is unique in that the patient focuses on body image or fears of obesity.

Treatment

Nonpharmacological

Multidisciplinary team including a primary-care physician, mental health counselor, and dietitian should be formed. Contracting has been found to be a useful strategy. The contract should include long-term weight goals, rate of weight gain/loss, amount of allowable exercise, strategies to reduce the number of bingeing/vomiting episodes, and the frequency of visits to the professionals.

Pharmacological

Imipramine, initiated at 50 mg and increased to 150–300 mg daily or until a satisfactory response is achieved, has had some success. Give at night to improve therapeutic levels. Do not give to persons with cardiac dysfunction.

Follow-up: Weekly visits with the team of health professionals to evaluate progress.

Sequelae: Gastric dilatation, esophageal tears, diarrhea, irregular menses are medical complications; approximately 5% commit suicide, and 80% are clinically depressed.

Prevention/Prophylaxis: Reduce the messages children get as to the "perfect" weight. Assist girls in forming a positive self-image. Educate teachers and coaches not to encourage poor habits such as fasting/bingeing cycles in children.

Referral: Consult with or refer patient to a primary-care physician for definitive diagnosis and admission to the hospital if necessary. Refer patient and family to a mental health counselor for family therapy. Refer patient to a dietitian for appropriate meal planning. Refer patient and parents to support groups.

Education: Instruct patient and family about the illness. Provide factual knowledge, not myths. Teach patient about eating and appropriate eating patterns; many have lost sight of what constitutes a normal eating pattern.

Depression

Depression is an intense, persistent state of unhappiness, often related to a recent event, that lasts for days or often weeks and interferes with the ability to experience pleasure or to be productive.

Etiology: There may be a genetic predisposition, as noted by occurrence secondary to depression in the mother; there may also be a familial tendency toward negative interpretations of life events, such as developmental situations (entering adolescence, going away to college) or chronic illness.

Occurrence: Occurs in 1–3% of preadolescent children and 3–6% of adolescents. Incidence is higher in children with a family history of depression.

Age: Any age.

Ethnicity: Not significant.

Gender: Probably occurs equally in males and females.

Contributing Factors: Rejection by peers, failure to achieve expectations, parent-child conflicts (may be "trigger" factors), history of abuse, and a poor home environment.

Signs and Symptoms: Child may present with any of the following clinical manifestations (Table 15–3):

Dysphoric mood: sad affect, slumped posture, and history of irritability, quick temper, and anger (adolescents often have difficulty talking about their sadness, rather exhibiting acting-out behaviors, particularly toward the parents).

TABLE 15–3 CLINICAL MANIFESTATIONS OF DEPRESSION IN CHILDREN AND ADOLESCENTS

Symptom	Clinical Manifestations
Dysphoric mood	Tearfulness; sad, downturned expression; unhappiness; slumped posture; quick temper; irritability; anger
Anhedonia	Loss of interest and enthusiasm in play, socializing, school, and usual activities; boredom; loss of pleasure
Fatigability	Lethargy and tiredness; no play after school
Morbid ideation	Self-deprecating thoughts, statements; thoughts of disaster, abandonment, death, suicide, or hopelessness
Somatic symptoms	Changes in sleep or appetite patterns; difficulty in concentrating; bodily complaints, particularly headache and stomachache

Source: Clark, RB: Psychosocial aspects of pediatrics and psychiatric disorders. In Hay, W, et al (eds): Current Pediatric Diagnosis and Treatment. Appleton & Lange, Stamford, Conn, 1994, p 170, with permission.

Anhedonia: Loss of interest and enthusiasm in school, social activities, and usual activities.

Fatigability, lethargy, and tiredness.

Morbid ideation: Thoughts of disaster, abandonment, death, and suicide; self-deprecation.

Somatic symptoms: Changes in sleep or appetite patterns, headaches, and/or stomachaches (Fig. 15–3).

Physical findings may be negative. Somatic symptoms must be investigated because they are often signs and symptoms of other organic disorders.

Diagnostic Tests: None. Behavioral checklists, such as the *Short Screening Scales for Anxiety and Depression* (Goldman et al, 1988), may be helpful for an initial assessment. Testing for diagnostic differentials includes the following:

CBC testing for anemia: Values less than 11 g/dL indicate anemia.

Thyroid panel: Low T_3 and T_4 levels and elevated TSH levels are indicative of hypothyroidism.

Epstein-Barr antibodies are elevated in chronic fatigue syndrome.

Drug screen for evidence of substance abuse.

Blood glucose levels: Levels less than 60 mg/dL indicate hypoglycemia; levels greater than 160 mg/dL indicate hyperglycenmia.

Before initiating treatment with tricyclic antidepressants, screen for cardiac problems, seizure disorder, and liver profiles. Monitor cardiovascular function via ECG with each dosage increase greater than 3 mg/kg per day.

Perform a general medical examination along with weight and blood pressure measurements before initiating treatment with selective serotonin reuptake inhibitors (SSRIs) and other types of medications.

Differential Diagnosis

Chronic fatigue syndrome is differentiated by low-grade fever, enlarged lymph nodes, sore throat, and an elevated Epstein-Barr antibody titer.

Hypothyroidism is differentiated by clinical laboratory findings and by clinical features such as dry skin and dry, brittle hair.

A concomitant *chronic illness* such as diabetes, hypoglycemia, anemia, or epilepsy may contribute to depression.

Substance abuse: Children often use/abuse chemicals to change the way they feel and as another way of "acting out," not realizing that a secondary effect is depression.

Treatment

Behavioral

Individual psychotherapy for the child, particularly cognitive therapy; family therapy to teach parents how to meet the child's emotional needs more effectively.

Pharmacological

Imipramine (tricyclic antidepressant): Starting dose is 1 mg/kg per day; increase by 0.25 mg every 4–5 days to 3 mg/kg per day. Contraindicated in cases of known

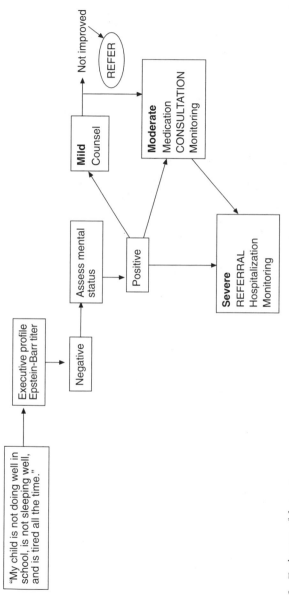

FIGURE 15–3   Evaluation of depression.

cardiac disease, seizure disorder, or electrolyte abnormalities; or a family history of cardiomyopathy.

Patients may experience anticholinergic effects, headaches, and sleep disorders. Interactions occur with antidepressants and stimulants: Plasma levels of antidepressants are lower in combination with barbiturates and cigarette smoking; plasma levels are increased in combination with phenothiazines, methylphenidate, and oral contraceptives.

Fluoxetine/sertraline/paroxetine (SSRIs): Usually once-daily dosing, in the morning. No known contraindications. Side effects may be increased psychomotor activity, headache, insomnia, and gastrointestinal (GI) distress. May interact with other antidepressants, leading to higher than expected blood levels.

Fluoxetine: Initially, 5–10 mg/day; increase by 5–10 mg every 2 weeks, as tolerated, to a maximum dose of 40 mg/day.

Sertraline: Therapeutic dose to 50–150 mg/day.

Paroxetine: Therapeutic dose to 100 mg–40 mg/day.

Bupropion (other category): Dosage range is 150–375 mg/day in divided doses. In adolescents, maximum dosage should be less than 450 mg/day. Contraindicated in seizure disorder. Few anticholinergic or cardiotoxic effects. Adverse effects include headache, increased psychomotor activity, anorexia, insomnia, and induction of seizures with doses greater than 450 mg/day.

Follow-up: Weekly follow-up until stabilized on medication, and then every 3–4 months. For patients on tricyclics, follow up every 3–4 months, taking height, weight, pulse, and blood pressure measurements and performing an ECG. For patients on SSRIs and other medications, follow up with a medical examination including weight and blood pressure measurements every 3 months.

Sequelae: Depressed children have school problems because depression interferes with memory and concentration, leading to failure and low self-esteem. Of children with an initial episode occurring between ages 8 and 13, 75% will have a recurrence later in life.

Prevention/Prophylaxis: Active listening to the child and awareness of "nuances" of behavior with appropriate interventions.

Referral: Consult/collaborate with a primary-care physician or psychiatrist before forming a definitive diagnosis and initiating pharmacological interventions. The child may require hospitalization for severe depression.

Education: Be supportive to parents as they learn to listen to their children and learn to meet the child's emotional needs more effectively. Instruct parents about the dosage, purpose, and side effects of medications.

Emotional Abuse

The rejection, ignoring, criticizing, isolation, or terrorizing of children resulting in loss of self-esteem. The most common form is verbal abuse or denigration.

Etiology: Child's failure to meet expectations of parents, teachers, and peers.

Occurrence: The abuse may occur at home, day care, or school, or during team sports.

Age: All pediatric age groups.

Ethnicity: Not significant.

Gender: Occurs equally in males and females.

Contributing Factors: Excessive expectations for age by parents, teachers, and significant others.

Signs and Symptoms: The child may present with a history of sleep disorders, somatic symptoms (stomachaches, headaches), or avoidance behaviors (refusal to go to school, running away).

Physical findings reveal a negative examination related to the somatic complaints. Observations of the child reveal a child with loss of self-esteem and hypervigilant behaviors.

Diagnostic Tests: None, except those in relation to the somatic complaints.

Differential Diagnosis: Evaluate the somatic complaints.

Treatment: No medical treatment; psychiatric treatment is not given unless the somatic complaints are accompanied by anxiety or depression.

Follow-up: Monitor child's progress in relation to somatic complaints.

Sequelae: May result in a chronic condition of low self-esteem and/or substance use and abuse.

Prevention/Prophylaxis: Parent effectiveness training.

Referral: Human services usually does not respond to these reports. Refer the child to mental health counseling and the family to family therapy.

Education: Involve parents in parent effectiveness training.

Failure to Thrive

Failure to thrive (FTT) refers to young children with inadequate weight gain, usually below the third percentile on a standard growth chart, and weight less than 80% of the median weight for height.

Etiology: The causes of FTT can be categorized as either nonorganic or organic:

Nonorganic causes relate to maternal factors, such as poor mother-child bonding; poor feeding techniques, including the child's excessive consumption of fruit juice; nutritional beliefs of the mother; errors in formula preparation; and child neglect.

Organic causes relate to a variety of chronic or serious childhood conditions, such as chromosomal disorders, fetal alcohol syndrome, immunodeficiency diseases, tumors, intestinal obstruction, renal failure, cystic fibrosis, celiac disease, and CNS pathology.

Occurrence: FTT accounts for 3–5% of admissions to teaching hospitals: 44% have environmental causes, 37% organic causes, and 19% no known cause.

Age: Infancy.

Ethnicity: Not significant.

Gender: Occurs equally in males and females.

Contributing Factors: Family dysfunction, maternal depression, and postpartum depression have been implicated in nonorganic FTT.

Signs and Symptoms: Child may have a history of poor feeding, vomiting, and/or diarrhea. Child may have a diagnosis of an organic illness.

Findings reveal inadequate weight gain and weight changes that are below norms for age-weight percentile on standard charts. Standardized charts are particularly useful when serial weights are not available. Child is observed to have frozen watchfulness, minimal smiling, decreased vocalization, resistance to being held, and self-stimulating rhythmic behaviors (Fig. 15–4).

Diagnostic Tests

Obtain a diet history that includes how the formula is prepared.
Observe parent-child interaction; watch the child being fed.
Investigate possibilities of environmental deprivation.
Obtain a CBC, urinalysis, serum electrolytes, erythrocyte sedimentation rate, calcium, T_4, and TSH.
If there are GI symptoms, order a stool culture and guiac.

Differential Diagnosis: To identify specific causes of organic FTT.

CNS pathology or neuromuscular disease should be suspected if child presents with the inability to suck or swallow.
If child presents with chronic diarrhea, cystic fibrosis, or celiac disease, suspect a maldigestion or malabsorption problem.
Poor nutrient utilization is observed with renal failure and inborn errors of metabolism.
Tumors, inborn errors of metabolism, and intestinal obstruction can cause vomiting.
Regurgitation is seen in gastroesophageal reflux or rumination syndrome.
Suspect an elevated metabolic rate in cases of thyrotoxicosis, chronic disease such as heart failure, inflammatory lesions, immunodeficiency diseases, and burns.
Patients with chromosomal disorders and fetal alcohol syndrome all have reduced growth potential.

Treatment: Increase caloric intake, record amount of feedings, and obtain before-breakfast weights daily. Involve parents in the interventions, particularly in planning an organized program of early-infant stimulation. Treat the underlying organic cause if one is found.

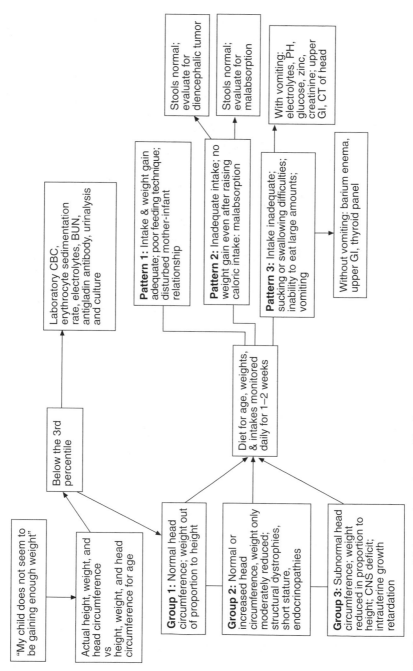

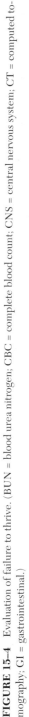

FIGURE 15–4 Evaluation of failure to thrive. (BUN = blood urea nitrogen; CBC = complete blood count; CNS = central nervous system; CT = computed tomography; GI = gastrointestinal.)

Follow-up: Regular monitoring of growth and development during the first 2 years of life. Initially, see child weekly for evaluation of weight gain; as weight gain stabilizes, follow up at 1- to 3-month intervals.

Sequelae: Children hospitalized for FTT exhibit mental retardation (15–67%), school learning problems (37–67%), and behavioral disturbances (28–48%) by 3–11 years of age.

Prevention/Prophylaxis: Emphasis in the prenatal period on infant nutrition, including formula preparation and parent-child interaction, will assist in preventing nonorganic FTT.

Referral: If outpatient treatment fails, refer child for hospitalization.

Education: Educate parents and caregivers in proper feeding techniques and daily requirements for adequate nutrition. Educate parents in parenting techniques to promote bonding.

Munchausen Syndrome by Proxy

Munchausen syndrome by proxy is a form of child abuse characterized by a parent, usually the mother, who induces signs and symptoms of illness in a child.

Etiology: Three types of parents are prone to be perpetrators:

Help seekers, who report illness in the child to convey distress in their personal lives.

Active inducers, who give the appearance of being perfect parents, resist treatment, and try to hide their psychological problems.

Doctor addicts, who because of their obsession with the child's health, become paranoid regarding the treatment team; these parents tend to change doctors and hospitals often.

Occurrence: Unknown. These children have a 9% mortality rate.

Age: Occurs mainly from infancy to age 2, rarely in children over 6.

Ethnicity: Not significant.

Gender: Occurs equally in males and females.

Contributing Factors: Often occurs in a nuclear family in which both parents live together, but the father is not typically involved in childrearing and the mother is very devoted to the child.

Signs and Symptoms: Diarrhea, neurological impairment, seizures, and vomiting are common presenting symptoms. A careful history reveals an unexplained persistent or recurrent illness whose signs and symptoms do not correlate with the history or appearance of the child. Furthermore, there will be evidence of the child's failure to respond to standard medical treatment, repeated hospitalizations, and parents' demand for vigorous medical evaluation.

The child's separation from the mother results in the absence of reported signs and symptoms.

Possible indicators of Munchausen syndrome by proxy include a mother who has had previous medical or nursing experience. The mother is calm, socializes with the staff, and appears not too concerned about child's illness. A history may reveal that the mother had an illness similar to that of the child. She is overprotective, not leaving the child alone; there are repeated requests for evaluation and care of the child. The physical examination focuses on the presenting complaint(s).

Diagnostic Tests

Video surveillance of parent-child interaction. Permission from the judicial system is required before videotaping.

Removal of parent from the room to see whether illness abates (evidenced by absence of GI complaints or apneic episodes).

Differential Diagnosis: Because of the often confusing findings, the differential diagnosis is focused on validating the presenting complaint. Close observation of parent-child interaction may require hospitalization in suspect cases.

Treatment: Confront the parent and advise her to undergo counseling. Treatment for the child may involve removal of the child from the home by protective services.

Follow-up: Follow up for remission of symptoms.

Sequelae: Depending on the degree of abuse and time until diagnosis, sequelae range from no long-term symptoms to death.

Prevention/Prophylaxis: Appropriate parenting skills.

Referral: Refer child to protective services. Refer parent and child to mental health services for counseling/psychotherapy.

Education: Educate the parent in parenting skills.

Nightmares

Nightmares are frightening dreams that occur during rapid eye movement (REM) sleep, followed by awakening in the latter part of the night; child is alert, can describe the images, and is sometimes able to recall and talk about them the following day.

Etiology: Unknown.

Occurrence: Occurs in 25–50% of children in the susceptible age group.

Age: Children aged 3–5 years.

Ethnicity: Not significant.

Gender: Occurs equally in males and females.

Contributing Factors: Stressful or frightening daytime events or anxieties may trigger nightmares; more frequently seen in sexually abused children.

Signs and Symptoms: Child is brought to clinic with the complaint of "having nightmares." Ask the parent about the frequency of the episodes, and about what is occurring at home, including the programs the child is allowed to watch on television that might trigger the dreams.

Physical findings are negative. Child is willing to talk about the dreams.

Diagnostic Tests: None.

Differential Diagnosis: Night terrors occur in 3% of 3- to 8-year-old children and in adolescents. They occur during non-REM sleep, and within 2 hours of sleep; they are associated with sleep walking, screaming, and other bizarre behavior. When awakened, the child is disoriented and incoherent and has no memory of the event the next day. These children often have Tourette's syndrome.

Treatment: Parental reassurance.

Follow-up: Some nightmares are normal; monitor the frequency of occurrence.

Sequelae: None.

Prevention/Prophylaxis: Attempt to keep the amount of stress in the home to a minimum. Monitor and guide television viewing in the susceptible age group.

Referral: In severe cases, refer the child for psychological help.

Education: Parents need to know that this condition is self-limiting and needs little treatment, and that the child will outgrow the problem.

Physical Abuse

Physical abuse is nonaccidental physical trauma usually inflicted by the child's caregiver.

Etiology: May be triggered by behaviors in the child such as persistent crying, toileting accidents, spilling, and disobedience.

Occurrence: Occurs in 1–2% of children in the United States; accounts for 2000 deaths per year.

Age: Occurs in all pediatric age groups, but primarily under age 6 years (one third of cases occur under age 1 year and one half between ages 1 and 6).

Ethnicity: Not significant.

Gender: Occurs equally in males and females.

Contributing Factors: Increased parental stress (less than 10% of parents have psychotic or criminal personalities) and parental substance abuse are among the factors implicated in physical abuse of children.

Signs and Symptoms: Child presents with a vague history of injuries. Indicators of abuse include a discrepant history (i.e., inconsistent with the injury) and a delay in seeking medical care. Pattern of increased severity of injury will be seen if no intervention occurs. Child has a history of multiple hospitalizations or multiple caretakers for injuries. Child may also have a history of behaviors that trigger the assaults.

Perform a careful, complete physical examination including height and weight. Record place, size, shape, and color of any bruises or burns. Bruising in cases of abuse is usually confined to the buttocks or lower back. Observe for distinctive patterns of bruising that suggest use of a belt, cords, pinches, and choke holds, for example. Some burns, such as those from irons, cigarettes, or submersion into scalding water, also have a distinctive pattern. Perform a funduscopic examination of the eye to look for retinal hemorrhages (particularly helpful in diagnosing shaken baby syndrome). Examine the eardrums, oral cavity, and genitalia for evidence of trauma. Evaluate the musculoskeletal system for tenderness and range of motion. Obtain color photographs of injuries, taking care to label with name, location, date, and time. Signs and symptoms of acute abdomen (e.g., rupture of the liver, spleen, intestines) may be the result of striking or squeezing the abdomen.

Diagnostic Tests

Perform radiographic studies of the skull, thorax, spine, and long bones in children under age 5 years in whom physical abuse is suspected. Periosteal tears will be noted in cases of shaken baby syndrome; coexistence of new and old injuries indicates long-term presence of abuse. If shaken baby syndrome is suspected, look specifically for subdural hemorrhages, as evidenced on CT scan or MRI.

When bruising is present, obtain a platelet count, bleeding time, prothrombin time, and partial thromboplastin time.

Investigate the family situation: Look for a caregiver who is stressed, has a history of abuse during childhood, has unrealistic expectations for the child, and is socially isolated.

Differential Diagnosis

Actual *accidental injuries* (accidental bruising is most common over the forehead, bony prominences, and anterior tibia).

Dermatological conditions such as impetigo and contact dermatitis may be confused with healing cigarette burns.

Unrestrained *motor vehicle accidents.*

Treatment: Inform the parents that the clinic is required to report the suspected abuse. Treat the specific injury. Develop a multidisciplinary plan along with the US Department of Health and Human Services for parents and children.

Follow-up: Follow up as indicated for the presenting injury. Follow up as part of the multidisciplinary team, providing services for the child and family.

Sequelae: Child is at risk for permanent injury or death.

Prevention/Prophylaxis: Identification and education of high-risk parents in proper parenting skills. Support groups such as Parents Anonymous.

Referral: Consult with child protection authorities to initiate a multidisciplinary investigation. Report suspected abuse to local authorities. Hospitalize the child while investigation continues to determine the safety of the home environment.

Education: Teach proper parenting skills. Educate parents, caregivers, and baby sitters as to the hazards of shaking babies and the need to support the head at all times.

Schizophrenia

Schizophrenia is any group of psychotic disorders characterized by withdrawal from reality and illogical thought patterns, such as delusions and hallucinations. In adolescents, it is a chronic disorder.

Etiology: Unknown. Genetic patterns, defects of the frontal lobe, and dopamine imbalance have been suggested as etiological factors.

Occurrence: Rare. Estimated incidence is 1–2 in 10,000 under age 15 years.

Age: Onset occurs in children over age 5 to under age 15.

Ethnicity: Not significant.

Gender: Occurs equally in males and females.

Contributing Factors: Dysfunctional family relationships and a family history of schizophrenia may be contributing factors.

Signs and Symptoms: Child is brought to clinic because of somatic complaints or behavioral problems. Findings include rambling or illogical speech patterns, bizarre thought content, and hallucinations and/or delusions. Physical findings are within normal limits.

Diagnostic Tests

Drug screen for presence of illicit substances.
Metabolic screen for endocrinopathies.
Ceruloplasma levels (normal values are 23–43 mg/dL). Elevated levels, as are found in Wilson's disease, may cause psychiatric symptoms.
MRI and EEG to assess for brain tumors.
Before initiating antipsychotic pharmacotherapy, obtain a baseline CBC, liver function tests, and an ECG if patient has a history of cardiac disease or arrhythmias.

Differential Diagnosis

Normal growth and development: Children under age 8 normally have a vivid fantasy life; however, rambling speech and bizarre thought content are differentiating characteristics.

In adolescents, *learning disabilities* may mimic schizophrenia.

Mania in adolescents is characterized by increased activity, energy, and irritability.

In *Wilson's disease,* there may be psychiatric symptoms as a result of hepatic degeneration.

Treatment: The goal of treatment is to ease psychotic symptoms, reduce risk of relapse, teach skills, and support parents.

Behavioral

Training child in appropriate life, social, and cognitive skills through a structured day treatment center.

Pharmacological

Haloperidol: Beginning dose of 0.5–1 mg/day increasing by 0.5 mg every 3–5 days until there are clinical effects or side effects, up to a maximum of 4 mg/day. Dosage is usually twice a day. Effects may take 2–3 weeks to become fully apparent. Before initiating drug regimen, examine for abnormal movements, and then watch for cognitive slowing and one or more extrapyramidal symptoms. Contraindicated in patients with poorly controlled seizures, cardiac arrhythmias, agranulocytosis, previous neuroleptic malignant syndrome, and tardive dyskinesia.

Clozapine: This drug is under investigation for children who do not respond to typical neuroleptics.

Follow-up: Monitor progress, in collaboration with the attending psychiatrist, every 3 months for signs of tardive dyskinesia.

Sequelae: Schizophrenia is a chronic disorder with remissions and exacerbations that impact on school and work performance as well as social interactions and relationships.

Prevention/Prophylaxis: None.

Referral: Consult with and refer patient to a psychiatrist.

Education: Provide support for family, emphasizing the provision of a calm environment and the importance of clear communication. Instruct parents about dosage, purpose, and side effects of medications.

Self-Injurious Behavior

Self-injurious behaviors range from the mild piercing of ears to the more severe suicidal behaviors.

Suicide is a self-injurious behavior that functions as a maladaptive attempt to actively solve a problem. It has been suggested that 70% of children have experienced a loss, a failure, or an arrest prior to attempting suicide. Prior to attempts, children may appear depressed and irritable, may withdraw from social activities, and show a loss of interest in usual activities. The incidence of suicide in adolescents and young adults tripled between 1952 and 1992.

Self-mutilation is the participation in the deliberate destruction of body tissue without suicidal intent; it is considered a form of self-directed violence.

Etiology

Suicide: Sadness, despair, and depression account for 50% of suicides; anger represents 20% of impulsive suicides; and substance abuse accounts for 20%. The remaining 10% are due to unknown causes. Firearms, hanging, carbon monoxide poisoning, and deliberate drug overdose are the most common methods in successful suicides.

Self-mutilation: A biologically driven behavior; a response to psychological and environmental stressors.

Occurrence

Suicide: Second leading cause of death in the 15–24 age group. Attempts outnumber success 100:1; under 14 years of age, for completed attempts, the rate is 0.7 in 100,000; for adolescents 15–19 years, the rate is 11.3 per 10,000; there are 50–100 attempts for every success.

Self-mutilation: Underreported, but some studies have found 750 cases per 100,000 in the general population of adolescents and adults. Becoming more common; it seems to parallel the increase in child abuse.

Age

Suicide: May occur in preschool children, but it is more common in adolescents.

Self-mutilation: Usually begins in adolescence.

Ethnicity

Suicide: Highest suicide rate is in white adolescent males.

Self-mutilation: Not known.

Gender

Suicide: Prepubertal males and adolescent females are the most likely to attempt/succeed. Females outnumber males in attempts, but males are more successful in completing the act.

Self-mutilation: Appears to be more frequent in females.

Contributing Factors

Self-injurious behaviors: Alcohol or drug abuse; psychosis; poor impulse control; parental conflict; previous attempts; family history of suicide; experiences that lead to guilt, shame, or humiliation; situations where the child feels trapped, helpless and hopeless; suicides among the circle of friends.

Self-mutilation: Organic conditions such as Lesch-Nyhan disease and Tourette's syndrome; severely retarded patients, particularly if they are institutionalized; overwhelming stress; pathological childhood experiences such as sexual and physical abuse. May be associated with substance abuse, bulimia, or anorexia.

Signs and Symptoms

History

Suicide: There may be a history of past or present suicide threats or gestures, reports of giving away personal possessions; or a written statement where life is described as futile.

Self-mutilation: Multiple episodes of nonlethal self-injury, usually with a razor blade, but any sharp object may be used. The forearm (opposite the handedness) is the foremost site, but any part of the body is subject of the self-cutting. Criteria for diagnosis has been suggested by Fovazza and Rosenthal (1993): (1) Preoccupation with physically harming self, (2) recurring failure to control impulse to do bodily harm (repetitive addictive acts), (3) feelings of tension that increase before the act, (4) feelings of gratification or relief during and after the act, (5) the act not associated with suicidal intent or in response to hallucinations or delusions.

Physical Examination

Suicide: Findings may reveal a child who appears depressed. Other physical findings are not significant. Questions to be asked during the interview for assessment of suicide risk should include: How have you been feeling (inside and outside) (feelings of hopelessness, helplessness, wanting to give up)? Have you been feeling "down" or discouraged (how often, how long, and how severe)? Do these feelings interfere with your life (school, home, eating, sleeping)? Have you ever thought of suicide? Have you ever made a plan (include means)? Is there someone to whom you can go for help? Inquire about any loss or a suicide attempt or success among the child's circle of friends.

Self-mutilation: Rule out organic disorders whose behaviors include self-injury. Typically, Tourette's syndrome manifests in head banging; in Lesch-Nyhan disease the manifestation is finger biting; mental retardation may take the form of scratching, biting self, and head banging. Rule out psychiatric disorders. Common manifestations in obsessive-compulsive behavior are hair pulling and skin picking; in schizophrenia the form taken is usually in response to the "voices." Assess for anxiety, depression, stressors, and family history of trauma. Explore with the patient other forms of addictive behavior such as substance abuse.

Diagnostic Tests: None.

Differential Diagnosis: None.

Treatment

Behavioral

Suicide

Consider any threat or attempt serious, and do not leave child alone.

Meet and discuss the situation with the parent and the child. Listen to the child and the parents as they describe their feelings and perceptions.

Individual counseling for suicide threats and attempts is often appropriate.

Admit to hospital immediately if you determine the potential for suicide is high, in severe depression and intoxication, and where concern for the child's safety is paramount.

Self-mutilation: Any behavioral interventions should include improving communication skills, raising self-esteem, identifying a support group, and finding persons the patient can turn to for individual support.

Follow-up: Monitor any medication with which an underlying depression or other behavior is being treated.

Sequelae: Actual death, either intended or accidental. Aborted or incomplete suicide attempts may result in permanent injury.

Prevention/Prophylaxis: Treatment for depression. Active life-skill education for those identified as high risk.

Referral: Refer child and parents to a mental health professional immediately.

Education: Reassure parents and child that the problem(s) are understood. Educate parents and general public in the signs and symptoms of at-risk behaviors.

Sexual Abuse

Sexual abuse is the engaging of a child in sexual activities that are not understood by the child (i.e., the child cannot give informed consent) and that violate sexual taboos. Activities include exhibitionism, fondling, child pornography, and oral, anal, and genital contact. The categories of sexual abuse may or may not include the following:

Incest: Sexual abuse by a close relative that includes sexual intercourse.
Molestation: Sexual abuse by a stranger that may or may not include penetration.
Rape: Forced genital contact.
Sexual assault: Violent or nonviolent manual, oral, or genital contact.

Etiology: Pedophilia or a family structure that considers incest normal.

Occurrence: There are 250,000 reported cases per year; severe and/or chronic cases of child abuse are found in 1–3% of children. Majority of offenders are male; adolescents constitute 20% of offenders.

Age: All pediatric age groups.

Ethnicity: Not significant.

Gender: The majority of victims are female.

Contributing Factors: Fear of perpetrator, low self-esteem, and ignorance of what is acceptable touching behavior by family members and/or strangers.

Signs and Symptoms: Child may be brought to the clinic because the parent suspects the child has been or is currently being sexually abused; for example, the parent may report a sexualized play in a developmentally immature child, or the child has related events that are compatible with such a diagnosis, such as "He plays with my bottom, and sticks his finger in there." Males may exhibit inappropriate sexual behavior, suicidal ideation, and concentration deficits.

The parent may report behavioral changes, such as sleep disturbances, nightmares, or night terrors; appetite disturbances (e.g., anorexia, bulimia); nocturnal enuresis; neurotic or conduct disorders; withdrawal, guilt, or depression; temper tantrums, aggressive behavior, suicidal ideation, or threats of running away; hysterical or conversion reactions; or excessive masturbation.

The school may have referred the child to the clinic because of inappropriate classroom behaviors.

Older children may be brought to clinic because of substance abuse, suspected promiscuity, prostitution, or sexual abuse of other children by the victim.

Medical conditions or complaints that might lead one to suspect sexual abuse are recurrent abdominal pain; genital, urethral, or anal trauma; sexually transmitted diseases; recurrent urinary tract infections; enuresis or encopresis; or pregnancy.

Referrals may also be made to the clinic by protective services or law enforcement, usually as a result of a complaint by a parent.

Any history taking—whether it is a discussion with the child to investigate a definite complaint or a direct discussion because of what is suspected—should be done in a compassionate, nonjudgmental manner, with consideration for the age and developmental level of the child. Issues to be discussed are who the perpetrator is or was, the relation to the victim, the duration of the abusive situation, and what was done to the child. Neither the NP nor the person accompanying the child should prompt the child by posing leading or suggestive questions. Use of a doll with body parts and a child's drawings of self and family may facilitate the history taking.

Physical findings may be negative or nonspecific for abuse. Possible indicators of sexual abuse include bruises to the hard or soft palate, grasp marks, and the presence of a foreign body in the vagina or rectum. Perform a vaginal examination in the young child; the knee-chest position is a good position for viewing. In the older child, use the lithotomy position. Findings that are consistent with sexual abuse are disruptions of hymenal tissue (e.g., clefts or notches, absence of hymen, scars), anal scars, or skin tags outside the midline. The anus may be dilated 15–20 mm, and there will be absence of stool in the ampulla. Children who have been previously abused may have labial adhesions, edema of the perineal tissues, and perianal fissures. In prepubertal males, maintenance of a penile erection during the examination may be seen.

Diagnostic Tests: The laboratory evaluation of the sexually abused child must include the collection of specimens that will be acceptable as forensic evidence. Obtain the following:

A wet mount of vaginal, oral, and rectal specimens for motile sperm.

An aspirate of cervical mucus for motile sperm.

Rectal, throat, urethral, vaginal, and/or endocervical cultures for *Neisseria gonorrhoeae.*

Throat, rectal, urethral, vulvovaginal cultures for *Chlamydia trachomatis.*

Blood for serological tests for syphilis; dark-field examination if chancre is present.

A wet mount and culture of vaginal discharge (if present) for *Trichomonas vaginalis.*

Wet mount of vaginal discharge for bacterial vaginosis.

Culture for herpes simplex virus and biopsy for human papillomavirus if herpetic lesion is present.

If possible, blood for hepatitis B and human immunodeficiency virus (HIV) from the perpetrator; blood for HIV from child at time of abuse and 3, 6, and 12 months later.

Blood or urine for pregnancy test if child is postmenarchal.

Specimens for police report, if indicated. If there was a struggle, fingernail scrapings for blood or fabric. Collection of loose hairs or threads of fabric from the body or clothing. Collection of air-dried specimens from the vagina, cervix, rectum, and mouth for testing for sperm antibodies, blood, and acid phosphatase. Inspection of the body and clothing for fluorescence of sperm using a Wood lamp.

Differential Diagnosis: Related to somatic complaints that may have brought the child to the clinic.

Normal Sex Play versus Sexual Abuse

Normal sex play occurs among children of the same developmental and cognitive levels. The children may play "house" or "doctor," touching their own or each others' genitals. The children have agreed to this infrequent activity. They feel guilty about their play, which is a normal response, and no physical injury results.

Suspect child abuse if there is an age gap in a relationship between a younger child and an older child (or young adult): for example, if the younger child is under 13, a 5-year age difference is suspicious; if the younger child is over 13, suspect a 10-year age difference. (*Note:* If the younger child has cognitive impairment, the age differences may be less.) In such cases, there is coercion either by force or emotional pressure to complete the act, and the activity is not consistent with the developmental levels of the participants. The victim has a negative response, such as anger or fear. There is documented evidence of a physical injury as a result of the activity.

Treatment

Nonpharmacological

Child and family need extensive counseling from a mental health professional.

Pharmacological

Infections:

Sexually transmitted diseases (see Chapter 11).

Recurrent urinary infections (see Chapter 10).

Nonspecific vaginitis (see Chapter 11).

Risk of pregnancy: Norgestrel and ethinyl estradiol (Oruval), two tablets at the time of examination and two tablets 12 hours later (may prevent pregnancy within 72 hours of sexual intercourse).

Empiric treatment if perpetrator cannot be found:

Ceftriaxone, 125 mg intramuscularly (IM), for gonorrhea or incubating syphilis.

Erythromycin, 40–50 mg/kg per day for 14 days, for *Chlamydia.*

Hepatitis B immunoglobulin, 0.5 mL IM for hepatitis B.

Follow-up: Patient should return in 10 days for evaluation of therapeutic response in cases of infection. Obtain a serological test for syphilis in 6 weeks.

Sequelae: Children who have a history of sexual abuse are at risk for becoming perpetrators. Some also develop low self-esteem and/or eating disorders, attempt or commit suicide, and engage in shoplifting and/or prostitution.

Prevention/Prophylaxis: Effective parental education in appropriate parenting skills. Teaching children about what constitutes inappropriate touching behavior by another person.

Referral: Referral/report to Department of Health and Human Services for follow-up of family. The police should also be notified. May wish to refer patient to a pediatrician specializing in sexual abuse cases for initial workup and court appearance as the expert witness.

Child may need to be admitted to the hospital for treatment of injuries and for personal safety. Refer the offender for treatment of psychological problems.

Education: Teach children what constitutes—and how to protect themselves against—inappropriate touching behavior from others. Teach parent effectiveness training. Educate the community regarding the prevalence of this problem and the ultimate outcomes.

Substance Abuse

Substance abuse is the use and misuse of habituating substances in a manner that deviates from social norms. Current drugs of choice are alcohol, marijuana, and cocaine. Substance abuse may be classified as follows:

Experimental: Infrequent, episodic use of a variety of drugs, with peers, that causes no problems at home, school, or work.

Recreational: Episodic use of tobacco, alcohol, or marijuana, with peers, with the intent to become accepted or feel at ease.

Circumstantial: Repeated use of drugs as a coping mechanism, because of a learned association between use and decreased feelings of stress and/or anxiety. Can lead to physical or psychological dependency.

Habitual: Substances and their use involves all areas of life; drug use is its own reward.

Compulsive: Physiologic addiction to the substance(s); child is unable to stop using without intervention. This type of addiction requires a multifaceted approach to treatment with multiple personal changes. Children and adolescents can become addicted in 1–4 years as compared to adult men, who may be social drinkers for 20–30 years before showing addictive behaviors.

Etiology: Failure to develop appropriate coping skills.

Occurrence: Before finishing high school, two thirds of teen-agers will have tried some illicit drug, almost 100% will have tried alcohol, and 40% will have tried a drug other than marijuana. Of high school seniors, 5% smoke cigarettes daily and/or drink daily. There are 3.3 million teen-agers who are problem drinkers.

Age: Adolescence primarily, but is occurring increasingly in younger age groups.

Ethnicity: Not significant.

Gender: Occurs equally in males and females. There is an increase in the use of diet pills in females and cocaine use in males.

Contributing Factors: Age at first use is correlated with a higher probability of continued use and abuse; low self-esteem, poor coping mechanisms, peer pressure, and a family history of substance abuse have been implicated. Other risk factors identified are friends who drink, a history of physical or sexual abuse, previous report of running away, threats, impulsivity, and the need for instant gratification.

Signs and Symptoms: The adolescent rarely comes to the clinic asking for help, but presents with symptoms related to organ systems affected by substance use or abuse. They may have presented previously in an emergency room because of intoxication and/or overdose states and have been referred for follow-up (Fig. 15–5).

The teen-ager is often in denial, as are the parents, so it is necessary to confront the family openly regarding the issue of drug use, when suspected. Use of alcohol and drugs is often considered by society normal experimentation for this age group. When taking the history of substance abuse, include questions related to types of drugs used, timing (e.g., daily, weekends), settings (e.g., alone, with friends), circumstances (e.g., to be accepted, to cope), and outcomes (e.g., problems with family, peers, school, law enforcement, work).

Few physical findings are associated with chronic use or abuse of substances in children. Alcohol use may cause gastritis and pancreatitis. Use of marijuana and tobacco is associated with bronchitis. Cocaine use may cause palpitations and chest pains. Serial observations that reveal changes in the teen-ager's appearance and emotional tone may be the first clue that he or she is using or abusing substances (Fig. 15–6).

Diagnostic Tests: The CAGE questionnaire is an easy screening tool for alcohol and substance abuse. (CAGE refers to the self-questions: "Have you ever

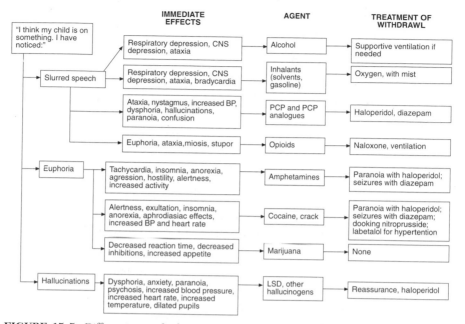

FIGURE 15–5 Differentiation of substances and treatment of withdrawal. (BP = blood pressure; CNS = central nervous system; LSD = lysergic acid diethylamide; PCP = phencyclidine hydrochloride.)

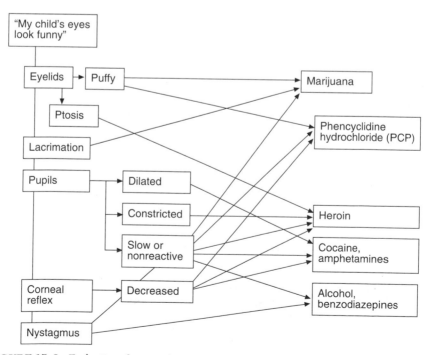

FIGURE 15–6 Evaluation of eyes to detect type of substance abuse.

felt you should **C**ut down on your drinking? Have people **A**nnoyed you by criticizing your drinking? Have you ever felt **G**uilty about your drinking? Do you ever have an **E**ye opener first thing in the morning?) Two or more positive responses indicate possible abuse. Drug screens are appropriate only when the patient presents with acute intoxication.

Differential Diagnosis: A variety of complaints related to substance abuse may bring the child to the clinic (unless they present as a result of overdose or withdrawal). Those complaints need to be evaluated and the child confronted as to the use of substances. The adolescent substance abuser is at risk for multiple problems. The normal risk-taking behavior of adolescents is enhanced by the addition of chemicals to the system (e.g., motor vehicle accidents due to driving under the influence [DUI]). Examples of medical complications are tachycardia in cocaine users, gastritis related to alcohol use, cerebral ataxia from the inhalation of toluene, and extreme fatigue after amphetamine use.

Treatment

   Mild (experimental): Anticipatory guidance as to future outcomes, education related to use and abuse, and exploration of drug-free alternatives.

   Moderate (recreational): Participation in a drug-free support group, and individual and family therapy. Continued relationship with patients as they participate in drug-free living.

   Severe (circumstantial, habitual, or compulsive): Participation in a formalized treatment program separated from drugs and drug-using peer group. Continued relationship with patients as they participate in drug-free living.

Follow-up: Weekly visits until stabilized. Let patients know that you are there to support them in their new behaviors.

Sequelae: Medical consequences of substance use and abuse include blackouts, trauma and accidental injury, intoxication, and overdose.

   Social consequences include conflicts with family, loss of friends, impulsive behavior (promiscuity, destruction of property, fighting), and automobile accidents. Disciplinary actions taken because of school problems, DUI incidents, and thefts are also negative outcomes.

Prevention/Prophylaxis: Collaborate with school officials to increase the awareness of the dangers of drugs in children from kindergarten through twelfth grade. Teach life skills programs for at-risk teen-agers to increase their self-esteem and to enable them to learn appropriate coping mechanisms.

Referral: Refer patient for outpatient or inpatient treatment or to an alcohol and drug rehabilitation service. Refer client and family to a 12-step program (e.g., Alcoholics Anonymous, Narcotics Anonymous, Al-Anon). Refer patient and family to a mental health professional for individual and family therapy.

Education: Teach programs in schools to educate teen-agers regarding the dangers and outcomes of substance abuse. Support parents as they work through their feelings of guilt and shame.

Temper Tantrums

Temper tantrums are a common expression of anger and frustration at ages 12 months to 4 years, as children attempt to gain mastery over their environment.

Etiology: In some children, temper tantrums seem to be related to their temperament, whereas other children innately have a higher tolerance for frustration and ability to cope with difficult experiences.

Occurrence: Occur weekly in 50–80% of children under 4; in 5–20% of these cases the tantrums are severe enough to be considered developmentally inappropriate.

Age: Occur primarily in children aged 1–4, but many occur in older age groups such as when children are immature for a particular age and have a developmental disorder.

Ethnicity: Not significant.

Gender: Occur equally in males and females.

Contributing Factors: Frustrations brought about by environmental conditions (e.g., crowding), physical limitations (e.g., hearing loss, speech or language delay, hyperactivity), or side effects of medications. Some tantrums appear to be related to the child's temperament. Poor parenting skills may be a factor in that the child learns to use the tantrums as a means of gain (i.e., negative behavior is continually reinforced).

Signs and Symptoms: Child presents with the following history: When demands are not met, child may kick, scream, and throw self on floor, or may throw objects. Physical examination is negative.

Diagnostic Tests: None.

Differential Diagnosis: None.

Treatment

Behavioral

Give parents guidelines for modifying their child's behavior, such as the following:

Construct an environment with a minimum of restrictions so that conflict will be reduced and the need to say "no" will be limited.

Use distraction when the child's frustration level increases.

Reward child's positive responses.

Present the child with choices and options within a developmental framework to help him or her gain mastery over such situations.

If the child loses control and needs time to regain it, use the "time out" technique.

Do not use threats, because they serve no purpose.

Do not allow the child to hurt self or others.

Do not give in to the child's demands.

Do not overreact to the episode, but set reasonable limits and provide direction for the child.

Pharmacological

None.

Follow-up: None.

Sequelae: Loss of control.

Prevention/Prophylaxis: No medical intervention. Behavioral intervention should be instituted (see Treatment).

Referral: None. If, however, tantrums exceed what is appropriate for age and developmental level, refer child to a pediatric developmental specialist.

Education: Teach parents effective behavior-modification techniques and parenting skills.

REFERENCES

General

Behrman, R, and Kliegman, R (eds): Nelson Essentials of Pediatrics. WB Saunders, Philadelphia, 1990.
Doenges, M, and Moorhouse, M: Nursing Diagnoses with Interventions, ed 4. FA Davis, Philadelphia, 1993.
Green, M: Pediatric Diagnosis: Interpretation of Symptoms & Signs in Infants, Children and Adolescents, ed 5. WB Saunders, Philadelphia, 1992, p 443.
Hay, W, et al (eds): Current Pediatric Diagnosis & Treatment, ed 12. Appleton & Lange, Norwalk, Conn, 1995.
Jarvis, C: Physical Examination and Health Assessment. WB Saunders, Philadelphia, 1992.
Stockman, J: Difficult Diagnosis in Pediatrics. WB Saunders, Philadelphia, 1990, p 142.

Anorexia

Danziger, Y, et al: Stunting of growth in anorexia nervosa during the prepubertal and pubertal period. Isr J Med Sci 30:581, 1994.
Kearney-Cooke, A, and Striegel-Moore, RH: Treatment of childhood sexual abuse in anorexia nervosa and bulimia nervosa: A feminist psychodynamic approach. Int J Eating Disorders 15:305, 1994.
Rosen, D: Eating disorders. Female Patient 20(9):12, 1995.
Vitousek, K, and Manke, F: Personality variables and disorders in anorexia nervosa and bulimia nervosa. J Abnorm Psychol 103:137, 1994.
Williams, R: Use of the Eating Attitudes Test and Eating Disorder Inventory in adolescents. J Adolesc Health Care 8:266, 1987.

Anxiety

Baughan, D: Barriers to diagnosing anxiety disorders in family practice. Am Fam Phys 52:447, 1995.

Attention Deficit/Hyperactivity Disorder

American Psychiatric Association: Diagnostic and Statistical Manual of Mental Disorders, ed 4. Washington, DC, 1994.
Buncher, P: Attention-deficit/hyperactivity disorder: A diagnosis for the '90s. Nurse Pract 21(6):43, 1996.
Fowler, M: Attention Deficit Disorder. NICHCY Briefing Paper. National Information Center for Children and Youth with Disabilities, Washington, DC, 1991.
Murphy, K: Coping strategies for ADHD adults. CHADDER Fall/Winter. 10, 1992.
Nahlik, J: New thoughts on attention-deficit/hyperactivity disorder. Hosp Pract 30(4):49, 1995.
Schnelle, E: Attention deficit disorder. Adv Nurse Pract 2(3);9, 1994.
Schvehla, TJ, et al: Clonidine therapy for comorbid attention deficit hyperactivity disorder and conduct disorder: Preliminary findings in a children's inpatient unit. South Med J 89(7):87, 1994.

Autistic Spectrum Disorder

American Psychiatric Association: Diagnostic and Statistical Manual of Mental Disorders, ed 4. Washington, DC, 1994.

Cascio, R, and Kilmon, C: Pervasive developmental disorder, not otherwise specified: Primary care perspectives. Nurse Pract 22:11, 1997.

Church, C, and Caplan, J: The high-functioning autistic experience; birth to preteen years. J Ped Health Care 9(1):22, 1995.

Fisman, S, and Steele, M: Use of risperidone in pervasive developmental disorders: A case series. J Child Adolesc Psychopharmacol 6:177, 1996.

Green, M: Pediatric Diagnosis: Interpretation of Symptoms & Signs in Infants, Children and Adolescents. WB Saunders, Philadelphia, 1992.

Hay, W, et al (eds.): Current Pediatric Diagnosis & Treatment, ed 12. Appleton and Lange, Norwalk, Conn, 1995.

Lotspeich, L, and Ciaranello, R: The neurobiology and genetics of infantile autism. Int Rev Neurobiol 35:87, 1993.

Mauk, J: Autism and pervasive developmental disorders. Pediatr Clin North Am 40:567, 1993.

McDougle, C, et al: Risperidone treatment of children and adolescents with pervasive developmental disorders: A prospective open-label study. J Am Acad Child Adolesc Psychiatry 36:685, 1997.

Peak, J, et al: Oral manifestation of Rett's syndrome. Br Dent J 172:248, 1992.

Shannon, M, and Graef, J: Lead intoxication in children with pervasive developmental disorders. J Toxicol Clin Toxicol 34:177, 1996.

Stockman, J: Difficult Diagnosis in Pediatrics. WB Saunders, Philadelphia, 1990.

Yirmiya, N, Sigman, M, and Freeman, BJ: Comparison between diagnostic instruments for identifying high-functioning children with autism. J Autism and Dev Disord 24(3):281, 1994.

Bulimia

Muscari, M: Primary care of adolescents with bulimia nervosa. J Ped Health Care 10:17, 1996.

Olsen, C, and Lemkau, J: The bulimic patient: Psychosocial and medical issues. Fam Pract Recert 13(1):93, 1991.

Rosen, D: Eating disorders. Female Patient 20(9):12, 1995.

Vitousek, K, and Manke, F: Personality variables and disorders in anorexia nervosa and bulimia nervosa. J Abnormal Psychol 103:137, 1994.

Williams, R: Use of the Eating Attitudes Test and Eating Disorder Inventory in adolescents. J Adolesc Health Care 8:266, 1987.

Depression

Green, M: Maternal depression: Bad for children's health. Contemp Pediatr 10:28, 1993.

Lizardi, H, et al: Reports of the childhood home environment in early-onset dysthymia and episodic major depression. J Abnorm Psychol 104:132, 1995.

Shaughnessy, A: Considerations in antidepressant therapy. Fam Pract Recert 17(4):31, 1995.

Failure to Thrive

Black, MM, et al: Randomized clinical trial of home intervention for children with failure to thrive. Pediatrics 95:807, 1995.

MacPhee, M, and Hoffenberg, E: Nursing case management for children with failure to thrive. J Pediatr Health Care 10(2):63, 1996.

Roesler, TA, et al: Factitious food allergy and failure to thrive. Arch Pediatr Adolesc Med 148:1150, 1994.

Schwartz, R, and Abegglen, J: Failure to thrive: An ambulatory approach. Nurse Pract 21(5):19, 1996.

Smith, MM, and Lifshitz, F: Excess fruit juice consumption as a contributing factor in nonorganic failure to thrive. Pediatrics 93:438, 1994.

Munchausen Syndrome by Proxy

Castiglia, P: Munchausen syndrome by proxy. J Pediatr Health Care 9:79, 1995.

Crouse, K: Munchausen syndrome by proxy: Recognizing the victim. Pediatr Nurs 18(3):249, 1992.
Wide, J, and Pedroni, AT: Privacy rights in Munchausen syndrome. Contemp Pediatr 10: 83, 1993.

Physical Abuse

Chiocca, E: Shaken baby syndrome: A nursing perspective. Pediatr Nurs 21(1):33, 1995.

Schizophrenia

Frazier, JA, et al: An open trial of clozapine in 11 adolescents with childhood-onset schizophrenia. J
    Am Acad Child Adolesc Psychiatry 33:658, 1994.
McKenna, K, et al: Looking for childhood-onset schizophrenia: The first 71 cases screened. J Am
    Acad Child Adolesc Psychiatry 33:636, 1994.
Towbin, KE, et al: Clozapine for early developmental delays with childhood-onset schizophrenia:
    Protocol and 15-month outcome. J Am Acad Child Adolesc Psychiatry 33:651, 1994.

Self-Injurious Behavior

Barstow, D: Self-injury and self-mutilation. Nursing approaches. J Psychosoc Nurs Ment Health Serv
    33:19, 1995.
Behrman, R, and Kliegman, R (eds): Nelson Essentials of Pediatrics. WB Saunders, Philadelphia, 1990.
Centers for Disease Control: Suicide among children, adolescents, and young adults—United States,
    1980–1992. MMWR Morbidity Mortality Weekly Report 44(15):289, 1995.
Dallam, S: The identification and management of self-mutilating patients in primary care. Nurse
    Pract 22(5):151, 1997.
Favazza, A, and Rosenthal, R: Diagnostic issues in self-mutilation. Hosp Comm Psychiatry 44(2):134,
    1993.
Faye, P: Addictive characteristics of the behavior of self-mutilation. J Psychosoc Nurs Ment Health
    Serv 33:36, 1995.
Green, M: Pediatric Diagnosis: Interpretation of Symptoms & Signs in Infants, Children and Adoles-
    cents, ed 5. WB Saunders, Philadelphia, 1992.
Hay, W, Groothuis, J, Hayward, A, and Levin, M. (eds): Current Pediatric Diagnosis & Treatment.
    Appleton and Lange, Norwalk, Conn, 1995.
Stockman, J: Difficult Diagnosis in Pediatrics. WB Saunders, Philadelphia, 1990.

Sexual Abuse

American Academy of Pediatrics: Guidelines for the Evaluation of Sexual Abuse of Children. Pedi-
    atrics 87:87, 1988.
Batash, A: What office-based pediatricians need to know about child sexual abuse. Contemp Pediatr
    11:83, 1994.
Elliott, A, and Peterson, L: Maternal sexual abuse of male children. Postgrad Med 94:169, 1993.
Elliott, D, and Smiljanich, K: Sex offending among juveniles: Development and response. J Pediatr
    Health Care 8(3):101, 1994.
Peterson, LW, et al: The use of children's drawings in the evaluation and treatment of child sexual,
    emotional, and physical abuse. Arch Fam Med 4:445, 1995.
Steele, R: The Clinical Handbook of Pediatric Infectious Disease. Parthenon, New York, 1994.

Substance Abuse

Brent, J: Drugs of abuse: An update. Emerg Med 27(7):56, 1995.
Caulker-Burnett, I: Primary care screening for substance abuse. Nurse Pract 19(6):42, 1994.
Fahey, P, and Gabel, L: Substance abuse in teens: Detection and early management. Fam Pract Re-
    cert 17(4):13, 1995.
Westreich, L, and Rosenthal, R: Physical examination of substance abusers. Postgrad Med 97(4):111,
    1995.

CHAPTER **16**

HEMATOLOGIC AND

IMMUNOLOGIC

ASSESSMENT

Infectious disorders are probably the most common reason that children require medical attention. Although hematologic and immune disorders are not as common, they should be considered in certain high-risk groups, such as those genetically predisposed to hematologic disorders, or children of mothers who are drug users or who engage in high-risk behaviors. Any suspected disorders require a thorough investigation.

Assessment for suspected hematologic, immunologic, or infectious disorders begins with a thorough history including the following information:

Past medical history: Particularly note the use of medications, chronic or recurrent symptoms or illnesses, previous blood transfusions and reactions, or history of nutritional deficiencies. Note any exposure to toxic substances, such as lead, or infectious agents including human immunodeficiency virus (HIV) and hepatitis.

Family history: Include history of anemia, excessive bleeding or bruising, or cancer.

Current history: Establish whether the current complaint is acute or chronic; the events surrounding the onset of the problem; what brings on the symptoms and what relieves them; the time course or the intensity of the problem; and related symptoms. Young children in day care have a greater frequency of exposure to infections. Also note any current medications (over-the-counter and prescription) the patient is taking. In the adolescent, ask about alcohol and/or drug use and participation in risky behaviors that can increase exposure to infectious agents. In the female adolescent, note excessive menstrual blood loss.

Nutritional history: Note normal dietary patterns.

The most common assessment findings associated with hematologic, immune, and infectious disorders include the following:

Abnormal bleeding or bleeding tendency (e.g., involving skin, mucous membranes, stool).

Dyspnea.

Edema.

Excessive bruising.

Fatigue and weakness.

Fever.

Headache.

Hypotension.

Joint pain.

Lymphadenopathy (swollen, enlarged, or tender lymph nodes).

Pallor (in dark-skinned patient, assess palpebral conjunctiva for pallor).

Paresthesia.

Skin rashes or changes.

Tachycardia or bradycardia.

Weight loss.

A basic evaluation of blood components is the first step in assessing hematologic conditions. A simple procedure, the complete blood count (CBC), may reveal clinical abnormalities and the presence of infection. If disorders are suspected, a peripheral smear will reveal changes in cell morphology. Recommendations for the timing of routine evaluation of blood components are included in the health screening recommendations. A hemoglobin or a hematocrit should be obtained from children at 6 months, 24 months, 8 years, and again at 18 years of age.

Blood disorders are usually manifested by an increase or decrease in cells, or are related to other blood factors. Changes in the values of the red blood cell number and size (RBCs) and white blood cells (WBCs) may indicate an underlying physical illness, such as an infection, as well as a condition specific to the blood component. Specific blood cell disorders are of two types: primary and secondary. Primary disorders involve those conditions related to mature cells, cell membranes, hemoglobin synthesis, or cellular enzymes. Secondary disorders are related to nutrition, the immune system, neoplasms, drugs, or genetics (Fig. 16–1).

The following normal variations are noted in the pediatric client:

Age: Blood cell counts rise above adult levels at birth and decline gradually throughout childhood.

Sex: Hemoglobin and hematocrit levels are slightly higher in males over age 12.

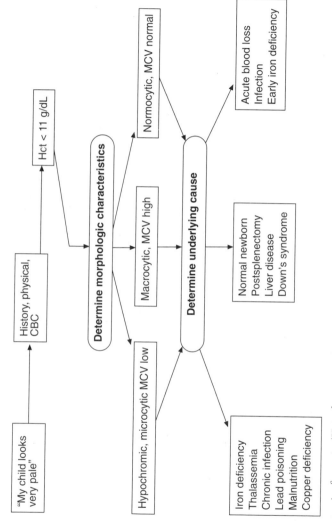

FIGURE 16–1 Diagnosis of anemia. (Hct = hematocrit; MCV = mean corpuscular volume.)

Race: African-American children generally have lower WBC counts.

Genetic screening may be indicated for children of parents who are at high risk for hemoglobinopathies (genetic disorders that affect the production and function of hemoglobin molecules, such as sickle cell disease and trait, the thalassemias, and other blood conditions). Genetic counseling should be provided, as indicated.

Iron Deficiency Anemia

Iron deficiency anemia (IDA) is a microcytic, hypochromic anemia resulting from an inadequate supply of iron for synthesis of hemoglobin. Anemia reduces the blood's capacity to combine with and transport oxygen to the peripheral tissues.

Etiology: A decreased hemoglobin concentration in RBCs, which in turn reduces the oxygen capacity of the blood, causes IDA. Inadequate stores of iron in the full-term infant can cause this problem in children under age 6 months. For some children, periods of rapid growth may also precipitate IDA.

Occurrence: The incidence is inversely proportional to socioeconomic status.

Age: IDA occurs in 17–44% of children between ages 6 weeks and 3 months; peak prevalence is found in children aged 10–15 months (25%).

Ethnicity: IDA is more prevalent among lower socioeconomic groups; a greater number of African-American children have IDA than other ethnic groups.

Gender: Not significant until puberty, at which point it is more frequent in females.

Contributing Factors: Preterm or low-birth-weight infants are at higher risk. If there has been fetal or perinatal blood loss without replacement, there is an increased likelihood of IDA. Children who consume large amounts of unfortified cow's milk or have poor dietary intake are also at risk, because these are low-iron-source food products.

Signs and Symptoms: The parent may relate any of the following risk factors: prematurity, low birth weight, or fetal or perinatal blood loss. They may also relate a history of irritability, decreased attention span, lethargy, anorexia, pica, headache, or learning problems.

On physical examination, there is mild to severe conjunctival pallor, mucous membranes are pale, poor growth or weight gain is noted, and palmar creases are pale. The child may appear small for age. The nails are flat, ridged, concave, and spoon-shaped, and they split easily. Splenomegaly may be noted on palpation or percussion. Hepatomegaly also may be noted. Auscultation reveals tachycardia and a systolic flow murmur.

Diagnostic Tests

Hemoglobin and hematocrit (H & H) will be decreased.

A hemogram can be performed; this will not only include an H & H, but also give the mean cell volume, reticulocyte count, WBC count, and platelet count.

Serum iron level is low.

Ferritin level is decreased.

Lead level may be elevated.

Free erythrocyte protoporphyrin level is increased.

Reticulocyte count is increased.

A peripheral blood smear can help determine the type of anemia.

Differential Diagnosis

Thalassemia, differentiated by hemoglobin electrophoresis.

Lead poisoning, differentiated by a lead level greater than 10.

Immune disorders that induce anemia, differentiated by a positive Coombs' test.

Sickle cell anemia, differentiated by electrophoresis.

Treatment: Supplemental iron is the most common treatment regimen, given at a dosage of 6 mg/kg per day in two divided doses. If this increases the hemoglobin by at least 1.0 g/dL in 1 month, this is considered diagnostic of IDA; therefore therapy is continued for at least 3 months.

Follow-up: Initially an H & H should be performed 1 month after treatment started, and then every month for no longer than 5 months to avoid iron overload.

Sequelae: Poor growth rate, learning problems, lethargy, and an increased incidence of infection are common. Iron overload can occur if the child is kept on supplemental iron therapy longer than 5–6 months.

Prevention/Prophylaxis: Routine screening should be done to identify children who have IDA or possibly other anemia. The schedule is as follows:

Ages 6–9 months.

Age 1 year and then yearly up to age 12.

Ages 13–20 every 2–3 years or if symptoms arise.

Referral: If hemoglobin does not increase at least 1.0 g/dL after 1 month of treatment, refer the child to a physician for further evaluation.

Education: Teach parents that absorption of iron is increased when taken on an empty stomach or given with vitamin C. Nausea, constipation, diarrhea, epigastric pain, and abdominal cramping are common side effects of iron therapy. If these occur, instruct them to administer iron after a meal. Teach parents safety precautions of iron administration, because iron overdose can be *fatal*. Teach them that iron can turn the stool black, and that they should administer the iron drops by putting the tip of the dropper in the back of the mouth to avoid staining the teeth.

Instruct parents to limit milk intake to 16 oz/day, limit empty caloric consumption, and increase age-appropriate, iron-rich foods.

Sickle Cell Anemia

Sickle cell disease is a term for a group of genetic disorders characterized by production of hemoglobin S (HbS), anemia, and acute and chronic tissue damage secondary to the blockage of blood flow produced by abnormally shaped cells. The sickling may develop spontaneously or may be precipitated by infection, exposure to cold, dehydration, low O_2 molecular tension acidosis, or localized hypoxia. Today 85% of all persons affected with HbSS will survive to age 20. The principle cause of death in infants with HbSS is overwhelming infections, cerebrovascular accident, and acute splenic sequestration crisis. Other sickle cell diseases include hemoglobin SC (HbSC) (1 in 835 African-Americans affected) and sickle beta-thalassemia (SB-thalassemia; 1 in 1667 African-Americans affected).

Etiology: Genetic causes as illustrated below are responsible for SS disease:

TRAIT (CARRIER)

Ss ss

Trait s _ Ss ss

(carrier) S _ SS Ss

FOR EACH BIRTH:

- 25% chance of having the disease.
- 25% chance of not having disease or being a carrier.
- 50% chance of being a carrier.

NO TRAIT OR DISEASE

Trait S _ Ss Ss

(carrier) s _ ss   ss

FOR EACH BIRTH:

- 50% chance of being a carrier.
- 50% chance of not being a carrier.

It is recommended that all infants at age 4 months, regardless of racial or ethnic background, be screened for sickle cell disease. There are three reasons:

1. Prophylactic penicillin can decrease mortality and morbidity.
2. It is impossible to define accurately a person's heritage by physical appearance or surname.
3. Screening should benefit all equally.

Screening should be linked to other newborn screening tests, if possible, to facilitate collection, identification, and handling. Clinical manifestations are minimal before age 4 months because of the presence of fetal hemoglobin.

Occurrence: Sickle cell anemia (HbSS) is the most common type of sickle cell disease, and it is estimated that it affects more than 50,000 Americans.

Age: Present at birth (genetically transmitted).

Ethnicity: Currently, approximately 1 in 375 African-Americans is affected with HbSS. Approximately 8% of the American population have sickle cell trait. Sickle cell anemia also affects persons from Mediterranean, Caribbean, South and Central American, Arabian, and East Indian descent.

Gender: Occurs equally in males and females.

Contributing Factors: Because HbSS is caused by an abnormal recessive mutation by the G-globin gene, the parents' genetic code is the most significant contributing factor.

Signs and Symptoms: The primary caregiver will report a history of poor growth with episodes of poor feeding and irritability. The child has a family history of sickle cell disease or trait. There may be periods of pain reported, which varies in severity. The parent may also give a history of frequent bouts of acute upper respiratory or gastrointestinal infections.

The health-care provider will observe that the child is small for age. There may be pronounced or mild scleral jaundice. Hands and feet may also be swollen. The child may appear pale, fatigued, or in pain. Splenomegaly and cardiomegaly (in older children) can be palpated. There may be pain on palpation of joints, abdomen, or sometimes in muscles. Severe abdominal pain with rebound may indicate gallbladder disease. When hemoglobin is extremely low, often a murmur is heard. Chest syndrome may also be heard—loose or dry hacking cough, and/or pneumonia.

In a vaso-occlusive crisis, there may be a painful, prolonged erection (priapism). The child may have fast or difficult breathing, chest pain, fever, rales, and decreased breath sounds. There may be loss of consciousness or dysfunction of an extremity (painful or not); for example, child may drag a foot or stop using a hand. The median age for stroke in these children is 7 years (Table 16–1; Fig. 16–2).

Diagnostic Tests

There is no one best method for screening. Several techniques are used. These include hemoglobin electrophoresis, isoelectric focusing, and high-performance liquid chromatography.

TABLE 16–1 SIGNS AND SYMPTOMS OF VASO-OCCLUSIVE CRISIS

Area	Signs and Symptoms
Hand-foot syndrome.	Patient under 5 years, painful swelling of hand and foot.
Bone crisis.	Painful bones, usually occurs at ages 3–4 years; rule out osteomyelitis.
Abdominal crisis.	Infarctions in liver, spleen, and lymph nodes.
Central nervous system crisis.	Convulsions, meningeal signs, cerebral infarction, blindness, vertigo, and acute mental syndrome.
Acute chest.	Pleuritic chest pain, dyspnea, fever; rule out pneumonitis.
Priapism.	Predisposing factors: sexual intercourse, masturbation, local trauma, and impotence.
Hematuria.	Mild, painless.
Interhepatic crisis.	Sudden onset of painful, enlarged liver; increase in bilirubin and liver enzyme levels.

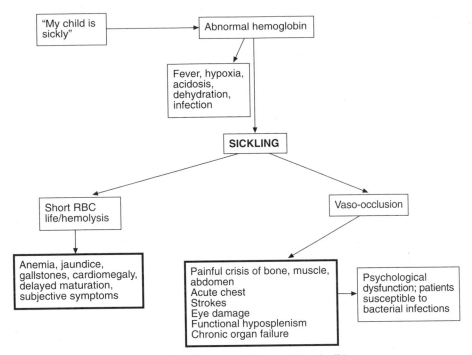

FIGURE 16–2   Evaluation of sickle cell anemia. (RBC = red blood cell.)

The initial screening sample should not be used to establish a definitive diagnosis: A second sample should be collected. Sickle cell trait should be identified to provide genetic counseling.

A baseline CBC, reticulocyte count, and peripheral smear should be done. A peripheral smear will contain target cells and sickled cells.

Erythrocyte sedimentation rates are slow, and platelet counts are increased.

Hemoglobin is decreased (usually less than 10).

Occasionally, liver function and renal function tests are done to reveal evidence of organ damage.

Differential Diagnosis

Rheumatoid arthritis produces an elevated antistreptolysin-O (ASO) titer.

Anemia (macrocytic or microcytic) is differentiated by CBC.

Thalassemia is differentiated by hemoglobin electrophoresis.

Pneumonia is seen on x-ray and not accompanied by other signs of sickle cell anemia.

Treatment: For children with sickle cell anemia, the well-child care should be provided on the same schedule as for disease-free patients; take each visit as an opportunity to reinforce previous teaching. Office visits are scheduled every other month for the first year of life, and then quarterly for the second year of life; the schedule after this depends on the severity of the disease. Penicillin prophylaxis should begin by age 2 months for infants suspected of definitive sickle cell disease (under age 3, 125 mg bid; over age 3, 250 mg bid). Fever in infants with sickle cell disease should be treated as an *emergency*. Parents should avoid giving aspirin, because it may increase acidosis; they should use acetaminophen.

Hydroxyurea, an antineoplastic drug, is currently being investigated for the palliative treatment of sickle cell disease. It is thought that because hydroxyurea increases the production of hemoglobin F, it will inhibit the polymerization of HbS.

Treatment of complications, specifically a vaso-occlusive crisis, includes the following:

Acute chest syndrome: Hospitalization, hydration, oxygen, antibiotics, and transfusions are indicated.

Stroke: Periodic RBC transfusions are the best therapy for preventing recurrence of stroke. Neurological workup should include magnetic resonance imaging (MRI) and transcranial ultrasound, if possible.

Hand-and-foot syndrome: Analgesics and hydration with application of warm compresses, massage, or warm baths may provide relief.

Priapism: Hospitalization, possible evacuation of pooled blood.

Severe abdominal pain: Hydration, analgesia, gallbadder x-ray, and hospitalization.

Acute splenic sequestration crisis: Immediate restoration of blood volume by RBC transfusion, possible splenectomy (after age 2 years).

Aplastic anemia: RBC transfusion.

Follow-up: Regular scheduled health care should be maintained, with all episodes of pain and fever being reported to the health-care provider.

Sequelae: Short stature or delayed physical growth and sexual maturation, stroke, pain, gallbladder disease, and multiple crises:

Acute splenic sequestration crisis: Sudden entrapment of a large portion of the blood volume in the spleen with cardiovascular compromise similar to hypovolemia (peak age, 6 months to 2 years).

Aplastic crisis: Temporary arrest of RBC production in the bone marrow, usually caused by a parvovirus infection (this is transient).

Prevention/Prophylaxis: None. This is a congenital, genetic disease.

Referral: Refer patient to a pediatric hematologist or the local sickle cell clinic for overall maintenance and during times of severe crisis. Otherwise, for routine care, the nurse practitioner can oversee the child's health regimen.

Education: Teach caregivers to recognize the signs and symptoms of the disease and to manage treatment on their own, provided the child is afebrile. Specific instructions should be given with regard to oral fluid therapy, analgesics, and antipyretics.

Teach caregivers the following precautions to minimize vaso-occlusive episodes: (1) Prevent dehydration (especially in warm weather); (2) shield child from the cold (slows circulation and increases stasis); and (3) make sure child avoids immersion in cold water, dresses warmly, gets adequate rest, and avoids wearing constrictive clothes.

Cat-Scratch Fever

Cat-scratch fever is characterized by regional lymphadenopathy following contact with cats or kittens who harbor the bacteria responsible for the disease. The nodes usually affected are the parotid, preauricular, axillary, epitrochlear, and inguinal. From the initial scratch to the primary cutaneous lesion to lymphadenopathy, there is a median incubation period of 12 days or in some cases as long as 50 days.

Etiology: A scratch from a cat harboring the causative agents, *Rochalimaea henselae* or *Afipier felis.*

Occurrence: Approximately 20,000 cases occur in the United States each year. Occurs more frequently in fall and winter.

Age: Occurs primarily in children and persons under 20.

Ethnicity: Not significant.

Gender: Occurs equally in males and females.

Contributing Factors: Contact with a cat or kittens.

Signs and Symptoms: Child presents with malaise, fatigue, and a low-grade fever. The parent or child provides information as to contact with a cat or kittens within the known incubation period.

Physical examination reveals a crusted papule, vesiculopustule, or ulcer at the site of the scratch or inoculation. There are enlarged, tender, single or multiple lymph nodes proximal to the scratch site.

Diagnostic Tests

Positive cat-scratch skin test (antigen may be difficult to obtain).

An incision and drainage should not be done because of the risk of chronic draining sinus. Thus, although not generally done, aspiration of the node and identification of the causative agent using Warther-Starry silver stain is a possible method.

Elevated erythrocyte sedimentation rate.

IgM–enzyme-linked immunosorbent assay (ELISA) for *Rochalimaea henselae* titers.

Differential Diagnosis: Infectious mononucleosis: presence of soft palate petechiae; enlargement of posterior and anterior cervical nodes.

Treatment: Trimethoprim-sulfamethoxazole, 20 mg/kg per day for 7 days, may be helpful; routine treatment not recommended.

Follow-up: Return in 1 week for evaluation of enlarged nodes and the primary lesion.

Sequelae: Rare complications include encephalitis, osteolytic lesions, hepatitis, or chronic systemic illness.

Prevention/Prophylaxis: None. All cat scratches should be cleansed thoroughly to decrease the risk of infection.

Referral: None, unless the progression of the recovery is not timely or the signs and symptoms of complications are observed.

Education: Teach children how to handle pets properly to reduce the risk of being scratched.

Cytomegalovirus

Cytomegalovirus (CMV) is a human herpesvirus transmitted by intrauterine transfer, maternal milk, secretions in the birth canal (incubation period 2–6 weeks), saliva of playmates, sexual partners, transfusions (incubation period of 2–4 weeks), and transplanted organs. Infection may range from acute, severe illness to a mild, self-limiting illness. The virus is harbored in the body and may be reactivated.

Etiology: CMV infection through intrauterine or milk transfer or contact with secretions harboring the virus, such as saliva and urine.

Occurrence: Estimated congenital infection is 1–2% of all newborns; 10% of these are symptomatic and an estimated 75% of day-care children are viral excreters.

Age: The infection may occur during the perinatal period; it can be found in newborns, older children, adolescents, and immunosuppressed children.

Ethnicity: Not significant.

Gender: Occurs equally in males and females.

Contributing Factors: Infection of the mother during the first half of pregnancy, infection in the birth canal, viral shedding in maternal milk, blood transfusions, contact with secretions of infected children.

Signs and Symptoms

Congenital infections: Hepatosplenomegaly, jaundice, purpura, microcephaly, cerebral calcifications, chorioretinitis, petechial rash with splenomegaly on first day of life, spasticity, and hypertonia.

Acquired infections: Pneumonia; paroxysmal, nonproductive cough; no chest pain; and fatigue, myalgia, and headache.

Diagnostic Tests

Newborn

CBC reveals anemia, thrombocytopenia, and lymphocytosis.
Spinal fluid reveals elevated protein and pleocytosis.
CMV can be isolated from urine, saliva, stool, and spinal fluid.
Presence of IgM antibodies is suggestive of the disease.
Skull films reveal microcephaly and periventricular calcification.
Long bone films reveal the "celery stick" pattern consistent with congenital CMV.
Chest films may reveal interstitial pneumonia.

Infants and Children

CBC reveals lymphocytosis, atypical lymphocytes, anemia, and thrombocy-
topenia.
Liver function is normal; there is a mild rise in aminotransferase levels.
CMV antibodies are elevated.
Virus is isolated from secretions.
X-rays may reveal diffuse interstitial pneumonia.

Immunosuppressed Children

CBC reveals neuropenia, thrombocytopenia, and atypical lymphocytosis.
Serum aminotransferase is elevated.
Virus is isolated from saliva, urine, and bronchial secretions.
Chest films reveal an interstitial pneumonia.

Differential Diagnosis

Infants

Toxoplasmosis is more likely to be associated with hydrocephalus, micro-
thalmia, and chorioretinitis.
Hepatitis B produces elevated serum glutamic oxaloacetic transaminase
(SGOT) above 800 µ/L

Children and Adolescents

Infectious mononucleosis produces pharyngitis and lymphadenopathy and is
caused by Epstein-Barr virus (EBV).

Immunosuppressed Children

Bacterial and fungal infections.
Radiation pneumonitis.

Treatment: For retinitis, give ganciclovir, 5 mg/kg intravenously (IV) bid for
14–21 days; or foscarnet, 60 mg/kg IV q 8 hours for 14–21 days.

Follow-up: For infants with congenital infection, observe growth and development closely.

Sequelae: Mortality rate in infants with congenital infection is 30%. Infection in
newborns may result in delayed development and hearing loss (5–15% of
asymptomatic infants born with the virus); during the perinatal period, severe

pneumonia may result from the infection. In immunosuppressed children, the possible retinitis may result in blindness.

Prevention/Prophylaxis: Screening of blood and milk donors for the presence of the virus.

Referral: Refer patient to a pediatrician for admission to the hospital for IV therapy.

Education: Teach parents to practice proper handwashing techniques and not to allow sharing of eating utensils. Emphasize the importance of CMV screening of donors of blood, milk, and organs for transplant.

Diphtheria

Diphtheria is an acute infection of the upper respiratory tract or the skin with an incubation period of 1–6 days. Laryngeal diphtheria is characterized by the formation of a gray membrane over the pharynx, causing respiratory difficulties, cervical lymphadenopathy, and edema of the neck ("bull neck").

Etiology: The causative agent is the toxin-forming *Corynebacterium diphtheriae,* a gram-positive, club-shaped rod.

Occurrence: Five or fewer cases are reported each year.

Age: All ages.

Ethnicity: Not significant.

Gender: Occurs equally in males and females.

Contributing Factors: Nonimmunized children and adults; the presence of carriers within the community.

Signs and Symptoms: Parent gives a history of a mild sore throat, moderate fever, and malaise that abruptly progresses to severe prostration. The child is usually taken to the clinic at this time.

Physical examination reveals an acutely ill child with a rapid pulse not related to the fever, and a pharyngeal grayish membrane surrounded by an area of erythema and edema. The cervical lymph nodes are swollen, resulting in an associated swelling of the neck. There is respiratory stridor.

Diagnostic Tests

Nasal smears from nose and throat, on Loeffler's and tellurite agar, require 16–48 hours for identification of organisms.

WBC is usually normal; there may be evidence of hemolytic anemia and thrombocytopenia, with rapid destruction of the RBCs.

Differential Diagnosis

Streptococcal pharyngitis is differentiated by the absence of a pharyngeal grayish membrane.

Infectious mononucleosis produces lymphedema and hepatosplenomegaly.

Laryngeal obstruction may be a result of epiglottitis; observe for characteristic posture and "drooling." In cases of suspected epiglottitis, do not examine the pharynx.

Treatment: Within the first 48 hours, administer diphtheria antitoxin. Administer penicillin G, 150,000 mg/kg per day IV for 10 days. If patient is penicillin-allergic, administer erythromycin, 40 mg/kg per day by mouth (PO), in three to four divided doses, for 10 days. Admit to the hospital, and isolate for 1–7 days; usual hospital stay is 10–14 days. Three consecutive negative throat cultures, beginning 24 hours after completion of antibiotic regimen, are required before lifting isolation.

Restrict carriers to the home. Administer erythromycin, 40 mg/kg per day PO in three or four divided doses, for 10 days; penicillin V, 50 mg/kg per day; or benzathine penicillin G, 600,000–1,200,000 units intramuscularly (IM). Three consecutive negative throat cultures, beginning 24 hours after completion of antibiotic regimen, are required before lifting isolation. For immunized household contacts, observe for signs of illness.

Follow-up: Weekly follow-up after hospitalization for cardiac and neurological evaluations.

Sequelae: Myocarditis occurs 2–40 days after the onset of the illness; it is characterized by a rapid, thready pulse, ST-T wave changes, dysrhythmias, hepatomegaly, and fluid retention. Polyneuritis occurs during the first or second week after onset. The nerves involving the palate and the pharynx, then the optic nerve, and later the peripheral motor nerves are affected. Bronchopneumonia is often fatal.

Prevention/Prophylaxis: Routine childhood immunizations.

Referral: Refer patient for hospitalization.

Education: Instruct parents in the importance of immunizations.

Human Herpesvirus 6

Human herpesvirus 6 (HHV-6) infection, formerly called roseola infantum or exanthem subitum, is a viral illness characterized by a very high fever lasting 3–7 days. The fever is followed by an erythematous, discrete, rose-pink macular or maculopapular rash, which lasts from 6 hours to 3 days.

Etiology: Infection caused by HHV-6.

Occurrence: Common; no seasonal variation.

Age: Occurs in children 3 months to 4 years of age; 90% of cases occur in children under age 2 years.

Ethnicity: Not significant.

Gender: Occurs equally in males and females.

Contributing Factors: Exposure to the virus; immunosuppression.

Signs and Symptoms: Child had a high fever for several days and now has a red rash reported to have started initially on the trunk. May have a history of vomiting and mild diarrhea. Physical examination reveals the presence of a small, discrete, rose-pink macular or maculopapular rash.

Diagnostic Tests: None.

Differential Diagnosis

Measles: No accompanying coryza, runny nose, cough, conjunctivitis, or Koplik spots present. The rash usually starts on the face.

Rubella: Incubation period is 14–21 days, with prodromal respiratory symptoms and postauricular and occipital nodes. The maculopapular rash begins on the face.

Scarlet fever: Usual age of onset is 2–10 years; the rash is erythematous and diffuse and has a sandpaper texture. Scarlet tongue and Pastia's sign are noted; there is no rash on the face.

Erythema infectiosum: Characterized by the "slapped cheeks" and by the distribution and lacy pattern of the rash.

Treatment: Supportive: acetaminophen, as needed, for fever control; increased fluid intake.

Follow-up: None.

Sequelae: Approximately 10% of these children experience febrile seizures. Reactivation of the virus occurs only in immunosuppressed patients. In rare cases, encephalitis can occur.

Prevention/Prophylaxis: None.

Referral: None.

Education: Teach parents the importance of adequate fluid intake and methods of fever control.

Human Parvovirus B19 (Erythema Infectiosum)

Infection with the human parvovirus B19, commonly called fifth disease, is a mild, contagious, erythematous illness characterized by mild flulike symptoms that diminish in about 3 days, followed in 7–10 days by a characteristic rash that is mildly pruritic. The rash fades, but may be exacerbated by sunlight (e.g., warm baths) or stress. The rash is considered to be an immune response to the virus.

The child is contagious until the eruption of the rash. Spread occurs via respiratory droplets.

Etiology: The causative agent is human parvovirus B19, not the canine variety.

Occurrence: Common, usually in winter or spring outbreaks.

Age: Usually occurs in school-age children, ages 5–15 years.

Ethnicity: Not significant.

Gender: Occurs equally in males and females.

Contributing Factors: Contact with the respiratory droplets (via coughing) of an infected person.

Signs and Symptoms: The child presents with a red rash that the parent states started on the face and spread to the trunk, buttocks, and extremities. There may be a recollection of contact with an infected person. There may be a history of a mild flulike illness (low-grade fever, malaise, sore throat, coryza) 7–10 days before the eruption of the rash (50%). The parent, depending on the timing of the visit, may report that the rash had faded and has now reappeared.

Examination of the skin reveals maculopapular lesions on the face ("slapped cheek"), trunk, buttocks, and extremities, especially the thighs. The palms, soles, and circumoral area are rash-free. The confluent lesions with central clearing give the characteristically lacy appearance. The rash may feel warm.

Diagnostic Tests

CBC reveals a mild leukopenia followed by leukocytosis and lymphocytosis. Serum IgM and IgG antibodies are elevated.
Viral cultures are of no clinical use.

Differential Diagnosis

Measles: No true prodromal symptoms.
Rubella: No lymphadenopathy.
Scarlet fever: Pharyngitis and other systemic symptoms.

Treatment: Comfort measures, such as cool baths. Avoidance of sunlight.

Follow-up: Usually none.

Sequelae: Children with chronic hemolytic anemia are at risk for the development of aplastic crisis. In immunosuppressed children, a pancytopenia may develop. If the child is pregnant, the fetus is at increased risk for hydrops fetalis. In late adolescence, the child may have a reactive arthritis for 2–4 weeks after the rash.

Prevention/Prophylaxis: None. By the time these children are examined, they are usually no longer contagious.

Referral: Refer child to a pediatrician in cases of suspected complications.

Education: Instruct parent and child about prolonged exposure to sunlight and other factors that may exacerbate the reappearance of the rash.

Infectious Mononucleosis

Infectious mononucleosis, known as the "kissing disease," is an acute, self-limiting, communicable disease caused by EBV. It is transmitted through nasal or oropharyngeal secretions. The incubation period is 30–50 days; recovery usually takes 3–6 weeks, and recurrence is rare. In most cases the disease is mild, but some fatalities have been noted when severe liver damage occurs or in otherwise immunocompromised individuals.

Etiology: Contact with EBV.

Occurrence: Common.

Age: Occurs primarily in adolescents.

Ethnicity: Not significant.

Gender: Occurs equally in males and females.

Contributing Factors: Contact with the saliva of playmates and family members; contact with symptomatic carriers.

Signs and Symptoms: Young children may have no symptoms or a mild, nonspecific febrile episode; older children complain of sore throat, malaise, anorexia, and swollen glands. Parents may not be able to identify the contact source.

Physical findings include enlarged, firm, mildly tender lymph nodes, particularly the posterior and anterior cervical nodes. Upon palpation, there may be an enlarged spleen (50% of cases) and an enlarged liver (30% of cases), which are frequently tender. Swelling of the eyelids is frequently observed, as are petechiae on the soft palate. A macular, scarlatiniform, or urticarial rash may be present.

Diagnostic Tests

Monospot test: positive if the titer is significant. Usually positive in 50% of cases by first weeks and in 90% of cases by fourth week. Usually negative in children under 5 years of age.

Anti-EBV antibodies: detection of IgM antibody to the viral capsid antigen, or the rise of IgG antibody after several weeks; detection of IgG–viral capsid antigen (VCA) antibody with absence of Epstein-Barr nuclear antigen late in the illness.

CBC: Leukopenia early, lymphocytosis. (*Note:* such changes may not be noted until after the third week of the illness.)

Heterophile antibodies: Positive in 90% of older children, but in less than 50% of children under age 5 years. Usually do not appear until after week 2 and may be noted for 1 year after recovery.

Liver function tests: Bilirubin is slightly elevated, but the SGOT may be as much as four times normal value.

If child is not allergic to penicillin, give penicillin or ampicillin, 250-mg single dose, and wait for the eruption of the characteristic rash.

Differential Diagnosis

Lymphadenopathy: More generalized adenopathy.

Pharyngitis/streptococcal infection. Absence of splenomegaly; neutrophilic leukocytosis.

Hepatitis: Absence of splenomegaly; liver function studies grossly abnormal.

Rubella: Atypical lymphocytosis, but pharyngitis unremarkable; there is no marked adenopathy and splenomegaly, and the illness has a shorter duration.

Adenoviruses: Conjunctivitis, mild adenopathy, upper respiratory symptoms (cough), and fewer atypical lymphocytes.

Leukemia: Differentiated by peripheral blood smear morphology.

Treatment: Symptomatic, as follows:

Increased fluid intake.

Fever control using acetaminophen.

Increased rest with children exhibiting fatigue.

Exclusion from school or on a part-time basis.

Exclusion from sports activities until danger of liver involvement is past.

Exclusion from sports in cases of splenomegaly for 6–8 weeks.

For pharyngitis symptoms, penicillin V, 250 mg qid for 10 days.

Follow-up: Two-week intervals for evaluation of splenomegaly and further hematologic and antibody evaluations.

Sequelae: Hepatitis, splenic rupture, and encephalitis are uncommon complications. For children with immunosuppression, induced either by genetics or chemotherapy, progressive EBV infections may develop.

Prevention/Prophylaxis: No kissing of known contacts or use of utensils that foster the transfer of infective agents through saliva.

Referral: Refer patients with liver, spleen, neurological or hematological involvement to pediatrician or internal medicine MD.

Education: Instruct parents in the importance of limiting activity of children with hepatic and/or splenic involvement. Instruct parents in the proper handling and cleaning of utensils used by the infected child.

Lyme Disease

Lyme disease is a tick-borne illness caused by the spirochete *Borrelia burgdorferi*.

Etiology: *Borrelia burgdorferi*, a spirochete that lives in the midgut of nymphal and adult deer ticks (*Ixodes dammini*, East and Midwest; *Ixodes pacificus*, West), is passed to humans by bites from infected ticks.

Occurrence: High occurrence in summer and early fall. In the United States, the highest incidence rates are in the Northeastern and Mid-Atlantic states;

lower rates occur in the North Central, Pacific, and Southeast, with the lowest incidence rates in the Great Plains and Mountain states. Lyme disease also occurs in horses, cattle, dogs, and cats.

Age: Age 2 and older.

Ethnicity: Not significant.

Gender: Slightly more prevalent in males.

Contributing Factors: Outdoor activity in an endemic area.

Signs and Symptoms: Client has a history of a tick bite.

There are three stages with different clinical manifestations that may overlap:

Stage 1

Skin rash (erythema chronicum migrans); rash usually appears 4–20 days after the bite and gradually expands to form a large, plaquelike, erythematous, non-scaly, annular lesion that may be as large as 20 cm. Central portion of lesion may be clear, erythematous, and indurated. Lesions are often hot and may burn, prickle, or itch. Lesions occur most commonly in warm, moist areas such as the popliteal spaces and the groin; lesions are not found in mucosal areas. In 50% of patients, smaller secondary annular lesions will appear in a few days. Duration of an average untreated initial lesion is 3 weeks; it often has a bluish hue and may recur for 1 year or more.

Other symptoms are fever, fatigue, headaches, myalgias, malaise, and arthralgias. Flulike symptoms include fever, malaise, neck pain, and no respiratory or gastrointestinal symptoms.

Stage 2

Occurs 1 week or months after the initial bite. Self-limiting cardiac symptoms are most common in males and last 3 days to 6 weeks. In untreated cases, there are neurological complications including meningitis, encephalitis, and cranial neuritis (15–31%). The seventh cranial nerve is the one most frequently involved. Other nerves may be involved, and symptoms may be migratory.

Stage 3

Arthritis begins 4 weeks after the skin lesion. Large joints (most commonly the knees) are affected. Attacks are intermittent, may last for days or weeks, and may recur over a 1-year period. May result in destruction of the joint. Fever may be high.

Diagnostic Tests: Diagnosis relies on clinical presentation and a careful history, especially of travel to an endemic area and outdoor activities. The following results confirm the diagnosis:

C-reactive protein positive.

Erythrocyte sedimentation rate elevated.

ELISA more sensitive, but antibodies not present until 3–6 weeks after the bite.

IgM ELISA titers positive at values less than 1 : 160.

IgG ELISA titers positive at values less than 1 : 320.

Blood cultures rarely identify the agent.

Rheumatoid factor is negative by latex agglutination.

Spinal fluid (in cases of possible meningitis) will show elevated protein level and pleocytosis.

Differential Diagnosis

Stage 1: Rash may be confused with cellulitis, erythema multiforme, or erythema marginatum rheumaticum as well a fungal infections or eczema. The syndrome may be confused with viral influenza.

Stage 2: May be confused with Bell's palsy, viral meningitis, lead poisoning, or rheumatic fever.

Stage 3: May be confused with arthritis.

Treatment: The earlier effective treatment is initiated, the better the prognosis. Table 16–2 provides an overview of appropriate antibiotic therapy.

Follow-up: Monitor treatment and progression of illness, being watchful for complications.

Sequelae: Inadequate treatment may result in cardiac complications and arthritis.

Prevention/Prophylaxis: The following precautions should be taken:

In wooded areas, wear light-colored clothing and tall socks, and tuck pants into boots.

Scan the body for ticks often, because ticks may take up to 24 hours to begin feeding.

Use repellents, but be careful with children because of their risk of systemic absorption.

TABLE 16–2   ANTIBIOTIC THERAPY FOR LYME DISEASE

Stage I	Amoxicillin	20–40 mg/kg per day for 10–21 days 250–500 mg tid for 10–21 days
	or Erythromycin	30 mg/kg per day for 10–21 days 250 mg qid for 10–21 days
Stage II	Amoxicillin	20–40 mg/kg per day for 1 month 250–500 mg tid for 1 month
	or Doxycycline	100 mg bid for 1 month
IV therapy may include:	Ceftriaxone (Rocephin)	50–80 mg/kg IV for 14 days 2 g/day IV for 14 days
	Penicillin G	250,000–400,000 units/kg per day IV for 14–21 days 20–24 million units/day IV for 14–21 days

Keep any suspicious ticks labeled with site at which they were obtained and body site.

If symptoms occur, tick may be checked by the Centers for Disease Control for the presence of the spirochete.

Referral: Consult and collaborate with a physician for confirmation of the diagnosis and plan of care. Report case to state epidemiologist.

Education: Teach parents and community about the tick, the cycle of the organism, and methods for prevention, such as wearing proper clothing and using repellents. Teach parents and children how to remove ticks properly.

Measles

Measles (rubeola) is an acute, highly contagious viral illness with an incubation period of 8–12 days. The disease can be transmitted from the first or second day before to the fifth day after the eruption of the rash.

Etiology: Morbillivirus, a genus in the Paramyxoviridae family.

Occurrence: Occurs more frequently in the winter and spring.

Age: Primarily infants and children.

Ethnicity: Not significant.

Gender: Occurs equally in males and females.

Contributing Factors: Some research has suggested that measles contracted from the opposite sex and transmission intensity (e.g., home exposure versus outside-home exposure) results in a more severe case.

Signs and Symptoms: Child may present to clinic with a history of exposure to measles in the past 9–14 days and a rash. The child had a fever, conjunctivitis, and cough before the rash appeared. The rash consists of discrete, brownish red macules progressing to papular or morbilliform. The rash is blotchy or confluent: The skin between the lesions is normal. Examination of the oral cavity reveals white lesions on the buccal mucosa from before the rash appeared and lasting 12–24 hours after the rash's appearance (Koplik spots). The rash began behind the ears and sides of neck, progressing to the trunk and extremities.

Diagnostic Tests: None.

Differential Diagnosis

Rubella: The incubation period is 14–21 days, with prodromal respiratory symptoms and postauricular and occipital nodes. The maculopapular rash begins on the face.

Scarlet fever: The usual age is 2–10 years. The rash is erythematous and diffuse and has a sandpapery texture; scarlet tongue and Pastia's sign are noted, and there is no rash on the face.

Erythema infectiosum: The "slapped cheeks" and the distribution and characteristically lacy pattern of the rash.

Treatment: Symptomatic for fever control.

Follow-up: Usually none.

Sequelae: Otitis media, bronchopneumonia, croup, and diarrhea often occur as a result of the measles. Encephalitis, which occurs in 1 in 1000 cases, can result in severe, permanent brain damage. Death can also occur in 3 in 1000 cases.

Prevention/Prophylaxis: Immunization at 15 months is recommended, with a second immunization between ages 4 and 6. The dose is 0.5 mL, administered subcutaneously (SC).

Referral: Usually none.

Education: Instruct parents in the importance of immunizations. Instruct pregnant adolescent females about the risks of fetal exposure to measles.

Mumps

Mumps is a systemic, acutely contagious disease characterized by swelling of the parotid gland; it is transmitted by nasopharyngeal secretions. The communicability time is 1 day prior to until 3 days after parotid swelling. The incubation period is 16–18 days or a range of 12–25 days. To reduce transmission, children should be excluded from school until 9 days after parotid gland swelling.

Etiology: The etiologic agent is Paramyxovirus.

Occurrence: Mumps is more common in late winter and spring. Since the use of mumps vaccine, the incidence has been greatly reduced.

Age: Peak age group is 10–14 years.

Ethnicity: Not significant.

Gender: Occurs equally in males and females.

Contributing Factors: Contact with Paramyxovirus.

Signs and Symptoms: Children complain of tenderness and pain in the jaw; may have had trouble swallowing. Parents have often done the "pickle test," stimulating the parotid and causing increased pain. Often there is no history of immunization (Fig. 16–3).

Enlargement of the parotid gland, usually bilaterally, is a significant sign. Approximately 30% of patients, however, have no apparent swelling of the glands. Severe tenderness and pain often accompany the swelling. On examination, the ear is displaced upward and outward, with obliteration of the angle of the jaw. Stenson's duct orifice is red and swollen, and yellow exudate may be expressed.

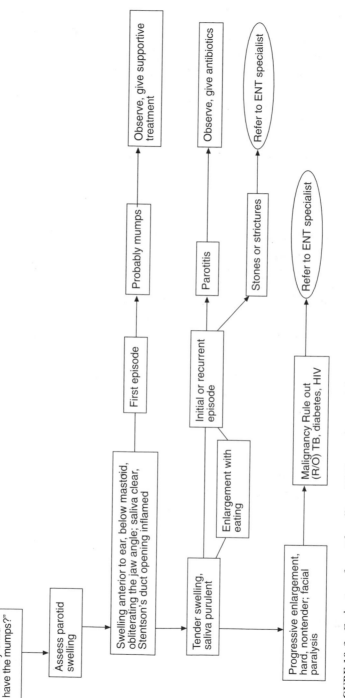
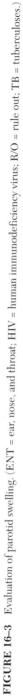

FIGURE 16-3 Evaluation of parotid swelling. (ENT = ear, nose, and throat; HIV = human immunodeficiency virus; R/O = rule out; TB = tuberculoses.)

Diagnostic Tests

To confirm infection or vaccination, tissue culture with urine, spinal fluid, and throat washings can be obtained for compliment fixation.

Hemagglutination tests or ELISA would indicate infection, but they are not usually done.

Leukocyte counts are usually normal.

Differential Diagnosis

Cervical adenopathy: The ear usually does not protrude.

Cat-scratch fever: Usually does not involve the parotid gland.

Pharyngitis/streptococcal infection: Leukocytosis is present, and the parotid gland is not usually involved.

Parotitis: The exudate from Stenson's duct is pustular; leukocytosis and neutrophilia are noted.

Tooth infection: Determined by examination of the oral cavity.

Enteroviral meningitis: Elevated serum amylase.

Pancreatitis: Serum amylase may be elevated in parotitis. Obtain lipase and amylase isoenzymes to evaluate pancreatic function; transient pancreatitis may be evident by the presence of abdominal pain.

Treatment: Symptomatic: Fluid should be increased; usually soft foods are tolerated better until the swelling begins to decrease.

Follow-up: Usually none.

Sequelae: Meningeal signs have been reported, with encephalitis occurring in 1 in 6000 cases. Unilateral orchitis is common when the infection occurs after puberty, but this rarely results in sterility and resolves in 1–2 weeks. Nerve deafness, which may be transient, causing the inability to distinguish high tones, may occur. Facial paralysis is a rare complication.

Prevention/Prophylaxis: Mumps vaccine, 0.5 mL SC at age 15 months and repeated at age 4–6. Mumps vaccine *cannot* be administered to immunocompromised children with the exception of HIV-positive children. Thus children receiving immunosuppressive therapy should not be immunized, but children with HIV should be immunized.

Referral: None, unless meningeal signs appear.

Education: None.

Pertussis

Pertussis (whooping cough) is an acute, highly contagious respiratory illness with an incubation period of 6–20 days. There are three stages:

Catarrhae stage (1–2 weeks): Rhinorrhea, conjunctival infection, lacrimation, mild cough, low-grade fever. Infants tend to have profuse nasal discharge.

Paroxysmal stage (2–4 weeks or longer): More severe, forceful, repetitive cough during which a characteristic "whoop" is produced due to increased respiratory effort. There is facial redness or cyanosis, bulging eyes, salivation, and distention of neck veins during the coughing episode. Post-tussive emesis often occurs. Exhaustion due to paroxysmal coughing spells is a common complaint.

Convalescent stage (1–2 weeks): paroxysmal coughing and vomiting decreasing. Leukocytosis (greater than 20,000–50,000) is characteristic.

Etiology: The causative agent is *Bordetella pertussis*. A similar disease, parapertussis, is caused by *Bordetella parapertussis*. The specific cause is the released toxin that causes the lymphocytosis and other symptoms.

Occurrence: Not as common now because of childhood immunizations.

Age: Most common in children under 1 year and in young adults.

Ethnicity: Not significant.

Gender: Occurs more frequently in females.

Contributing Factors: Unrecognized symptomatic family members.

Signs and Symptoms: Parents describe the characteristic whoop of, and the exhaustion after, the coughing spells; vomiting may occur after a coughing episode. There is an associated low-grade fever. Patient has no history of immunization.

On physical examination, the coughing episodes are observed to be accompanied by cyanosis and sweating. The coughing is severe, having the characteristically loud inspiration (whoop) after 10–30 coughs. The child is listless and exhausted. Mild respiratory symptoms, such as rhinitis and sneezing, may be present.

Diagnostic Tests

Catarrhal stage: 20,000–30,000 WBCs with 70–80% lymphocytes.

Nasapharyngeal swabs: culture for *Bordetella pertussis* using chocolate agar or Bordet-Gengou agar containing an antimicrobial agent.

Chest x-ray: Thickened bronchi and sometimes a "shaggy" heart border indicative of bronchopneumonia and patchy atelectasis.

Serum agglutinins, positive late in the illness, are of no diagnostic value.

Differential Diagnosis

Bronchitis: No characteristic cough or marked elevation in WBC count.

Pneumonia: Cough is not as severe and WBC count not as elevated.

Aspiration of foreign body: Chest x-ray usually reveals the foreign body; no characteristic cough or marked elevation in WBC count.

Parapertussis: A milder illness, usually found in Europe.

Treatment: Administer erythromycin, 40–50 mg/kg per day in four divided doses for 14 days. If patient is allergic to erythromycin, give ampicillin 100 mg/kg in four divided doses. Increase hydration, and give frequent, small feedings. Avoid respiratory irritants. Albuterol dosage (tachycardia is a common side effect, and aerosol methods may improve a paroxysmal episode) for ages 2–5 years is 0.1 mg/kg tid PO (not to exceed 2 mg tid); for ages 6–11 years it is 2 mg/kg tid or qid PO. Cough suppressants are not useful in decreasing paroxysmal coughing episodes.

Follow-up: Weekly during the severest part of the illness, and then as needed.

Sequelae: Pneumonia is the most common complication of pertussis. Atelectasis, aspiration pneumonia, subconjunctival hemorrhage, umbilical or inguinal hernia, and rarely intracranial hemorrhage can occur. Death occurs in 10 in 1000 cases.

Prevention/Prophylaxis: Immunization is the most important method of prevention. Pertussis vaccine, given in combination with diphtheria and tetanus (DPT), is administered at 2, 4, 6, and 15 months of age. In newborn infants whose mothers have pertussis, erythromycin can be given (50 mg/kg per day) for 14 days.

Family and hospital contacts should be treated with erythromycin prophylactically.

Referral: None, unless complications develop.

Education: Emphasize the importance of immunizations.

Rocky Mountain Spotted Fever

Rocky Mountain spotted fever is a tick-borne illness characterized by fever and a rash. There is an incubation period of 2–8 days. The offending tick is the dog tick in the East, the lone star tick in the Southwest, and the wood tick in the West.

Etiology: *Rickettsia rickettsii* is the causative organism. The organism multiplies within the endothelial lining and smooth muscle cells of blood vessels, causing generalized vasculitis.

Occurrence: Most often occurs in the Eastern half of the United States, Arkansas, Texas, and Oklahoma, but rarely in the West. It is a seasonal illness that usually occurs from April to September.

Age: All ages, but particularly in children aged 5–9 years.

Ethnicity: Not significant.

Gender: Occurs equally in males and females.

Contributing Factors: Rural, wooded areas most often in the spring and summer. Tick must be attached for at least 4 hours.

Signs and Symptoms: History reveals outdoor activities and a history of a tick bite. Patient presents with a high fever of abrupt onset, myalgia, and a headache that is severe and persistent. Vomiting and diarrhea occur 2–6 days after fever. Rose-red macular or maculopapular rash appears on palms, soles, and extremities; becomes petechial and spreads centrally; blanches on pressure; and is exacerbated by warmth in 95% of cases. Conjunctivitis, splenomegaly, muscle tenderness, edema, and meningism.

Diagnostic Tests

WBC count may be normal or slightly decreased with a shift to the left during the first week; leukocytosis is reported in the second week.

Platelets are depressed.

Urinalysis reveals hematuria.

Rocky Mountain spotted fever complement fixation titers (convalescent titers) may increase after 14 days of illness.

Fibrinogen is depressed, and there is disseminated intravascular coagulation.

Creatinine levels are increased.

Liver function tests reveals elevated aspartate transaminase and alanine transaminase; bilirubin and total protein and albumin are depressed.

Weil-Felix reaction reveals a *Proteus* Ox-19 and Ox-2 single titer of greater than 1 : 160 (fourfold increase).

Immunofluorescent biopsy of the skin may yield an early diagnosis.

Differential Diagnosis: Differential diagnosis includes a large variety of illness ranging from measles to collagen diseases. The epidemiological data of the season, the history of a tick bite, and the type of rash should facilitate making the diagnosis.

Treatment: Remove tick by gentle upward traction with forceps to avoid contaminating self or patient with material from the crushed tick. Administer antibiotic therapy: chloramphenicol (100 mg/kg per day) or tetracycline (25 mg/kg per day) IV in divided doses q 6 hours for 10 days. To restore circulation, consider fluid management with replacement if needed. Presence of noncardiogenic pulmonary edema may require mechanical ventilation with positive and expiratory pressure to correct hypoxemia.

In cases of intravascular coagulation and hemorrhage, replacement of platelets and clotting factors will be necessary.

Follow-up: Weekly follow-ups to evaluate disease status and efficacy of therapy.

Sequelae: Complications and death may occur from severe vasculitis in brain, heart, and lung. The mortality rate is estimated at 5–7%.

Prevention/Prophylaxis: Give patient and family the following instructions:

Remove tick early.

In wooded areas, wear light-colored clothing and long socks, and tuck pants into boots.

Scan body for ticks often.

Use repellents, but be careful with children because of the risk of systemic absorption.

Keep any suspicious ticks labeled with site at which they were obtained and body site.

Referral: Refer patient for hospitalization.

Education: Teach parents the importance of wearing protective clothing and using insect repellents. Teach parents and children the proper technique for tick removal.

Rubella

Rubella (German or three-day) is an acute, viral infection with an incubation period of 14–21 days, that usually presents as a mild illness. Communicability is 2 days before to 7 days after the appearance of the rash. The characteristic rash begins on the face and lasts 3 days or less. Asymptomatic illness occurs in 25–50% of cases.

Etiology: The Rubivirus, family Togaviridae, is the causative agent.

Occurrence: The peak incidence is in early spring or late winter. Incidence has decreased due to the increase in immunized children.

Age: Any pediatric age group.

Ethnicity: Not significant.

Gender: Occurs equally in males and females.

Contributing Factors: Exposure to infected children; nonimmunized status. Fetuses exposed to rubella at 1–4 months' gestation have an increased risk of congenital rubella.

Signs and Symptoms: Child presents with the complaint of "red rash" that started on the face; child is usually afebrile. There may have been nonspecific respiratory symptoms before the onset of the rash (prodromal phase). Adolescents and adults (usually women) may complain of transient polyarthralgia and polyarthritis, but this is less common in young children.

There is a fine, pink, discrete, macular rash that becomes punctate or scarlatiniform on the second day, with fine desquamation as rash fades. Postauricular and occipital nodes may be noted early, progressing to generalized lymphadenopathy.

Diagnostic Tests

CBC reveals leukopenia and a low platelet count.

Congenital rubella is characterized by a low platelet count, abnormal liver function studies, and hemolytic anemia with pleocytosis. There is an elevated rubella IgM antibody titer, total serum IgM level is elevated, and IgA and IgG levels are depressed.

In the pregnant woman, a fourfold rise in antibody titer obtained 1–2 weeks apart is diagnostic; the fetus is considered at risk, particularly in the first trimester.

Differential Diagnosis

Measles: No accompanying coryza, runny nose, cough, conjunctivitis, or Koplik spots present.

Scarlet fever: The usual age at onset 2–10 years. The rash is erythematous and diffuse and has a sandpaper texture. Scarlet tongue and Pastia's sign are present. There is no rash on the face.

Erythema infectiosum: Differentiated by the "slapped cheeks" and the distribution and the characteristically lacy pattern of the rash.

Contact dermatitis: Rash not characteristic of rubella.

Lymphadenopathy: More nodes are usually involved.

Treatment: Symptomatic.

Follow-up: None, unless the patient is pregnant or has any other evidence of complications.

Sequelae: Encephalitis and thrombocytopenia are rare complications. Congenital rubella usually is associated with anomalies that involve the cardiac, ophthalmic, auditory, and neurological systems.

Prevention/Prophylaxis: Immunization is the most effective method of control. If a pregnant woman is exposed, a blood specimen is obtained to measure the rubella titer as soon as possible. If negative, a second specimen is obtained 3–4 weeks later; if positive, infection is assumed to have occurred and the risk to the fetus increases. Although immunization should ensure against fetal exposure, it is wise to do the titers.

Referral: None.

Education: Teach the importance of immunizations.

Scarlet Fever

Scarlet fever is an acute, infectious bacterial infection involving the respiratory system, skin, soft tissue, and blood. There is a characteristic rash that begins within 12–48 hours of onset of symptoms and a scarlet-colored tongue preceded by the complaint of a severely sore throat. The incubation period is 24–48 hours.

Careful treatment is necessary to reduce the risk of cardiac and renal complications.

Etiology: Infection with Group A β-hemolytic streptococcus.

Occurrence: Fairly common.

Age: Any pediatric age group.

Ethnicity: Not significant.

Gender: Occurs equally in males and females.

Contributing Factors: Exposure to the bacteria.

Signs and Symptoms: Child presents with a history of acute onset of fever (greater than 103–104°F) accompanied by chills, vomiting, headache, and sore throat. The characteristic rash may or may not be present, depending on how long family waited before seeking medical services.

Physical examination reveals a hyperemic, edematous pharynx covered with a gray-white exudate; pharynx is inflamed. The tongue is white with projections of red, edematous papillae (early sign), progressing to a scarlet-colored tongue with prominent red papillae ("strawberry tongue"). The rash is red, punctate, or finely papular and blanches when touched; rash begins in the axillae, groin, and neck but becomes generalized, except on the face, within 24 hours. Circumoral pallor and Pastia's sign are noted. The skin will desquamate as illness resolves.

Diagnostic Tests

Throat culture is positive.
Quick streptococcal test is positive.

Differential Diagnosis

Rubella: The incubation period is 14–21 days; patient has prodromal respiratory symptoms and postauricular and occipital nodes. The maculopapular rash begins on the face.

Erythema infectiosum: Differentiated by the "slapped cheeks" and the distribution and characteristically lacy pattern of the rash.

Measles: No accompanying coryza, runny nose, cough, conjunctivitis, Koplik spots present.

Infectious mononucleosis: Positive EBV titers and generalized lymphadenopathy.

Enterovirus: Usually the WBC count is normal; often the rash is more prominent on the soles and palms.

Roseola: Usually seen in children under age 2 years; patient has upper respiratory symptoms and abrupt onset of fever, followed by the rash.

Treatment: The treatment of choice is penicillin: long-acting benzothine penicillin G: 600,000 units IM for children less than 60 lb, 1.2 million units IM for children greater than 60 lb. If patient is allergic to penicillin, administer erythromycin, 40 mg/kg per day for 14 days.

Follow-up: Repeat throat culture in 1 week.

Sequelae: When the infection is severe, bacteremia, pneumonia, meningitis, deep soft tissue infections, or streptococcal toxic shock syndrome may result. Inadequately treated infections can result in rheumatic fever, cardiac involvement, and renal problems.

Prevention/Prophylaxis: Throat cultures should be done for all who are in close contact with infected persons. Prophylactic penicillin should be administered: 400,000 U/dose qid for 10 days or 600,000 U IM (single dose), or erythromycin 40 mg/kg per day for 14 days.

Referral: None.

Education: Instruct parents and children not to use eating or drinking utensils after the infected person. Stress the importance of completing the treatment regimen.

Varicella

Varicella (chickenpox) is a viral, highly contagious, acute disease with an incubation period of 14–21 days. Communicability begins 1 day before eruption of vesicles until 6 days after the last lesion appears or when all crusts have formed.

Etiology: Infection with varicella-zoster virus, a member of the herpesvirus group.

Occurrence: More common in spring and winter.

Age: All pediatric age groups.

Ethnicity: Not significant.

Gender: Occurs equally in males and females.

Contributing Factors: Contact with infected children; common in day-care centers and schools.

Signs and Symptoms: Child presents with a history of exposure to other infected children, usually mild fever, the presence of the characteristic, pruritic rash, which usually begins on the scalp.

Physical examination of the skin reveals macules or papules: small, red, elevated vesicles shaped like a tear drop, with an erythematous ring ¼–½ inches in diameter. The rash occurs in "crops"; that is, all stages are present as new lesions appear.

Diagnostic Tests

Tzanck smear.
Immunofluorescent staining of vesicular lesions.

Differential Diagnosis

Impetigo bullosa: Characterized by fewer lesions, no typical vesicles, and response to antibiotic agents.
Coxsackievirus: Fewer lesions and less crusting.
Insect bites: No typical vesicles.

Treatment: Symptomatic for fever and itching. Avoid administering aspirin because of the association between the use of aspirin and the development of Reye's syndrome. For itching, prescribe diphenhyramine (Benadryl), 1.25 mg/kg (4–6 mg/kg per day), q 6 hours; and/or hydroxyzine (Atarax), 0.5 mg/kg (10 mg) q 6 hours per day.

Some research has recommended administration of acyclovir, 80 mg/kg per day in four divided doses, for children aged 3–24 months to reduce symptoms, interrupt vesicle formation, and accelerate the healing process. Acyclovir must be administered within the first 24 hours after the onset of the illness. Cool oatmeal baths (Aveeno) are often soothing.

Follow-up: Usually none.

Sequelae: Bacterial superinfection of lesions can occur. Encephalitis, pancreatitis, hepatitis, or pneumonia can develop in immunocompromised children. Older persons who acquire chickenpox are at risk for pneumonia.

When the infection is reactivated from a latent form following the primary infection, it is called herpes zoster, also known as shingles.

Prevention/Prophylaxis: Isolation of infected children from other children can prevent the spread of the disease. Varicella vaccine, given at 15 months, produces immunity.

Referral: None for well children. Refer infected immunosuppressed children and neonates, in whom varicella is a life-threatening illness, to a pediatrician or infectious disease specialist.

Education: Teach the importance of hygienic measures, such as keeping the nails short, to reduce the risk of superinfections.

Human Immunodeficiency Virus (HIV) Infection & Acquired Immunodeficiency Syndrome (AIDS)

HIV infection, with acquired immunodeficiency syndrome (AIDS) being the end of its clinical course, causes the slow demise of the body's immune system, affecting the renal, cardiac, integumentary, respiratory, neurological, and gastrointestinal systems. When the body's immune system is unable to thwart any form of infection, AIDS results. AIDS is fatal in nearly all cases. There are a few long-term survivors, but their ultimate outcome is still uncertain.

Etiology: AIDS is caused by the human immunodeficiency virus type 1 (HIV-1) and less commonly by HIV-2. It is an RNA cytopathic retrovirus.

Occurrence: Childhood AIDS is the ninth leading cause of death in children aged 1–4 years and seventh in adolescents and adults aged 15–24. Childhood AIDS constitutes 2% of all reported cases of AIDS in the United States. Approximately 8–10% of infants HIV-positive at birth will remain positive and succumb to AIDS when both mother and infant have received appropriate prophylaxis.

Age: Infancy and adolescence are the most common age groups.

Ethnicity: Not significant.

Gender: Occurs equally in males and females.

Contributing Factors: Transplacental transmission of HIV, contact with bodily fluids of HIV-positive persons, unprotected sexual activity with multiple partners, transfusions of contaminated blood, and sharing of needles among persons with needle-dependent drug addiction.

Signs and Symptoms: Infant may be brought to clinic because of feeding problems, recurrent diarrhea, persistent or recurrent diaper rashes or generalized rash, or respiratory problems.

Clinical manifestations of HIV infection include generalized lymphadenopathy, hepatomegaly, splenomegaly, oral candidiasis, parotitis, and cardiomyopathy. There may also be developmental delay, failure to thrive, and pneumonia (most serious cases caused by *Pneumocystis carinii*). Chronic parotid swelling is common in children with AIDS. Kaposi's sarcoma and B-cell lymphoma are very uncommon in children with AIDS.

Diagnostic Tests

Western blot is positive.

Currently, the polymer chain reaction (PCR) is the gold standard of diagnosis. A PCR should be done at birth to detect the viral load of the infant. This is repeated at 3 months and at 6 months. If two negative tests are received, the child is considered seronegative. Unfortunately, if a child remains seropositive for 3 years, the immune system will be irreparably damaged with a permanent loss of antiviral antibodies.

Laboratory abnormalities include the following: reversal of T4-helper–suppressor cell (T8) ratio (T4 : T8), elevated erythrocyte sedimentation rates, anemia, lymphocytosis, leukopenia, neutropenia, lymphopenia, thrombocytopenia (which actually precedes other findings), and an elevated lactate dehydrogenase.

Differential Diagnosis

Failure to thrive: Evaluate for feeding problems related to poor parenting skills or other physical causes.

Central nervous system disorders: Atrophy and calcification in the basal ganglion and the frontal lobe may be demonstrated on imaging studies in patients with brain infections.

Anemias: Low leukocyte count and elevated erythrocyte sedimentation rate.

Systemic candidiasis: Evaluate for diabetes.

Pneumonia: Observe for evidence of atypical findings on chest x-ray. Lymphoid interstitial pneumonitis produces diffuse interstitial reticulonodular infiltrates, often with hilar adenopathy.

Treatment: Treatment of presenting systemic manifestation. Predominant drug used for treatment of AIDS is zidovudine (AZT). After 1 month of age Bactrim is added.

Follow-up: Follow-up for "well-baby" care should be done at routine intervals. Coordinate activities with an AIDS health-care treatment center.

Sequelae: Ultimately death occurs. In children with perinatal infections, survival ranges from 2.5 months to 10 years. In those infected later—through blood transfusions, unprotected sex, and/or the sharing of needles—incubation is longer, and thus the survival period is longer.

Prevention/Prophylaxis: Use of a latex condom, especially one with nonoxynol 9, is important in breaking the chain of the spread of disease. Avoidance of exchange of any and all bodily fluids helps to decrease the risk of HIV infection. Needle-dependent drug addicts should not share needles. An AIDS vaccine is not available at this time.

Referral: Refer HIV-positive patients and those children with a presumptive diagnosis of AIDS to an AIDS treatment facility for treatment.

Education: Provide education for patients, their families, and the community related to resources and treatment options. Educate the parents regarding the overall disease process and survival rates. Caution the parents to report all health changes to the health-care provider immediately. This should be done because often opportunistic infections can worsen the prognosis when left untreated. Make counseling available to both the child and the parents.

REFERENCES

General

Behrman, R, and Kliegman, R, (eds): Essentials of Pediatrics. WB Saunders, Philadelphia, 1990.
Doenges, M, and Moorhouse, M: Nursing Diagnoses with Intervention, ed 4. FA Davis, Philadelphia, 1993.
Hay, WW, et al: Current Pediatric Diagnosis and Treatment, ed 12. Appleton & Lange, Norwalk, Conn, 1995.
Peter, G, et al: The Red Book: Report of the Committee on Infectious Diseases. American Academy of Pediatrics, Elk Grove Village, Ill, 1994.

Iron Deficiency Anemia

Bushnell, FK: A guide to primary care of iron deficiency anemia. Nurse Pract 17(11):68, 1992.
Francis, EE, et al: Anemia as an indicator of nutrition in children who are enrolled in a Head Start program. J Pediatr Health Care 7:156, 1993.
Hathaway, WE, et al: Current Pediatric Diagnosis and Treatment. Appleton & Lange, Norwalk, Conn, 1993.
Kline, N: A practical approach to a child with anemia. J Pediatr Health Care 5:99, 1996.
Roberts, J: Assessing iron poisoning. Emerg Med 25(10):6, 1993.
Uphold, R, and Graham, MV: Clinical Guidelines in Family Practice. Barrmarrae Books, Gainesville, Fla, 1994.
Wellborn, JL, and Meyers, FJ: A three-point approach to anemia. Postgrad Med 89:179, 1991.

Sickle Cell Anemia

Barker, LR, et al: Principles of Ambulatory Medicine, ed 4. Williams & Wilkins, Baltimore.
Burke, S: Hydroxyurea in sickle cell disease. Matern Child Nurs 21(4):210, 1996.

Day, S, et al: A successful education program for parents of infants with newly diagnosed sickle cell disease. J Pediatr Nurs 7(1):52, 1992.

Frush, K, et al: Current Pediatric Diagnosis and Treatment, ed 12. Appleton & Lange, Norwalk, Conn, 1995.

Graham, MV, and Uphold, CR: Clinical Guidelines in Child Health. Barrarrae Books, Gainesville, Fla, 1994.

Smith, JA, and Kinney, TR: Sickle cell disease: Screening and management in newborns and infants. Am Fam Phys 48:95, 1993.

U.S. Department of Health and Human Services: Sickle cell disease: Screening diagnosis, management and counseling in newborns and infants. (AHCPR publication no. 93-0562). Agency for Health Care Policy and Research, Rockville, Md, 1993.

Infectious Mononucleosis

Bailey, RE: Diagnosis and treatment of infectious mononucleosis. Am Fam Phys 49:879, 1994.

Lyme Disease

Feder, H, and Hunt, M: Pitfalls in the diagnosis and treatment of Lyme disease in children. JAMA 274:66, 1995.

Lumpkin, T: A great imitator: Lyme disease. J Am Acad Phys Assist 4:284, 1991.

Measles

Aaby, P: Assumptions and contradictions in measles and measles immunization research: Is measles good for something? Soc Sci Med 41:673, 1995.

Mumps

vanLoon, FP, et al: Mumps surveillance—United States, 1988–1993. MMWR CDC Surveill Summ 44(3):1, 1995.

Pertussis

Deen, JL, et al: Household contact study of *Bordatella pertussis* infections. Clin Infect Dis 21:1211, 1995.

Deville, JG, et al: Frequency of unrecognized *Bordatella pertussis* infections in adults. Clin Infect Dis 21:639, 1995.

Rocky Mountain Spotted Fever

Steele, R: The Clinical Handbook of Pediatric Infectious Disease. Parthenon, New York, 1994.

Rubella

Centers for Disease Control: Rubella and congenital rubella syndrome—United States, January 1, 1991–7 May, 1994. MMWR 43:391, 1994.

Human Immunodeficiency Virus

Ellaurie, M, et al: IgE levels in pediatric HIV infection. Ann Allergy Asthma Immunol 75:332, 1995.

Manerd, J, et al: Recent advances in pediatric HIV. J Ark Med Soc 92:165, 1995.

CHAPTER **17**

ENVIRONMENTAL

ASSESSMENT

For a child, the environment is an exciting place for exploration, full of new and different things from which to learn. On the other hand, the environment has the potential to be a threatening, dangerous place that may cause harm. It is the responsibility of the caregiver to protect and to bring no harm not only by insulating the child from danger, but also by teaching the child self-help skills.

The place of residence, that place where one should feel the safest, is full of things to pique the curiosity of a small child: the medicine cupboard with pretty pills, the kitchen cabinets with bottles of variously colored liquids, buckets of water, the toilet, and the bathtub; windowsills to chew on, paint chips to peel with little fingers (and what goes on the fingers goes in the mouth), stairs to climb, and rooms to explore. Outside is another world that is full of wonderful "critters," and children have little sense of danger.

Is it any wonder that more than 60% of deaths in children aged 1–3 years are attributed to injuries? To help parents and providers prevent accidents, the American Academy of Pediatrics has established The Injury Prevention Program (TIPP). The program includes questionnaires to assess risk, as well as parent information sheets on prevention. The materials can be obtained from the American Academy of Pediatrics, Publications Department, 141 Northwest Point Boulevard, PO Box 927, Elk Grove Village, IL 60007; phone 1-804-433-9016.

456

Animal/Human Bites

Animal and human bites are injuries that cause disruption of skin integrity. A true bite may be occlusional or the result of a clenched fist injury, which results from the impact of a fist on teeth.

Etiology: Animal bites are most frequently caused by dogs (90%) and cats (10%), but other mammals, including rodents (1%), bite humans. Human bites are usually caused by children, but some forms of child abuse include bites by adults.

Occurrence: One to two million Americans are bitten each year, of which 70% are children under age 10 years. Bites constitute 1% of emergency room visits, and 90% of pets involved are owned by the victim's family or neighbors. Bites among children are common but rarely serious.

Age: Occurs in all pediatric age groups.

Ethnicity: Not significant.

Gender: Dogs bite males more often than females; cats bite females more often.

Contributing Factors: Being ignorant of potential dangers is a primary factor, as well as provoking animals and engaging in fist fights.

Signs and Symptoms

Victim

The history is important prior to initiating treatment. The following questions should be asked:

What was the source of the bite—animal or human (Fig. 17–1)?
If animal, what kind, and is the animal known to the family?
What is the health status of the animal?
Was the attack provoked?
Can the animal be observed over the next 10–14 days?
How old is the wound?
What home treatment, if any, was initiated?
When was the last tetanus immunization?
Was the human bite from a child or an adult? If from an adult, was the bite part of an abusive cycle, or the result of a physical altercation?

Assessment of the wound includes the following:

Assessing for bleeding and signs of infection.
Determining the type of wound: puncture or laceration.
Determining the presence of infection.

Infection is usually clinically evident within 24 hours. Clenched-fist injuries usually result in lacerations over the fourth and fifth metacarpal joints.

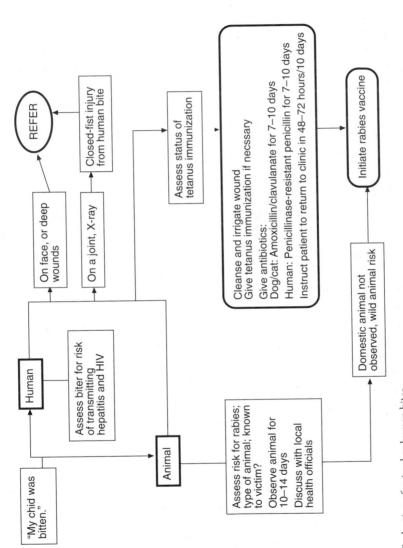

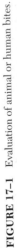

FIGURE 17–1 Evaluation of animal or human bites.

Diagnostic Tests

Radiographic studies may be indicated if there is a suspicion of a fracture or of a foreign body, such as a tooth, embedded in the wound.

Culture the wound area for identification of pathogenic bacteria.

Differential Diagnosis: None.

Treatment

Victim

Initial treatment includes irrigation of the open wound with normal saline, debridement of the area, assessment for possible presence of foreign body, and assessment of the need for surgical closure.

Systemic treatment includes tetanus prophylaxis, antibiotics, and postexposure rabies management.

The following are the recommendations for tetanus prophylaxis put forth by the Advisory Committee on Immunization Practices:

If the wound is minor and clean, the history of tetanus immunizations is unknown, or the client has had less than three doses, administer tetanus and diphtheria toxoids (Td).

If last tetanus immunization was given more than 10 years earlier, administer Td.

Immunization is not required if the patient received three or more doses, nor is tetanus immune globulin (TIG).

For all other wounds, if history of tetanus immunizations is unknown or the patient has had less than three doses, administer Td and TIG; administer Td if immunization occurred less than 5 years earlier. The administration of TIG is not required.

Initiate broad-spectrum antibiotic therapy:

Amoxicillin-clavulanate: amoxicillin 40 mg/kg per day in divided doses q 8 hours.

Penicillin V, 50 mg/kg per day in divided doses q 6–8 hours.

Doxycycline 2–4 mg/kg per day in divided doses q 12 hours. Not for children under age 8 years.

Ceftriaxone 50 mg/kg per day. Not for children under age 12 years.

If indicated, postexposure rabies prophylaxis. For wild animals or domestic animals not observed or tested, administer human rabies immunoglobulin (HRIG) 20 IU/kg total dose (10 IU/kg infiltrated around wound and 10 IU/kg IM), or human diploid cell vaccine (HDCV) 1 mL on days 0, 3, 7, 14, and 28.

Perpetrator

Dogs, cats, wild carnivores, and bats are potentially rabid. Rodents and rabbits are usually not considered potentially dangerous. The following guidelines should be followed in dealing with the animal:

Assess, if possible, the immunization status of the animal.

Do not destroy the animal.

Pen the animal and observe for 10–14 days.

Report strays and other unknown animals; discuss with local health officials.

Humans

Human perpetrators should be tested for hepatitis (A and B) and human immunodeficiency virus (HIV).

Follow-up: Examine the wound in 48 hours, and reassess at the end of antibiotic therapy for signs of infection. If rabies immunization initiated, obtain a follow-up rabies antibody titer on day 42.

Sequelae: If not treated appropriately, infection and/or sepsis may result.

Prevention/Prophylaxis: Educate children in the proper care and treatment of animals.

Referral: Refer child for surgery if the lacerations are massive, involve the face, or require hospitalization. It is mandatory to report cases of suspected child abuse.

Education: Teach the child to be wary of unknown animals, and not to provoke family pets or neighborhood animals. Instruct the child that any wild animal is to be considered dangerous, and therefore direct contact is to be avoided.

Heat Cramps

Heat cramps are brief muscle contractions, without rigidity of skeletal and abdominal muscles, as a result of sodium loss.

Etiology: Excessive sodium chloride loss from sweating.

Occurrence: Common in areas where climate factors indicate risk.

Age: Occurs primarily in adolescents and young adults.

Ethnicity: Not significant.

Gender: Occurs equally in males and females.

Contributing Factors: Athletic activity and drinking excessive water in response to sweating are factors to be considered.

Signs and Symptoms: The patient presents with complaints of painful muscle contractions and cramping of skeletal or abdominal muscles following exertion. Physical examination reveals painful muscles (Fig. 17–2).

Diagnostic Tests: None.

Differential Diagnosis: None.

Treatment: Supportive treatment including rest, muscle massage, and oral replacement of sodium chloride. Severe cases may require administration of intravenous (IV) normal saline solution.

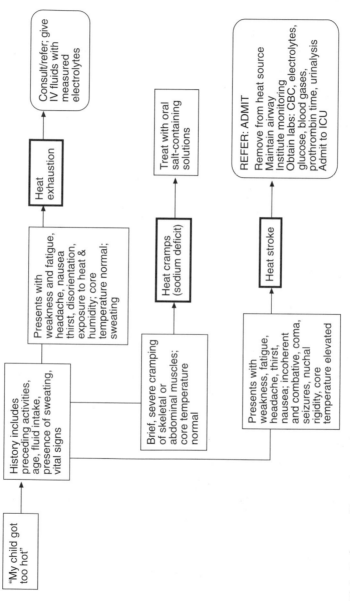

"My child got too hot"

History includes preceding activities, age, fluid intake, presence of sweating, vital signs

Presents with weakness and fatigue, headache, nausea thirst, disorientation, exposure to heat & humidity; core temperature normal; sweating

Heat exhaustion

Consult/refer; give IV fluids with measured electrolytes

Brief, severe cramping of skeletal or abdominal muscles; core temperature normal

Heat cramps (sodium deficit)

Treat with oral salt-containing solutions

Presents with weakness, fatigue, headache, thirst, nausea; incoherent and combative, coma, seizures, nuchal rigidity; core temperature elevated

Heat stroke

REFER: ADMIT
Remove from heat source
Maintain airway
Institute monitoring
Obtain labs: CBC, electrolytes, glucose, blood gases, prothrombin time, urinalysis
Admit to ICU

FIGURE 17–2 Evaluation of hyperthermia. (CBC = complete blood count; ICU = intensive care unit; IV = intravenous.)

Follow-up: As warranted.

Sequelae: None.

Prevention/Prophylaxis: At times of excessive sweating, patients should take salt tablets.

Referral: None.

Education: Teach parents and patients ways to keep electrolytes balanced during times of excessive sweating.

Heat Exhaustion

Excessive sweating due to exertion in a hot and humid environment.

Etiology: Depletion of plasma volume.

Occurrence: Common in adolescents and young adults in conducive environments.

Age: Primarily in adolescents and young adults.

Ethnicity: Not significant.

Gender: Occurs equally in males and females.

Contributing Factors: Overexertion in a hot and humid environment, often during athletic activities or in the workplace.

Signs and Symptoms: History of exposure to heat. Patient presents with complaints of general malaise, weakness, headache, anorexia, nausea, and vomiting. The body core temperature rises to more than 100°F but less than 104°F. There is hypotension and tachycardia, and the patient continues to sweat (see Fig. 17–2).

Diagnostic Tests: None.

Differential Diagnosis: In heatstroke, the central nervous system (CNS) dysfunction is increased (e.g., the heatstroke patient is incoherent and combative).

Treatment: Supportive treatment, such as rest in cool environment and restoration of fluids and salt. In severe cases, patient may need hospitalization for cooling and intravenous rehydration.

Follow-up: None; patient usually recovers in 2–3 hours.

Sequelae: Usually none.

Prevention/Prophylaxis: Can be avoided by acclimatization and increased fluid and salt intake.

Referral: In severe cases, refer patient for hospitalization.

Education: Teach parents and the general public of the dangers of fluid depletion in hot weather.

Heatstroke

Heatstroke is the failure of thermoregulation. Exertional heatstroke affects young, healthy persons who are not acclimated to heat and/or humidity. Classic heatstroke affects the elderly and debilitated.

Etiology: Exertional heatstroke is a result of engaging in strenuous muscular activity; classic heatstroke is a failure of thermoregulation that occurs during limited activity.

Occurrence: Common; responsible for approximately 4000 deaths in the United States each summer (adults and children) and is the third leading cause of death among high school athletes.

Age: Occurs in all pediatric age groups; more common in adolescent athletes.

Ethnicity: Not significant.

Gender: Occurs equally in males and females.

Contributing Factors: Debilitating chronic illness, alcohol, medications (diuretics, β-blockers, antipsychotic drugs [e.g., haloperidol, chlorpromazine], major tranquilizers, anticholinergics), sports activities, and failure to acclimatize to hot and humid environments.

Signs and Symptoms: Patient presents with a history of strenuous activity in a climate of high heat and humidity, complains of lack of sweating, and has a rectal temperature greater than 40°C (104°F). There is marked CNS dysfunction, and the patient is often incoherent and combative. The patient may lapse into a coma or have seizures and nuchal rigidity (see Fig. 17–2).

Diagnostic Tests

Dehydration may result in an elevated hematocrit and an elevated blood urea nitrogen (BUN).

Urinalysis may reveal an increase in urine-specific gravity due to dehydration; usually reveals proteinuria; and may reveal the presence of red blood cells and casts.

Electrocardiogram (ECG) tracings show changes consisting of conduction abnormalities and nonspecific ST-segment and T-wave changes.

Differential Diagnosis: Hyperthyroid storm, neuroleptic malignant syndrome, pheochromocytoma, and CNS injury. Patients who have ingested a variety of drugs can present with hyperthermia and mental status changes.

Treatment

Nonpharmacological

Remove patient from the heat source and cool the body using cool water, cool mist, or fans. Maintain airway. Monitor cardiac function, urinary output, and temperature.

Pharmacological

Administer IV fluids.

Follow-up: As warranted.

Sequelae: Transient personality changes occur when initiation of treatment is slow. If treatment is not prompt and appropriate, death may occur.

Prevention/Prophylaxis: *Do not* administer salt tablets. Fans are helpful in low-humidity and ambient temperatures less than 90°F. However, fans can increase heat stress when ambient temperature is greater than 100°F. Offer patient the following guidelines:

Visit air-conditioned areas, such as malls or libraries.
Avoid excessive activity in extreme temperatures.
Take scheduled rest periods.
Wear lightweight and light-colored clothing, wear a hat, and use an umbrella.
Increase fluid intake.
Allow children to play in tub of cool water (59–61°F) during the summer.
Hydrate well before and during outdoor activities.

Referral: *Immediate transfer to hospital.*

Education: Teach preventive measures as listed above.

Insect and Arthropod Bites and Stings

Insect and arthropod bites and stings cause a toxic reaction due to the saliva, venom, or injury. Reactions may be classified as immediate or delayed. Immediate reactions are classified as follows:

Normal: Localized swelling, erythema, and transient pain.
Toxic: Produced by exogenous vasoactive amines in the venom; usually occurs with multiple stings.
Large local: Contiguous swelling that lasts more than 24 hours.
Systemic: Generalized symptoms remote from sting site.

Delayed reactions are systemic, with varied manifestations such as serum sickness–like reactions, myocarditis, transverse myelitis, and nephrosis.

Etiology: Bees and wasps and ants cause the majority of insect bites and stings. Common arthropods that bite and/or sting include spiders, scorpions, ticks, centipedes, and millipedes.

Occurrence: Common worldwide.

Age: All age groups.

Ethnicity: Not significant.

Gender: Occurs equally in males and females.

Contributing Factors: Lightweight clothing; conducive environmental factors (e.g., wooded areas) and hiding places (e.g., dark closets).

Signs and Symptoms: Patient presents with skin lesion with or without specific knowledge of the time of bite or the specific agent. If the agent was an insect, patient will report that there was immediate local pain with variable redness and later itching. Physical findings depend on the type of sting reaction.

Insect Bites and Stings

Patients with insect bites and stings present with skin lesions of varying sizes; the stinger may still be embedded, and redness and erythema are noted around the lesion site.

Spider Bites

Black widow (Latrodectus mactans): Within 1 hour of bite, there is local erythema and pain in regional lymph nodes and local muscle groups. Classic severe cramping pains in the abdomen, thorax, and back.

Brown recluse (Loxosceles reclusa): Local symptoms of itching, redness, and tenderness, with a target lesion, enlarging to form a necrotic central region that heals slowly. Systemic symptoms, often occurring as late as 72 hours after the initial bite, may include fever, chills, headache, and malaise. Severe cases may involve a self-limited hemolysis.

Scorpion (members of the Vaejovis, Hadrurus, Anuroctonus, and Centruroides groups): The first three produce local edema and pain; the latter produce burning paresthesia at the sting site. Other symptoms include hyperventilation, abdominal cramps, urinary incontinence, and respiratory failure.

Diagnostic Tests

None for insect stings.

For a brown recluse spider bite, obtain a urinalysis and a complete blood count (CBC); monitor for hemodialysis.

Differential Diagnosis: None.

Treatment

Insect Stings and Bites

Initial treatment involves removing the stinger, cleansing the site with skin disinfectant, and giving supportive measures (e.g., cool compresses, elevation of the body part, if possible).

For mild allergic symptoms, systemic therapy includes diphenhydramine, 1–2 mg/kg intramuscularly (IM) or by mouth (PO), one dose. Large local reactions may need a short course of prednisone.

For generalized urticaria, wheezing, chest or throat tightness, syncope, or dizziness, give epinephrine (1 : 1000, 0.01 mL/kg, to maximum of 0.3 mL) subcutaneously.

Spider Bites

Initial treatment for black widow spider bites includes thorough cleansing of the wound, application of ice to the wound to impede the effects of venom, checking for current tetanus immunizations, and supportive measures (e.g., rest, elevation of body part, cool compresses to the area).

Scorpion: Sedation is the usual therapy. Maintain a patent airway. Most clinical signs subside within 48 hours.

Follow-up: Follow up in 1 week if patient is prescribed antibiotics or prednisone, or if he or she requires hospitalization.

Sequelae: Anaphylaxis is always a possible sequela. If this occurs, give subcutaneous epinephrine (1 : 1000) 0.01 mL/kg up to 0.5 mL and nebulized β-adrenergic agents for bronchospasm.

Prevention/Prophylaxis: Provision of anaphylaxis kits for children at high risk. Automatic injectors, such as EpiPen, deliver 0.3 mg epinephrine; EpiPen Jr. delivers 0.15 mg epinephrine. Avoid wearing lightweight clothing, and exterminate contaminated areas.

Referral: In cases of upper airway obstruction, refer patient immediately for intubation.

Insect Stings

Refer high-risk patients to an allergist. Those with moderate or severe systemic symptoms should be admitted to the hospital.

Spider Bites

Refer patients for antivenom therapy. Black widow antivenom is available; it has significant side effects, such as anaphylaxis, but it can be used in children. Always test for hypersensitivity to horse serum before administering the drug. There is no antivenom for brown recluse spider bites.

Scorpion: Scorpion antivenom may be necessary for severe cases. Contact local poison control center for availability of specific antivenom.

Education: Ensure that parents know the dangers of insect and arthropod bites and stings, and teach them to call 911 when necessary. Educate parents and children to recognize stinging insects and venomous spiders and to avoid potential danger areas.

Lead Poisoning (Plumbism)

Lead poisoning is toxicity caused by ingestion of lead; likely to occur when more than 0.05 mg of lead is absorbed.

Etiology: Ingestion of lead. Potential sources include lead-based paints, leaded gasoline, leaded objects, lead-based pottery glazes, leaded crystal, battery casings, and the occupations or hobbies of family members (e.g., painting, stained glass making, ceramics).

Occurrence: One in six children is at risk; one in two inner-city children is at risk. Those most at risk are primarily disadvantaged children from decaying neighborhoods.

Age: Usually affects children under age 5 years; those most at risk are aged 1–3 years.

Ethnicity: Not significant.

Gender: Occurs equally in males and females.

Contributing Factors: Older homes painted before 1960 with lead-based paint, lead water pipes, pica, and parental hobbies.

Signs and Symptoms: Child has been found chewing on window sills or crib, or family is remodeling an older house. Assessment of the child at risk involves a simple questionnaire that asks questions such as, Does your child:

> . . . live in or regularly visit a house with peeling or chipping paint that was built before 1960? This might be a day-care center, a preschool, or the home of a babysitter or relative.
> . . . live in or regularly visit a house built before 1960 with recent, ongoing, or planned renovation or remodeling?
> . . . have a brother or sister, housemate, or playmate being followed or treated for lead poisoning (i.e., blood lead level greater than 15 μg/dL)?
> . . . live with an adult whose job or hobby involves exposure to lead?
> . . . live near an active lead smelter, battery recycling plant, or other industry likely to release lead? (sample, CDC, 1991).

The assessment should be completed at each early preventive screening diagnostic testing (EPSDT) visit of children covered by Medicaid. Check with your local health department for the questionnaire developed by your state.

Physical examination reveals the following:

Early stages: Weakness, irritability, weight loss, vomiting, constipation, headache, colicky abdominal pain, burtonian blue lines, and bluish discoloration at the gingival margin.

Late stages: Bradycardia, ataxia, lethargy, retarded mental and physical development, convulsions, and coma.

Diagnostic Tests

> Children at low risk should be screened for lead poisoning yearly until age 4 years.
> Children at high risk should be screened at age 6 months and every 6 months thereafter.
> Children should have a CBC, serum iron levels, serum ferritin, whole blood lead level test (PbB), and erythrocyte photoporphyrin taken when lead levels are greater than 20 μg/dL.
> Radiographic studies of the abdomen should be done.
> Levels of essential metals such as calcium, magnesium, and zinc should be monitored to determine the effects of chelating agents.

Differential Diagnosis: Gastroenteritis, if the early symptoms are vomiting and diarrhea. Attention deficit with hyperactivity.

Treatment

Nonpharmacological
Chelation is not recommended for levels of 25–45 μg; treatment consists of elimination of source, the removal of children from contaminated areas.

Pharmacological
Children with blood lead levels greater than 45 μg/dL (class IV) should be hospitalized for chelation. Chelating agents include the following:

Succimer (Chemet), initial dose 10 mg/kg (350 mg/m^2) q 8 hours for 5 days, and then every 12 hours for 14 days; wait at least 2 weeks before reinitiating therapy.

Dimercaprol (British antilewisite[1] BAL) 4 mg/kg per dose (not preferred therapy).

Edetate calcium disodium (edathamil), usually given with dimercaprol.

Treatment of an associated iron deficiency anemia includes supplemental iron 4–6 mg/kg per day.

Follow-up

Low-Risk Children
Children at low risk are screened at age 12 months. If lead levels are less than 10 μg, screen yearly. If levels are 10–14 μg, recheck every 3–4 months. Obtain a detailed environmental history when levels are 15–19 μg. Begin educational and nutritional counseling. Recheck in 3–4 months; if level is still high, investigate the environment.

High-Risk Children
Children at high risk (positive answers to the risk questionnaire) are screened at age 6 months. If blood levels are less than 10 μg/dL, recheck every 6 months; if greater than 10 μg/dL, recheck every 3–4 months, begin educational and nutritional counseling, and obtain an environmental history. If blood lead level is equal to or greater than 20 μg/dL, recheck every 3–4 months and obtain a detailed history, including clinical symptoms, environmental sources, hand-to-mouth activities, pica, and family history of lead poisoning.

Sequelae: Effects of lead at levels of 35–40 μg/dL or less include learning disabilities, developmental delays, decreased hearing, and impaired growth. There will also be impairment in vitamin D metabolism and hemoglobin synthesis. At blood lead levels above 70 μg/dL encephalopathy, cerebral edema, seizures, coma, and even death may occur.

Lead is teratogenic to the fetus via placental transfer; it causes reduced birth weight and reduced gestational age.

Prevention/Prophylaxis: Use paint containing less than 1% lead for interior use. Remove other sources of lead. Remove the child from areas of environmental pollution.

Referral: Refer patient to a physician for chelation therapy when blood lead levels are greater than 45 μg/dL. Contact social services and health department for environmental assessments and family assistance.

Education: Teach parents the following protective measures for dealing with household lead dust:

Place furniture in front of peeling paint to make it less accessible to children.

Use sticky-backed tape to cover small peeling areas.

Damp dust and mop with a high-phosphate cleaner two times per week to decrease the amount of lead dust. Examples of such cleaners are trisodium phosphate cleaners and some dishwasher detergents.

Remove paint chips with a disposable cloth dampened with the phosphate cleaner and dispose in an appropriate manner.

Do not dry sweep or vacuum: This only spreads the dust.

Do not scrape, sand, or burn lead paint off the surfaces.

Provide a diet high in calcium and iron, as well as a daily vitamin with iron.

Wash and dry toys and pacifiers frequently.

Wash hands frequently, especially before meals and bedtime.

Near Drowning

Near drowning is the survival for 24 hours or more after suffocation by submersion; there is aspiration and apnea resulting in hypoxemia. Illness and death are a result of hypoxic-ischemic injury to the brain. Of the children who survive, 5–20% will have permanent and severe neurologic sequelae. Children who are conscious after resuscitation have an excellent prognosis.

Etiology: Activities such as bathing and swimming place children at risk for drowning. The major sites for children under age 2 years are bathtubs and large buckets of water; for children over age 2, private swimming pools are the major site.

Occurrence: Near drowning is a frequent emergency; children aged 1–3 years have the highest rate of drowning.

Age: Occurs in any age group.

Ethnicity: African-American children are six times more likely to drown in a bucket than white children. Industrial-type, 5-gallon buckets are half the height (14 in.) of an average toddler.

Gender: Occurs equally in younger boys and girls, but more often in adolescent boys than in adolescent girls.

Contributing Factors: Poor supervision of young children, failure to teach children how to swim, swimming in unsupervised waters, and swimming alone. Children with epilepsy or developmental delays are at higher risk.

Signs and Symptoms: Child presents with a history of submersion in water. Child may be or may not be awake or oxygenated. Child may present in a coma. Evaluate state of consciousness, pupils, size, and reaction to light. Whether the child is hypothermic or not depends on the temperature of the water and the length of time submerged. The longer the child is in coma, the poorer the prognosis. The following are some predictors of a poor prognosis:

Submersion greater than 10 minutes.
Delay in providing cardiopulmonary resuscitation (CPR).
Severe metabolic acidosis: pH less than 7.1 after correction for partial pressure of carbon dioxide (PCO_2).
Fixed, dilated pupils.
Glasgow coma score less than 5.
Asystole.

Diagnostic Tests

Arterial blood gases to determine extent of hypoxemia.
Neck and skull films to determine associated injuries; many cases are diving accidents.

Differential Diagnosis: None.

Treatment: The goal is to correct acidosis and hypoxia as soon as possible. Closed chest massage is initiated if no pulse is present. Intubation and positive end-expiratory pressure are often helpful to improve oxygenation. Treat hypothermia with warm blankets. Hyperventilate to maintain PCO_2 in the range of 25–28 mmHg; use fluid restriction and osmotic diuresis. Drainage of ventricular fluid may be required to prevent cerebral ischemia due to intracranial hypertension.

Follow-up: Patient should return to the clinic after release from the hospital for evaluation of progress.

Sequelae: Cerebral edema may result from hypoxia. Pneumonia may result if the water was grossly contaminated. Treat with antibiotics.

Prevention/Prophylaxis: A child under age 3 years should never be left unattended in a bathtub or wading pool or near a swimming pool. Children aged 3–8 years should take swimming lessons. Parents should provide a fence for pools and hot tubs, and if they have a home pool, they should learn CPR.

Referral: Refer patient to a primary-care physician for immediate admission to the hospital; near drowning is always an emergency.

Education: Instruct parents never to leave a child under age 3 years unattended in a bathtub or wading pool, or near a swimming pool. Advise parents to arrange for swimming lessons for children aged 3–8 years. Instruct parents to provide a fence for pools and hot tubs and to learn CPR if they have a home pool.

Poisoning

Poisoning is the accidental or purposeful ingestion of hazardous substances.

Etiology: Any hazardous substance: chemical, medicinal, or botanical.

Occurrence: Common.

Age: Peak age range is 2 years to under 5 years. (*Note:* 25% of children with an initial case of poisoning will have a second episode within 1 year.) In adolescents, such incidents are purposeful and usually represent either "acting out" behavior or a genuine suicide attempt.

Ethnicity: Not significant.

Gender: More common in males than females.

Contributing Factors: Complex issue related to familial and environmental factors, such as (1) inadequate storage of drugs and chemicals in the home (prime factor in childhood poisonings); and (2) lack of knowledge that some house plants, as well as common garden and wild plants, are poisonous when ingested. Occurs most frequently in kitchen, bathrooms, and garages.

Signs and Symptoms: Child presents with a history of either known or suspected ingestion of a poisonous substance (Fig. 17–3). Caregiver has often found the child engaged in the harmful activity. Adolescents may purposely ingest toxic substances as a means of attempting suicide. Gather information related to time of ingestion (noting time elapsed before parents began to seek health care), how the event happened, possible substance, where the event occurred, any previous episodes of drug abuse, possibility of suicide attempt, and what has already been done (e.g., home remedies) to help the patient. Also, obtain a past medical history and a list of the substances that were present and accessible to the patient. (*Note:* this history may not be reliable; patient may be asymptomatic or may present in an unconscious or agitated state.)

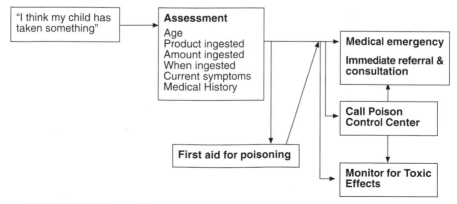

FIGURE 17–3 Evaluation of poisoning.

A thorough physical examination can provide clues as to the substance as well as confirm the history. Conduct a review of systems, taking into consideration the following:

Vital signs: Blood pressure may be increased (amphetamine, lysergic acid diethylamide [LSD], cocaine, rhododendron) or decreased (barbiturates, imipramine, tricyclic antidepressants, monk's hood); pulse may be increased (atropine, aspirin) or decreased (digitalis, narcotics, organophosphates); respirations may be increased (aspirin, amphetamines) or decreased (alcohol, narcotics, yellow jasmine). Check for pattern of respirations (Kussmaul's, apneustic) and body temperature, hyperthermia or hypothermia.

Breath odors: Alcohol (ethanol); bitter almonds (cyanide); acetone (salicylate, methanol); garlic (arsenic, organophosphates); wintergreen (methyl salicylate); violets (turpentine).

Skin: Diaphoretic (aspirin, cocaine, organophosphates); dry (anticholinergic agents); mottled and/or track marks (heroin, phencyclidine [PCP], amphetamine); discoloration (lobster red, boric acid; red, belladonna alkaloids; yellow, delayed jaundice in acetaminophen toxicity).

Mouth: Dry (amphetamines, antihistamines); increased secretions (organophosphates, corrosives).

Eyes: Pupils characterized by miosis, mydriasis (irritant gases, organophosphates); conjunctivae injected, pale, and yellow (delayed jaundice, acetaminophen toxicity).

CNS: Ataxia (alcohol, narcotics, phenytoin); coma (sedatives, salicylate, carbon monoxide, cyanide, poison hemlock); altered behavior (LSD, PCP, alcohol, cocaine, camphor).

Gastrointestinal system: Increased or decreased bowel sounds, constipation, colic (arsenic, lead); diarrhea (arsenic, iron, boric acid, castor bean, foxglove, lily of the valley); vomiting (larkspur, castor bean).

Diagnostic Tests: Laboratory tests can provide clues toward determining the substance ingested. The following are commonly ordered tests:

Hematocrit, arterial blood gases, pulse oximetry, and serum electrolytes.

Carboxyhemoglobin (suggests carbon monoxide poisoning).

Urine ferric acid provides evidence of ingestion or salicylate of phenothiazine, or isoniazid.

Blood calcium reveals oxalates, fluoride, and ethylene glycol.

Radiographic studies (radiopaque substances are visualized on kidney, ureter, and bladder); ingestion of chloral hydrate, heavy metals, iron, Play-Doh is also revealed.

ECG: prolonged Q–T intervals suggest phenothiazine. Widened QRS complexes suggest ingestion of quinidine or tricyclic antidepressants; sinus bradycardia suggests digoxin, cyanide, or β-blocker ingestion.

Differential Diagnosis: If the child presents with altered mental status, consider metabolic disorders, with ketoacidosis; infectious problems, such as meningitis; and structural diseases, such as an intracranial mass. An in-depth history will rule out these problems.

Treatment (Detoxification)

Cutaneous Exposure

Remove the clothing and wash the exposed areas to decontaminate. In cases of ocular exposure, rinse the eye with copious amounts of normal saline, paying particular attention to the conjunctival fornices.

Ingestion

Gastric emptying: Syrup of ipecac, 15 mL for children over 1 year and 30 mL for adolescents (ipecac induces vomiting in about 20 minutes). Home ipecac administration, under the supervision of a physician or poison control center, is indicated for ingestion of acetaminophen, aspirin, toxic plants, and iron-containing substances, such as multivitamins. Induced vomiting within 30 minutes of ingestion can eliminate about 30% of the substance. Ipecac is contraindicated in children who are comatose or who have ingested caustic agents or volatile petroleum distillates (Figs. 17–4, 17–5, and 17–6).

Lavage: Use a tube that approximates the size of the child's thumb and use 50 to 100 aliquots of fluid. Always protect the airway, as vomiting does occur during the procedure. The effectiveness of lavage is inversely proportional to the length of time since toxic ingestion. Do not initiate lavage when the substances contain caustics and solvents because of the risk of damage to the esophagus. Having the patient drink water or milk is a reasonable measure in these cases.

Absorbents: Activated charcoal, 1 g/kg. Mix the powder with enough liquid to make a drinkable slurry. Have the patient drink the solution, or administer it via a nasogastric tube. If ipecac was administered, wait 20 minutes before giving the charcoal. Not recommended for pure caustics, solvents, or iron. Serum concentrations of theophylline, salicylates, and barbiturates are reduced with multiple doses of activated charcoal.

Alkalinization of the urine to a pH of 7.8, combining fluid loading and diuresis (the principle of ion trapping), enhances the excretion of phenobarbital and salicylates.

Follow-up: Return in 24 hours for evaluation.

Sequelae: Permanent tissue injury or even death.

Prevention/Prophylaxis: Proper storage of chemicals and medicines.

Referral: Call the Regional Poison Control Center for definitive antidotes. If necessary, refer patient immediately to a primary-care physician for definitive treatment and hospitalization. Refer patients who have attempted suicide to a mental health center for counseling.

Education: Increase awareness to the dangers of childhood poisoning through parent education. Remind parents that children are curious and investigative.

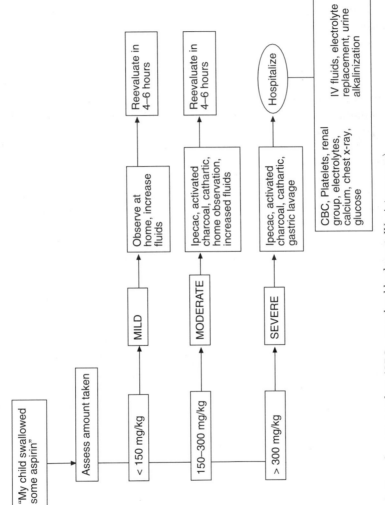

FIGURE 17–4   Evaluation of aspirin overdose. (CBC = complete blood count; IV = intravenous.)

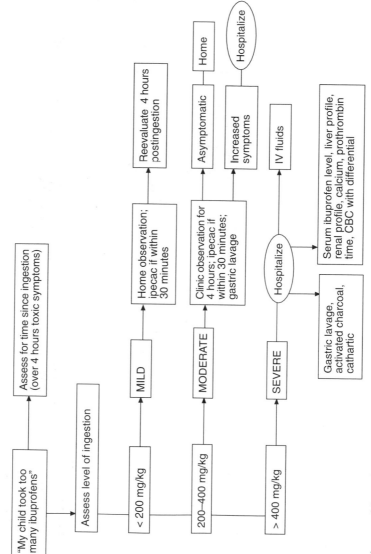
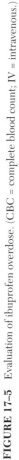

FIGURE 17–5   Evaluation of ibuprofen overdose. (CBC = complete blood count; IV = intravenous.)

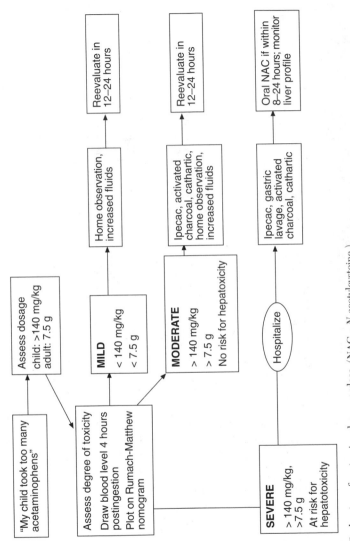

FIGURE 17–6 Evaluation of acetaminophen overdose. (NAC = *N*-acetylcysteine.)

Instruct parents of young children to keep hazardous products out of sight and out of reach—under lock and key, if possible. Teach parents never to store medicine and chemicals in a cabinet used to store food, and not to store such substances in a container normally used for food. Instruct parents to learn to use safety closures on packages, to read the labels on products, to avoid taking medicine in the presence of children, and never to tell a child that medicine is "candy." Advise parents to keep emergency phone numbers—doctor, hospital, police department, fire department, and emergency rescue squad—by the telephone.

Snake Bites

A snake bite is any puncture of the skin by the fangs of a snake, possibly with envenomization.

Etiology: Of bites by venomous snakes in the United States, 98% are caused by rattlesnakes, water moccasins, copperheads (pit vipers), coral snakes (elapids), and occasionally by exotic, imported snakes. No envenomation occurs in 25% of all bites.

Occurrence: Rare to common, depending on the area.

Age: All pediatric age groups.

Ethnicity: Not significant.

Gender: Occurs equally in males and females.

Contributing Factors: Living or participating in activities in rural, wooded areas.

Signs and Symptoms: Patient reports having been bitten by a snake. Determine the time elapsed from the bite to the patient's arrival at the health-care facility. Determine the type of snake; most bites are from nonvenomous varieties.

> *Pit vipers:* There is a double puncture wound surrounded by ecchymosis, pain, discoloration, and edema.

> *Elapids:* Initially there is little local pain, swelling, or necrosis around the double-puncture wound. In 5–10 hours, however, bulbar paralysis, dysphagia, and dysphoria may develop.

Diagnostic Tests

Obtain baseline studies: CBC, platelets, glucose, blood urea nitrogen (BUN), creatinine, serum electrolytes, transaminases, bilirubin, creatine kinase, prothrombin time, partial thromboplastin time, thrombin time, and fibrinogen. Cross-type in cases of hemolytic anemia.

Differential Diagnosis: Venomous snakes, in contrast to nonvenomous snakes, have a triangular head, elliptical pupils, and long fangs. If there are no fang marks, envenomation did not occur.

Treatment: Observe for 4 hours for progression of local or systemic symptoms. Assess for tetanus immunization status.

Emergency

Apply tourniquet loosely, proximal to edema, and splint the extremity. Transport patient to a medical facility. When transport will take more than 1 hour and the bite is from a venomous variety, clean the wound, make a 5-mm incision over the fang marks, and apply suction. *Do not* use a tight tourniquet or pack with ice.

Inpatient Treatment

Observe for development of severe symptoms of envenomation. Antivenom therapy should be started within 2 hours of the bite. Perform a skin test for sensitivity before initiating antivenom. Local envenomation includes bites involving digits and other tight fascial compartments; bites that are swelling rapidly; swelling involving more than half of the bitten limb; and bites from pit vipers, whose venom is known to be necrotic. Systemic envenomation is manifested by hypotension, shock, cardiac arrhythmias, impaired consciousness, neurotoxic signs, dark urine, tender and stiff muscles, and bleeding (spontaneous or excessive).

The dose of the antivenom is individualized based on the degree of envenomation. In moderate cases, give 3–5 vials IV; in severe cases, give 10–20 vials IV. Monitor for allergic reactions: Serum sickness is common 4–7 days after treatment.

Follow-up: Depends on the severity of illness.

Sequelae

Pit vipers: In severe cases, respiratory difficulty, shock, and death (within 6–8 hours).

Elapids: In severe cases, total peripheral paralysis and death (within 24 hours).

Prevention/Prophylaxis: Teach patients to wear boots and long pants, not to go barefoot, and not to explore under logs or crevices when walking in wooded areas.

Referral: Refer patient for immediate hospitalization. Consult with surgeon if bite is on a distal extremity. Consult the Antivenom Index, Tucson, AZ; 24-hour hot line, 1-520-626-6016.

Education: Teach children the difference between venomous and nonvenomous snakes in their areas. Instruct them to wear appropriate clothing when engaging in activities in wooded areas.

REFERENCES

General

Behrman, R, and Kliegman, R (eds): Nelson Essentials of Pediatrics. WB Saunders, Philadelphia, 1990.

Doenges, M, and Moorhouse, M: Nursing Diagnoses with Interventions, ed 4. FA Davis, Philadelphia, 1993.

Hay, W, et al: Current Pediatric Diagnosis & Treatment, ed 12. Appleton & Lange, Norwalk, Conn, 1995.

Lee-Chiong, T, and Stitt, J: Heatstroke and other heat-related illnesses. Grad Med 98:26, 1995.

Animal and Human Bites

ACIP: Recommendations of the Immunization Practices Advisory Committee (ACIP). MMWR 88:55, 1991.

Dinman, S, and Jarosz, D: Managing serious dog bite injuries in children. Pediatric Nursing 22(5):413.

Gluckman, S, et al: Acute care for bite wounds: Mammalian bites—watch for infection. Patient Care 29(8):146, 1995.

Lewis, K, and Stiles, M: Management of cat and dog bites. Am Fam Phys 52:479, 1995.

Steele, R: The Clinical Handbook of Pediatric Infectious Disease. Parthenon, New York, 1994.

Heatstroke

Starr, C: Preventing heat-related tragedies. Patient Care 29(13):8, 1995.

Insect and Arthropod Bites and Stings

Gluckman, S, and Talley, J: Venomous spiders: Think black or brown. Patient Care 29(8):170, 1995.

Lead Poisoning

Castiglia, P: Lead poisoning. J Pediatr Health Care 9:134, 1995.

Centers for Disease Control: Preventing lead poisoning in children: A statement. Centers for Disease Control, Atlanta, 1991.

Chao, J, and Kikano, G: Lead poisoning in children. Am Fam Phys 41:113, 1993.

Jonides, L, et al: Three year old child with elevated lead level. J Pediatr Health Care 9:40, 1995.

Needham, D: Diagnosis and management of lead-poisoned children: The pediatric nurse practitioner in a specialty program. J Pediatr Health Care 8:268, 1994.

Near Drowning

Bross, M, and Clark, J: Near-drowning. Am Fam Phys 51(6):1545, 1995.

Castiglia, P: Drowning. J Pediatr Health Care 9:185, 1995.

Poisoning

Foltin, G, and Goldfrank, L: Emergency care of the poisoning victim. Hosp Med 29(12):33, 1993.

Snake Bites

Gluckman, S, and Talley, J: Poisonous snake: Shy but deadly. Patient Care 29(13):162, 1995.

CHAPTER **18**

SYMPTOM-BASED

PROBLEMS

The previous chapters in this volume have focused on the clinical approach to patients using an organ-system approach. The nurse practitioner gathers information—through taking a history and performing a physical examination, analyzing that information in terms of the organ system or illness involved, and synthesizing that data into a working diagnosis that determines additional data required—and then makes a preliminary treatment plan. However, because children are seldom able to verbalize their complaints or describe their symptoms as adequately as adults, the reliability of their comments is often questioned, as are the comments of sometimes overwrought caregivers.

Often the child is brought to the clinic with vague complaints (e.g., fever, pain) focusing on a symptom, rather than a specific illness, that may affect several organ systems. Therefore, the ability to sort through not only the limited information given, but the bulk of data available, and to select from multiple options for treatment is the trademark of a good clinician.

The monographs and decision trees presented in this chapter focus on such vague complaints as a means of outlining how to select and gather appropriate data from the history, the physical, and the laboratory in order to make an acceptable diagnosis and determine the plan of care. The decision trees serve as aids to the problem-solving process in terms of clinical decision-making.

Febrile Seizures

Febrile seizures are generalized tonic-clonic episodes, associated with high fevers; patients have little postictal confusion or weakness. Seizures usually last less than 15 minutes and occur once in a 24-hour period.

Etiology: Unknown, but the rapidity of onset of fever, 101°F or higher, appears to be related.

Occurrence: Febrile seizures occur in 3–4% of all children; 25–30% will have a second occurrence and less than 9% will have more than three. Seizure recurrences occur within 6–12 months of the initial seizure.

Age: Onset typically occurs before age 3 years but may continue in children as old as 6 years.

Ethnicity: May be higher in African-Americans.

Gender: More common in males.

Contributing Factors: Any underlying illness that increases body temperature.

Signs and Symptoms: Child is brought to the clinic, and parent reports that a seizure occurred when the child's temperature went up. Child has a history of a sudden increase in body temperature to greater than 101°F, onset of generalized tonic-clonic seizure activity, and loss of consciousness. Child had little or no postictal confusion (Fig. 18–1).

Diagnostic Tests

None for the initial episode or repeated episodes when preceded by a fever and when the source of the fever is identified.

Lumbar puncture may be performed if meningitis is suspected.

Electroencephalography (EEG) performed 2 weeks after the seizure may help to rule out seizure disorder. Related episodes unrelated to fever require additional workup for seizure disorder.

Differential Diagnosis: Focus on determining the underlying cause. Differentiate febrile seizures from seizures due to epilepsy or a primary injury or disease of the central nervous system (CNS), such as head trauma or aneurysm, respectively. A description of the seizure may assist in the diagnosis: Complex seizures are focal, last longer than 15 minutes, and occur more than once in a 24-hour period.

Treatment: Acetaminophen or ibuprofen can reduce the fever. Further treatment depends on the underlying cause. See Tables 8–6a and 8–6b for dosing.

Follow-up: Have caregiver report any further seizures. Consider initiating anticonvulsant therapy if patient has more than three episodes, if the seizures last longer than 15 minutes, if there is a family history of nonfebrile seizures, or if neurological abnormalities are present or persist.

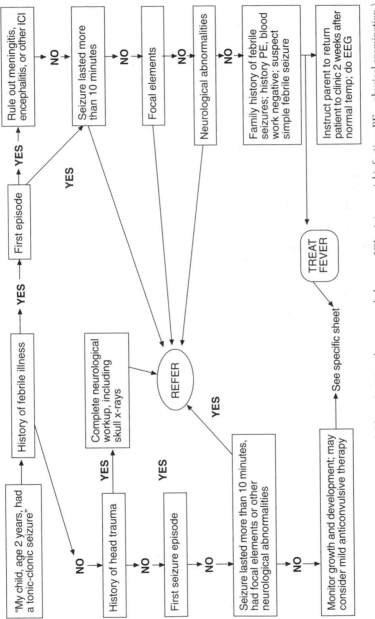

Sequelae: A seizure episode that lasts for a long time may result in Todd's paralysis. The paralysis is transient (1 hour to 1 month) and affects one side and the extremities.

Prevention/Prophylaxis: Children with a history of febrile seizures may be given diazepam 0.033 mg/kg at the onset of a fever (one dose) and should be treated with Advil or Tylenol appropriate for age.

Referral: For repeated episodes, consult with or refer patient to a primary-care physician or neurologist for definitive diagnosis and treatment.

Education: Explain to caregivers that, although frightening, febrile seizures are usually self-limiting with little or no significant sequelae. Most children have no more than one episode.

Fever

Fever is a rectal temperature greater than 38°C (100.4°F), oral temperature greater than 37.5° (99.5°F), and axillary temperature greater than 37° (98.6°F). The three categories of fever are as follows:

Fever of short duration with localizing signs.
Fever without localizing signs and with a duration of less than 1 week.
Fever of unknown origin (FUO), with a duration of more than 14 days, that remains undiagnosed; in adolescents, an FUO is a sustained fever lasting more than 21 days with 7 days' hospitalization that remains undiagnosed.

Fever should be distinguished from hyperthermia, which is an abnormal rise in body temperature that is not due to a disease process.

Etiology: The body's natural response to infection or certain disease processes.

Occurrence: Common.

Age: Any age group.

Ethnicity: Not significant.

Gender: Occurs equally in males and females.

Contributing Factors: Contributing factors include the child's immune status (e.g., nonimmunized, immunosuppressed, diagnosed with sickle cell anemia); and environmental factors, such as enrollment in a day-care center, history of family illness, presence of pets, and recent travel.

Signs and Symptoms: Child presents with a history of fever, or parent complains that the child feels hot. The history should include queries related to the immune system, recent hospitalizations, environmental factors, and the presence of rashes (Figs. 18–2, 18–3, and 18–4).

Specific physical findings may or may not be present; they are not present in cases of nonspecific fever. The presence of rashes, organomegaly, painful

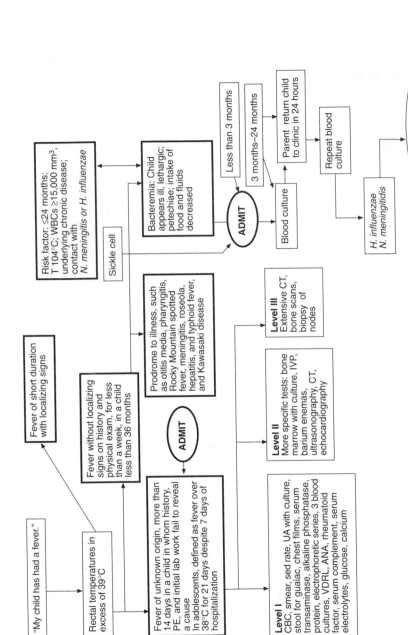

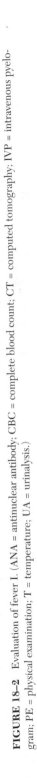

FIGURE 18–2 Evaluation of fever I. (ANA = antinuclear antibody; CBC = complete blood count; CT = computed tomography; IVP = intravenous pyelogram; PE = physical examination; T = temperature; UA = urinalysis.)

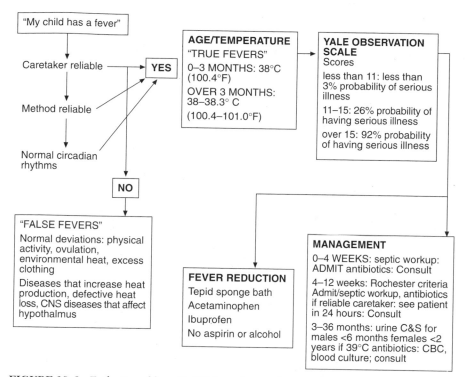

FIGURE 18–3   Evaluation of fever II. (C&S = culture and sensitivity.)

joints, and murmurs may provide clues to diagnosis. Assess the level of illness (Tables 18–1 and 18–2). The Yale Observation Scale and the Rochester Criteria are useful for determining who can be treated as an outpatient.

Diagnostic Tests

Complete blood count (CBC) with differential, peripheral smear, and erythrocyte sedimentation rate less than 15,000 cells/mm^3 and 10% bands.

Urinalysis with culture (particularly for boys under 6 months and girls under 2 years).

Blood culture (takes 24–48 hours for results).

Spinal tap to rule out meningitis.

Stool for blood and culture to rule out enteric causes.

Chest radiograph to rule out pneumonia.

Serum transaminase, alkaline phosphatase.

Serologic tests: Venereal Disease Research Laboratory (VDRL); tests to rule out collagen diseases include antinuclear antibodies, rheumatoid factor, and complement.

Differential Diagnosis: True fevers are usually due to viral infections; other causes are bacterial infections, leukemia, lymphoma, juvenile rheumatoid arthritis, and enteric fever. Differentiate between true fevers and the following:

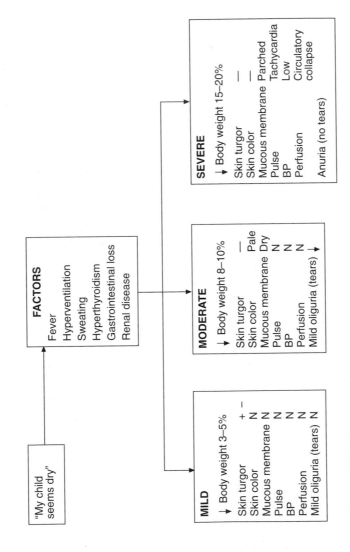

FIGURE 18–4 Classification of dehydration.

TABLE 18–1 YALE OBSERVATION SCALE

Observation Item	1: Normal	2: Moderate Impairment	3: Severe Impairment
1. Quality of cry	Strong or none	Whimper or sob	Weak or moaning; has high-pitched, continuous cry or hardly responds
2. Reaction to parent stimulation	Cries briefly, or does not cry and is content	Cries off and on	Persistent cry with little response
3. State variation	If awake, stays awake; if asleep, awakens quickly	Eyes close briefly when awake or awakens with prolonged stimulation	No arousal and falls asleep
4. Color	Pink	Pale extremities or acrocyanosis	Pale, cyanotic, mottled, or ashen
5. Hydration	Skin and eyes normal; moist membranes	Skin and eyes normal and mouth slightly dry	Skin doughy or tented; dry mucous membranes and/or sunken eyes
6. Response to social overtures	Smiles or alert (consistently)	Brief smile or alert	No smile, anxious, dull; no alertness to social overtures

A total score of less than 11 signifies a less than 3% probability of serious illness.
A total score of 11–15 signifies a 26% probability of serious illness.
A total score of greater than 15 signifies a greater than 92% probability of serious illness.

"Fevers" reported by unreliable caretakers.

Elevations in body temperature due to normal deviations, such as physical activity, ovulation, environmental heat, and excess clothing.

Temperature elevations due to diseases that increase heat production or cause defective heat loss, or CNS diseases that affect the hypothalamus.

"Fevers" reported as a result of an incorrectly taken temperature or a thermometer that is unreliable.

Treatment: Take immediate measures to reduce fever in the following cases:

Child is less than 2–3 months old.

Child is having an active seizure.

Temperature is greater than 106–107°F.

Child has altered mental status.

Child is immunocompromised.

There is an alteration in vital signs: hypotension or extremely fast pulse and respiratory rate.

There is a suspicion of non–interleukin-1 fever as a result of underlying CNS disease.

TABLE 18-2 ROCHESTER CRITERIA

Previously healthy febrile infants less than 60 days of age are considered at low risk for serious
bacterial infection if all of the following criteria are met:
1. Infant appears generally well and nontoxic
   Activity, hydration, and perfusion normal*
2. **Infant has been previously healthy:**
   Born at term (37 weeks' gestation)
   No antenatal or perinatal antimicrobial therapy
   No treatment for unexplained hyperbilirubinemia
   Not hospitalized longer than mother
   Has not received and not currently receiving antimicrobial therapy
   No previous hospitalization
   No chronic or underlying illnesses
3. Infant has no evidence of skin, soft tissue, bone, joint, or ear infection on physical examination.
4. **Infant meets the following laboratory parameters:**
   Peripheral white blood cell count of 5000–15,000 cells/mm³ (5.0–15.0 × 10⁹/L)
   Absolute band cell count of less than 1500 bands/mm³
   Less than 10 white blood cells per high-power field on microscopic examination of spun urine
   sediment†or gram-stained smear*
   Less than 5 white blood cells per high-power field on microscopic examination of a stool smear
   (in infants with diarrhea)†
5. **Social situation:**
   Parents/caregiver mature and reliable
   Reliable transportation available
   Thermometer and telephone at child's home
   Travel time to care facility less than 30 minutes*

*Adapted from Baraff, LJ, et al: Practice guidelines for the management of infants and children 0–36
months of age with fever without source. Pediatrics 92:1, 1993.
†From McCarthy et al: Predictive value of abnormal physical examination findings in ill appearing
and well appearing febrile children. Pediatrics 76:167, 1985.

Fever is a result of burns or exposure.

Tepid sponges reduce the temperature by 0.5–1.0°F and may induce a rise as a
result of the shivering. *Do not give* alcohol sponges baths. *Do not give aspirin.*
Initiate pharmacologic measures to reduce fever. Alcohol may cause the fever to
drop too rapidly; the use of aspirin has been linked to Reye's syndrome. Dosages
for acetaminophen and ibuprofen are provided in Tables 8–6a and 8–6b.

Management

Infants aged 0–28 days: Order septic workup and admit to hospital. Direct antibiotics at apparent focus; if none, give ampicillin and a third-generation
cephalosporin.

Infants aged 4–12 weeks: If Rochester Criteria are met, order septic workup
and give ceftriaxone 50 mg/kg intramuscularly (**IM**) if spinal tap and blood
culture were obtained; recheck in 12–24 hours (severe bacterial infection
will develop in only 1%).

Toxic infants: If infant is toxic and fails Rochester Criteria, order septic workup, admit, and direct antibiotics at apparent focus; if none, give ampicillin and a third-generation cephalosporin pending culture results.

Nontoxic child with temperature greater than 39.9°C (102.2°F): Order septic workup, give empiric antibiotics, and instruct parents to return child to clinic in 24 hours.

Follow-up: Routine postinfection follow-up after the administration of antibiotics.

Sequelae: Depend on the underlying cause and the appropriateness of the treatment; "false fevers" can be harmful if steps are not taken to recognize the basis of the "fever" and eliminating its cause (e.g., removing excess clothing).

Prevention/Prophylaxis: Reduction of environmental risks and initiation and maintenance of appropriate immunization status.

Referral: Refer patient to pediatrician for admission in the following cases:

Any child under age 28 days.

Any child in whom the cause cannot be determined.

Sickle cell anemia patients with fever.

Any level II or III evaluation.

Education: When child is sent home to be observed, instruct the parent or caregiver to assess the child every 4 hours for temperature, activity, and skin color. Have parent call immediately if there are changes such as poor feeding, the presence of a rash, cyanosis, jerky movements (including eye movements), bulging fontanelle, and any difficulty in arousing or comforting. Instruct parents in the proper method of taking a temperature. Teach parents the definition of fever and how to properly use and read a thermometer. Instruct parents in ways to reduce environmental factors and to avoid overreporting of false fevers.

Pain

Pain is the objective response to a traumatic event that occurs with varying degrees of severity.

Etiology: Trauma, infection, burns, lesions, and tumors.

Occurrence: Common.

Age: All age groups.

Ethnicity: Not significant.

Gender: Occurs equally in males and females.

Contributing Factors: Individual responses to pain may be culturally determined, especially as related to appropriate gender responses. A person's pain threshold determines the reported severity of the pain.

Signs and Symptoms: Signs and symptoms may vary from stoicism to crying; from verbalization of the area of discomfort to guarding of the body part.

Diagnostic Tests

Self-report (children aged 5 years and older are considered reliable reporters).

Observed behavioral and physiologic changes, such as crying, changes in facial expression, and changes in pulse rate, blood pressure, and skin color.

Pain assessment tools such as the following:

Simple descriptor scales: Severity rating is selected by words ranging from "very little" to "a whole lot." Words can be changed to fit the age of the child.

Numeric scales: Severity is rated using a scale from 0 to 10 or 100. The tool can be easily constructed using a ruler, using 1 inch per degree of severity of pain.

Visual analog scales: Severity is rated on scale from 0 to 10. A rating of 10 is twice as severe as a rating of 5.

Color analog scales: The colors used are either a gradation of one color or gradation of several colors, with the highest intensity of pain related to the most intense color. The clinician then matches this scale with a numerical scale.

Pain thermometer: Severity of pain is described by matching the perceived pain to the drawing of a thermometer.

Faces scales: Severity of pain is described by matching the perceived pain to the facial drawing that most matches the feeling.

The Oucher: An adaptation of the Faces scale that allows children to select the photograph that most adequately describes the severity of their pain.

Poker chip tool: The degree of severity is measured by the number of poker chips chosen from a group of 10.

Differential Diagnosis: Assess the child for the degrees of fear and anxiety, because these factors relate to the intensity of the pain (Fig. 18–5).

Treatment: Specific pain management depends on the causative event. Refer to other chapters on each causal event. Table 18–3 lists recommended dosages of controlled substances (opiates) used to control pain.

Follow-up: Monitor the child to assess efficacy of treatment.

Sequelae: Unrelieved pain may result in increased anxiety, panic, or combativeness.

Prevention/Prophylaxis: Elicit from parent and child their expectations of the visit, as well as a history of past painful experiences and the child's usual coping mechanisms.

Referral: Refer patient to a physician if it is necessary to administer opiates.

Education: Counsel parents to assist the child in approaching new experiences in a realistic manner, and not to use scare tactics as related to health-care pro-

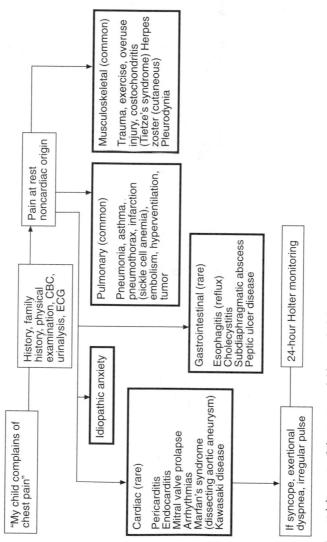

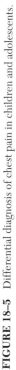

FIGURE 18–5 Differential diagnosis of chest pain in children and adolescents.

TABLE 18-3   RECOMMENDED DOSAGES FOR SELECTED
CONTROLLED SUBSTANCES USED FOR PAIN MANAGEMENT

Drug	Persons Greater Than 50 kg Body Weight		Persons Less Than 50 kg Body Weight (over age 6 months)	
	Oral	Parenteral	Oral	Parenteral
Morphine	30 mg q 3–4 h	10 mg q 3–4 h	0.3 mg/kg q 3–4 h	0.1 mg/kg q 3–4 h
Codeine	60 mg q 3–4 h	60 mg q 2 h IM, SC	1 mg/kg q 3–4 h	Not recommended
Meperidine (Demerol)	Not recommended	100 mg q 3 h	Not recommended	0.75 mg/kg q 2–3 h
Hydrocodone (Lorcet, Lortab, Vicodan)	10 mg q 3–4 h	Not available	0.2 mg/kg q 3–4 h	Not available
Oxycodone (Percocet, Percodan, Tylox)	10 mg q 3–4 h	Not available	0.2 mg/kg q 3–4 h	Not available

vider visits, such as "Behave or they will give you a shot." Instruct parents in the proper administration of analgesics via a syringe or graduated dropper.

Vomiting

Vomiting is a common symptom of many disease processes, gastrointestinal and nongastrointestinal, described as the forceful ejection of gastric contents often preceded by nausea. Vomiting is differentiated from regurgitation, which is a passive ejection of gastric contents due to reflux.

Etiology: Caused by the coordination of gastric atony, relaxation of the gastroesophageal junction, and increased abdominal pressure; mediated by the medullary emesis center in the floor of the fourth ventricle and influenced by visceral afferent and chemoreceptive trigger zone stimuli. Less common causes are ear infections, brain tumor, hepatitis, and increased intracranial pressure.

Occurrence: Common.

Age: Any age.

Ethnicity: Not significant.

Gender: Occurs equally in males and females.

Contributing Factors: Various stimuli, including drugs and motion, affect the emesis center.

Signs and Symptoms: Patient presents with a history of nausea and forceful ejection of gastric contents. Assessment of the child with vomiting includes a history of time (i.e., since last feeding and number of times vomited); character of vomiting (forceful, projectile); description of the vomitus (color and amount); and other associated symptoms, such as abdominal pain, fever, and headache (Fig. 18–6).

On palpation, there may be epigastric tenderness; auscultation may reveal increased bowel sounds. Nausea is assumed to be present in infants if, after vomiting they do not want to feed but do drool. Obtain an accurate weight.

Diagnostic Tests

CBC to determine whether underlying cause is viral or bacterial.
Urinalysis to check for urinary tract infection and dehydration.
Screen for sodium, potassium, calcium, magnesium, and blood urea nitrogen to identify metabolic disorders and acidosis.
Amylase screen to rule out pancreatitis.
Erythrocyte sedimentation rate to determine presence of inflammatory bowel disease.

Differential Diagnosis: Investigation of the complaint of vomiting, the age of the child, and the characteristics of the vomiting, along with the physical examination, can lead to the differentiation of the illness (Tables 18–4 and 18–5).

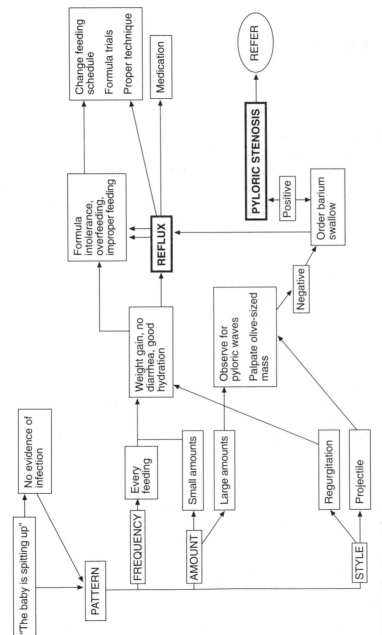

FIGURE 18-6 Vomiting in infants.

TABLE 18–4 DIAGNOSTIC SIGNS IN VOMITING

Color	Quality	Suspect
Gastric contents	Passive	Reflux
	Forceful	Overfeeding
		CNS lesions
		Peptic ulcer
		Chronic UTIs
		Chronic otitis
	Projectile	Pyloric stenosis
Bile-colored		Obstruction
		Gastroenteritis
Mucus/blood		Intussusception
		Toxic colitis

CNS = central nervous system; UTIs = urinary tract infections.

Treatment: Goal is to treat underlying cause and to restore hydration.

Nonpharmacological

No solid foods: only clear liquids for 24 hours.

TABLE 18–5 COMMON AGE-SPECIFIC CAUSES OF VOMITING

Infancy	
Disease or Symptom	**Etiology**
Volvulus intussusception	Congenital malformations
Gastroenteritis	Bacterial or viral infection
Formula intolerance	Milk-protein intolerance
Overfeeding	Not true vomiting
Reflux	Not true vomiting

Children/Adolescents	
Disease or Symptom	**Etiology**
Gastroenteritis	Bacterial or viral infection
Systemic diseases	Inflammatory bowel disease, ulcers, appendicitis
Signs of toxic ingestion	Ingestion of poisons, drugs, medications
Abdominal pain	Appendicitis
Bulimia	Self-induced vomiting immediately after meal

Less common causes of vomiting: ear infections, brain tumor, hepatitis, and increased intracranial pressure

Pharmacological

Promethazine (Phenergan) suppositories, 25 mg, ½ to 1 suppository q 6 hours for vomiting.

Intravenous fluid replacement if patient is severely dehydrated.

Follow-up: Follow up in the first 24 hours and again in 72 hours to evaluate progress.

Sequelae: Child may become dehydrated, depending on the underlying cause.

Prevention/Prophylaxis: None.

Referral: Consult with or refer patient to a primary physician in case of dehydration or suspicion of a complex underlying disorder. Refer to a surgeon if appendicitis is suspected.

Education: Reassure parents that most cases are self-limiting and that vomiting is a symptom, not a disease.

REFERENCES

General

Behrman, R, and Kleigman, R: Nelson Essentials of Pediatrics. WB Saunders, Philadelphia, 1990.
Berman, S: Pediatric Decision Making. Decker, Philadelphia, 1991.
Doenges, M, and Moorhouse, M: Nursing Diagnosis with Interventions. FA Davis, Philadelphia, 1993.
Green, M: Pediatric Diagnosis, ed 5. WB Saunders, Philadelphia, 1992.
Hay, W, et al: Current Pediatric Diagnosis and Treatment. Appleton & Lange, Norwalk, Conn, 1995.

Febrile Seizures

Freeman, J: What have we learned from febrile seizures? Pediatr Ann 21:355, 1992.
Monson, R, and Snell, G: Febrile seizure: Caring for patients—and their parents. Postgrad Med 90:217, 1991.
Rosmasn, N, et al: A controlled trial of diazepam administered during febrile illnesses to prevent recurrence of febrile seizures. N Engl J Med 329:79, 1993.

Fever

Daaleman, T: Fever without source in infants and young children. Am Fam Phys 54:2503, 1996.
Kruse, J: Management of the young child with fever. Am Fam Phys 54:2362, 1996.
McCarthy, P, et al: Predictive value of abnormal physical examination findings in ill appearing and well appearing febrile children. Pediatrics 76:167, 1985.

Pain

Carr, D, et al: Treat pain as a medical emergency. Patient Care 29(13):60, 1995.
McGrath, PA: Pain in the pediatric patient: Practical aspects of assessment. Pediatr Ann 24:126, 1995.
McGrath, PJ, and McAlpine, L: Psychologic perspectives on pediatric pain. J Pediatr 122:22, 1993.
Schechter, NL: Common pain problems in the general pediatric setting. Pediatr Ann 24:139, 1995.

APPENDIX 1

RESOURCES

ADD Advocacy Group
15772 E. Crestridge Cir.
Aurora, CO 80015
1-303-690-7548

AIDS Hotline
Atlanta, GA
1-800-551-2728

Alpha Line
1-800-425-7421

Alpha-1 National Association
1829 Portland Ave.
Minneapolis, MN 55404
1-612-871-1747

American Lung Association
1740 Broadway
New York, NY 10019-4371
1-800-LUNG-USA

American Pseudo-Obstruction &
   Hirshsprung's Disease Society
P.O. Box 772
Medford, MA 02155
1-617-395-4255

American Sleep Disorder Association
1610 14th St., NW, Suite 300
Rochester, MN 55901
1-507-287-6006

American Speech-Language-Hearing
   Association (ASHA)
10801 Rockville Pk., Dept. MO
Rockville, MD 20852
1-800-638-8255

American Sudden Infant Death
   Syndrome Institute
Atlanta, GA
1-800-232-7437

Association of Birth Defect
   Children
827 Ima St.
Orlando, FL 32803
1-407-245-7035

Autism Society of America
7910 Woodmont Ave. #650
Bethesda, MD 20814-3015
1-800-328-8476
Fax 1-301-657-0869

BASH—Bulimia Anorexia
  Self-Help
St Louis, MO
1-800-227-4785

Candlelighters Childhood Cancer
  Foundation
7910 Woodmont Ave. #460
Bethesda, MD 20814-3015
1-800-366-2223

Capital Area Pediatric Heartburn
  Reflux Assoc
P.O. Box 1153
Germantown, MD 20875-1153
1-301-972-6128

Children and Adults with Attention
  Deficit Disorder
499 N.W. 70th Ave. #109
Plantation, FL 33317
1-305-587-3700

Clearinghouse on Disability
  Information
The Council for Exceptional
  Children
1920 Association Dr.
Reston, VA 22091-1589
1-703-620-3660

Cystic Fibrosis Foundation
6931 Arlington Rd.
Bethesda, MD 20814
1-301-951-0902

800 Cocaine Information
Summit, NJ
1-900-262-2463

Epilepsy Foundation of America
4351 Garden City Dr.
Landover, MD 20785
1-800-332-1000

ERIC Clearinghouse on Handicapped
  and Gifted Children
1920 Association Dr.
Reston, VA 22091-1589
1-703-336-4797

Food Allergy Network
4744 Holly Ave.
Fairfax, VA 22030-5647
1-800-929-4040

Juvenile Diabetes Foundation
New York, NY
1-800-223-1138

Learning Disabilities Association of
  America
4156 Library Rd.
Pittsburgh, PA 15234
1-412-341-1515

Medic Alert Foundation
Turlock, CA
1-800-344-3226

National Asthma Educational Program
National Heart Lung/Blood Institute
1-301-251-1222

National Attention Deficit Disorder
  Association
1-800-487-2282

National Center for Education in
  Maternal and Child Health
38th and R St., N.W.
Washington, DC, 20057
1-202-625-8400

National Center for Learning Disabilities
381 Park Ave. #1420
New York, NY 10016
1-212-545-7510

National Down Syndrome Congress
Park Ridge, IL
1-800-232-6372

National Easter Seal Society for
   Crippled Children & Adults
70 East Lake St.
Chicago, IL 61601
1-312-726-6200

National Hemophilia Foundation
The SOHO Bldg
110 Greene St. #303
New York, NY 10012
1-800-424-2634

National Herpes Hotline
1-919-361-8488

National Information Center for
   Children & Youth with Handicaps
P.O. Box 1492
Washington, DC 20013
1-703-893-6061

National Marfan's Foundation
382 Main St.
Port Washington, NY 11050
1-800-862-7326

National Multiple Sclerosis Information Hotline
New York, NY
1-800-227-3166

National Organization on Fetal
   Alcohol Syndrome
1815 H St. NW #1000
Washington, DC 20006
1-800-666-6327

National Scoliosis Foundation
72 Mount Auburn St.
Watertown, MA 02172
1-617-926-0397

National STD Hotline
1-800-227-8922

National Stuttering Project
2151 Irving St., Suite 208
San Francisco, CA 94122-1609
1-800-364-1677

ODPHP National Health Information
   Center
P.O. Box 1133
Washington, DC 20013-1133

Office of Special Education and
   Rehabilitative Services
US Department of Education
Room 3132 Switzer Building
Washington, DC 20202-2524
1-202-732-1241

Overeaters Anonymous
World Service Office
P.O. Box 44020
Rio Rancho, NM 87174-4020
1-505-891-2664

Pediatric Crohn's & Colitis
   Association
P.O. Box 188
Newton, MA 02168-0002
1-617-290-0902

Sickle Cell Disease Association of
   America
3345 Wilshire Blvd. #1106
Los Angeles, CA 90010-1880
1-800-421-8453

Spina Bifida Association
Chicago, IL
1-800-621-3141

Stuttering Foundation of America
P.O. Box 11749
Memphis, TN 38111-0749
1-800-992-9392

TEF/Vater
15301 Grey Fox Dr.
Upper Marlboro, MD 20772
1-301-952-6837

Tourette's Syndrome Association
Bayside, NY
1-800-237-0717

United Cerebral Palsy Association, Inc.
1522 K Street, Suite 1112
Washington, DC 20006
1-202-842-1266
1-800-USA-5UCP

Wish Upon a Star
Visalia, CA
1-800-821-6805

APPENDIX 2

REPORTABLE

DISEASES AND

INFECTIONS

(CDC, 1995)

AIDS
Anthrax
Botulism
Brucellosis
Chancroid
Chlamydia trachomatis (genital infections)
Cholera
Coccidioidomycosis
Diphtheria
Escherichia coli O157:H7
Gonorrhea
Haemophilus influenzae
Hansen's disease
Hantavirus infection
Hemolytic-uremic syndrome
Hepatitis A
Hepatitis B

Hepatitis C/non-A, non-B
Invasive Group A streptococcus
Legionellosis
Lyme disease
Malaria
Measles
Meningococcal infection
Mumps
Pertussis
Plague
Poliomyelitis, paralytic
Psittacosis
Rabies, animal
Rabies, human
Rocky Mountain spotted fever
Rubella
Salmonellosis
Shigellosis

Streptococcus pneumoniae (drug-
   resistant)
Syphilis, primary and secondary
Tetanus
Toxic shock syndrome

Trichinosis
Tuberculosis
Typhoid fever
Yellow fever

INDEX

An *f* following a page number indicates a figure; a *t* indicates a table.